Receptors, antibodies and disease

Receptors, antibodies and disease

Ciba Foundation symposium 90

1982

Pitman
London

12/1982
Biol.

© Ciba Foundation 1982

ISBN 0 272 79654 9

Published in August 1982 by Pitman Ltd, London. Distributed in North America by CIBA Pharmaceutical Company (Medical Education Administration), Summit, NJ 07006, USA

Suggested series entry for library catalogues:
Ciba Foundation symposia

Ciba Foundation symposium 90
x + 312 pages, 49 figures, 35 tables

Evered, David
  Receptors, antibodies and disease.—(Ciba
  foundation symposium; 90)
  1. Immune response—Congresses
  2. Immunoglobins—Congresses
  I. Title   II. Whelan, Julie   III. Series
  616.07'95   QR186

Text set in 10/12 pt Linotron 202 Times, printed and bound
in Great Britain at The Pitman Press, Bath

Contents

Participants

L. BITENSKY   Division of Cellular Biology, The Mathilda and Terence Kennedy Institute of Rheumatology, 6 Bute Gardens, London W6 7DW, UK

M. BLECHER   Department of Biochemistry, Georgetown University School of Medicine, Washington, DC 20007, USA

G. F. BOTTAZZO   Department of Immunology, Arthur Stanley House, Middlesex Hospital Medical School, 40–50 Tottenham Street, London W1P 9PG, UK

M. J. CRUMPTON   Imperial Cancer Research Fund Laboratories, PO Box 123, Lincoln's Inn Fields, London WC2A 3PX, UK

T. F. DAVIES   Thyroid Section, Division of Endocrinology, The Mount Sinai Medical Center, One Gustave L. Levy Place, New York, New York 10029, USA

D. B. DRACHMAN   Neuromuscular Unit, Johns Hopkins University School of Medicine, c/o 317 Traylor Bldg., Baltimore, Maryland 21205, USA

A. G. ENGEL   Department of Neurology, Mayo Clinic, Rochester, Minnesota 55901, USA

H. G. FRIESEN   Department of Physiology, University of Manitoba Faculty of Medicine, 770 Bannatyne Avenue, Winnipeg, Canada R3E OW3

S. FUCHS   Department of Chemical Immunology, The Weizmann Institute of Science, Rehovot, Israel

R. HALL   Department of Medicine, Welsh National School of Medicine, Heath Park, Cardiff CF4 4XN, UK

L. C. HARRISON   Endocrine Laboratory, Department of Diabetes and Endocrinology, c/o Post Office, The Royal Melbourne Hospital, Victoria 3050, Australia

S. J. JACOBS Wellcome Research Laboratories, Burroughs Wellcome Co., 3030 Cornwallis Road, Research Triangle Park, North Carolina 27709, USA

C. R. KAHN The Joslin Diabetes Center, 1 Joslin Place, Boston, Massachusetts 02215, USA

J. G. KNIGHT MRC Autoimmunity Research Unit, Otago University Medical School, PO Box 913, Dunedin, New Zealand

J. M. LINDSTROM The Salk Institute, PO Box 85800, San Diego, California 92138, USA

S. McLACHLAN Department of Medicine, Wellcome Research Laboratories, Royal Victoria Infirmary, Newcastle upon Tyne NE1 4LP, UK

N. A. MITCHISON Tumour Immunology Unit, Department of Zoology, University College London, Gower Street, London WC1E 6BT, UK

J. NEWSOM-DAVIS Department of Neurological Science, The Royal Free Hospital, Pond Street, London NW3 2QG, UK

M. A. RAFTERY Division of Chemistry and Chemical Engineering, The Chemical Laboratories, California Institute of Technology, Pasadena, California 91125, USA

B. REES SMITH Department of Medicine, Welsh National School of Medicine, Heath Park, Cardiff CF4 4XN, UK

M. RODBELL Institut de biochimie clinique, Sentier de la Roseraie, 1211 Genève 4, Switzerland

I. M. ROITT Department of Immunology, Arthur Stanley House, Middlesex Hospital Medical School, 40–50 Tottenham Street, London W1P 9PG, UK

J. C. VENTER Department of Biochemistry, School of Medicine, State University of New York at Buffalo, 102 Cary Hall, Buffalo, New York 14214, USA

A. VINCENT Department of Neurological Science, The Royal Free Hospital, Pond Street, London NW3 2QG, UK

Introduction

N. A. MITCHISON

Tumour Immunology Unit, Department of Zoology, University College London, Gower Street, London WC1E 6BT, UK

We all know why we are here at this symposium, and we know where this subject of receptor antibodies started. I think it actually began in two places: first, when a group of persevering, patient people in New Zealand started pulling Long Acting Thyroid Stimulator apart. It is therefore particularly good to have John Knight from Duncan Adams' team here. The other place where it began was the Salk Institute, when some rabbits' ears started drooping and a trick was found to get those ears to perk up—I am thinking here of the work of Patrick and Lindstrom. Then we knew we were in business! So that is where we go on from. It has become quite clear that the discovery of antibodies against receptors, and of how important they are in clinical autoimmune disease, is now a central topic in the sense that it has all sorts of implications for cell biology and biochemistry (which are actually the same subject) on one side, and for immunology on the other. The cell biology that we shall hear about will include studies on the structure of receptors— molecular biology proper—and how they mediate transmembrane signalling. It is very interesting to see how these clinically important antibodies turn out also to be probes which provide insight into how transmembrane signalling works and clues about deep questions in endocrinology. On the other hand, in immunology, the fact that an antibody appears is really the *end* of the story. One wants to know how the antibody came to be there to begin with, and also how it can be regulated once it has begun to be produced—how it can be turned on and off. That will take us right into the central questions of regulatory control in the immune system. I suspect we shall hear a great deal about two things: firstly, idiotypes and the idiotype network, because that is one exciting current idea about immune regulation; and secondly, perturbations in the regulatory T cell system, or T cell circuits, which is a second exciting idea at present.

It is a pleasant occasion that brings endocrinologists and immunologists

1982 Receptors, antibodies and disease. Pitman, London (Ciba Foundation Symposium 90) p 1-2

together like this, because endocrinology and immunology are subjects that have much in common. They are both very 'conceptual' parts of science, set a little apart from mainstream physiology and biochemistry. We are living in a time of technical revolution for both these subjects. The major revolution is in recombinant DNA, and although we may not talk much about that here, we know it will be looking over our shoulders all the way through this meeting. A second revolution going on in immunology at present is in cloning. In the past year or two, the immune system, which essentially consists of sets of parallel clones of cells all interacting with each other (competing for antigens and suppressing or helping one another), has been systematically pulled apart by cloning. Immunologists are basically divided into T cell people and B cell people, and the two groups got round to cloning at about the same time but more or less independently of one another. The hybridoma, an innovation due to César Milstein, has completely changed the world of antibodies, and equally we know that T cells are also being cloned—sometimes by hybrids; sometimes by viral transformation; sometimes simply by repeated antigenic stimulation, or by using growth hormone; there is a whole range of available techniques. A technical revolution of that sort doesn't immediately change our concepts. What it does is to make much of the work that has already been done semi-obsolete, in that much has now to be repeated, using cloned cells. All the problems in immune regulation that we shall be discussing have to be thought of from that point of view.

Structure–function relationships in adenylate cyclase systems

MARTIN RODBELL

National Institutes of Health, Bethesda, Maryland 20205, USA

Abstract Hormone-sensitive adenylate cyclase systems are composed of hormone-recognition units (R), a nucleotide-regulatory unit (N) for reaction with GTP and divalent cations, and the catalytic unit (C). From the reported sizes of purified R and N subunits and target analysis of functional sizes of these units, the functions of the components for the binding and actions of hormones and GTP require minimally dimers, homologous or heterologous. It is proposed that the catalytic unit exists in the membrane also as a dimer and that its transition to the active state with MgATP as substrate involves corresponding transitions in linked dimers of the hormone-recognition and nucleotide-regulatory units. It is postulated that hormones trigger the activation process by inducing in concert with GTP and divalent cations the appropriate dimer structure of the holoenzyme. In large aggregates of such structures, realignment of only a few occupied holoenzyme units may be sufficient to induce activation of the total aggregate enzyme. This theory serves to explain the synergistic actions of hormones, and how several hormones can activate a common enzyme. It also provides an explanation for 'spare' receptors, and for the efficacy of hormone action.

Most hormones act on their target cells through receptor molecules located on the outer surface membrane. The principal functions of these receptors are to concentrate their specific hormones by a reversible process and to transduce this process into the regulation of cellular responses. The recognition process has been more intensively studied than the transduction process because of the availability of labelled hormones, antagonists, drugs, toxins, cross-linking agents, and receptor antibodies with which to monitor and quantify the presence of receptor molecules. As will be discussed in other papers, through such agents and with the aid of affinity chromatography,

---

1982 Receptors, antibodies and disease. Pitman, London (Ciba Foundation symposium 90) p 3-21

Present address: Department of Medical Biochemistry, University of Geneva Medical School, 1211-Geneva 4, Switzerland

receptors for acetylcholine and insulin have been purified, the components analysed and, in the case of the cholinergic receptor, even biological function has been reconstituted from purified components. The latter studies indicate that transduction and recognition are achieved by a composite of distinct macromolecules. I have recently reviewed (Rodbell 1980) evidence that hormone receptors involved in the regulation of adenylate cyclase systems are also composed of distinct subunits for hormonal recognition and transduction. Here I will discuss certain aspects of the structure–function relationships in the cyclase components and then suggest how these components may be organized and the enzyme may be regulated by hormones and other regulatory ligands.

Components of adenylate cyclase systems

A large body of evidence has accumulated to show that binding or recognition components (abbreviated R) involved in the hormonal activation of adenylate cyclase are separate molecules from the transduction components that directly induce activation of the catalytic components (C). The transduction process involves proteins (abbreviated variously as N, G/F, or G) that contain sites for the binding of GTP and divalent cations, key elements in the transduction process. The N unit is required also for activation of C by fluoride ion and by cholera toxin. The toxin catalyses ADP-ribosylation of the N unit, a process that with labelled NAD has enabled investigators to identify and purify to near homogeneity a functional N unit (Northup et al 1980). Toxin-labelled proteins with relative molecular masses (M_r) of 42 000 and 53 000 have been detected in purified N units from liver membranes; only the 42 000 M_r protein is seen in certain other membranes. These proteins appear to contain homologous structures but it is not clear that they function identically in the transduction process. In addition to toxin-labelled proteins, the purified N unit contains a 35 000 M_r protein, the function of which remains unknown but which co-purifies in equal quantity with the toxin-labelled proteins. Possibly it is the site of binding and action of divalent cations (Mg or Mn). The functional mass required for hormonal activation of adenylate cyclase is 130 000, suggesting that two or more N units are minimally involved in the transduction process.

The N unit and the C unit are situated on the inner face of the plasma membrane and have sufficiently hydrophobic properties to suggest that they are bound to the membrane through hydrophobic forces, possibly with lipids. The N unit forms complexes with C; these complexes can be activated by fluoride ion or by non-hydrolysable guanine nucleotides such as 5′-guanylylimidodiphosphate (Gpp(NH)p). As judged from the ability of hormones to promote the binding and degradation of GTP and the ability of the latter to affect the binding of hormones, the N unit also forms complexes with R units (Lad et al 1980). It is likely that such interactions take place in the membrane and that such complexes span the plasma membrane. As with the linkages of N with C, the linkages of N with R are also reversible: the latter are stabilized when R is occupied by hormone. The different properties of RN and NC complexes toward phospholipases, detergents, metal ions, organic mercurials and guanine nucleotide analogues argue for N having differing domains for its interactions with C and R. Studies with cell variants also suggest differing complex-forming domains on N (Schleifer et al 1980). Given the complex subunit structure of N and the possible heterologous structures of both the C and R units, it is not possible at this time to give a detailed view of how the units are organized in the membrane and what forces are involved in their interactions. From what little is known, lipids and SH groups are strong candidates for some of the interacting forces.

The 'coupling' problem

Because R, N and C form reversible associations, it is possible that associations between the units may be rate-limiting steps during the activation process. However, our current inability to quantify the number of functional R, N and C units required for activation, combined with the experimental difficulties of directly measuring interactions in membranes, make it difficult to establish that such interactions are indeed involved in the regulatory process. By the same token, there must be an explanation for findings that different hormones can activate, through distinct receptors, the same enzyme through what appear to be identical N units. Such findings have been cited as arguments for receptors being 'mobile' and capable of interchanging with one another in their interactions with N. Moreover, it has been shown that R or RN complexes can be inserted by fusion techniques into membranes with functional consequences in the hormonal activation process (Schramm 1979). The kinetics of hormonal activation can be accommodated by a concept of a step-wise cascade of events in which R, N and C units interact sequentially in response to the actions of hormones and guanine nucleotides (DeLean et al 1980). Nonetheless, despite what appear to be convincing arguments for ligand-induced associations, there is no convincing evidence against the possibility that the cyclase units are already complexed in the membrane in a form subject to regulation by hormones and guanine nucleotides. A relatively slow equilibrium between complexed and free components might affect the extent and duration of the stimulatory process but not the immediate triggering actions of the activating ligands. If the rate-limiting steps do not involve associations between the macromolecular components, what other steps or processes have been or should be considered?

The GTPase cycle

In some systems it has been shown that dissociation of tightly bound GDP is a rate-limiting step in the overall activation process by hormones and GTP (Cassel & Selinger 1978). Depending on the system examined, GDP formed by hydrolysis of GTP (presumably at the N unit) can be either a potent inhibitor or a partial activator. In either case, GDP inhibits the activating effects of GTP, the presumed natural activator of the system. In systems in which hormones stimulate release of tightly bound GDP, this action permits activating ligands to enter the site. If it is occupied by GTP, rapid hydrolysis occurs and activation of the enzyme system is dependent on the continued occupation of the R unit by the hormone. This so-called GTPase regulatory cycle can satisfactorily explain the kinetic behaviour of some cyclase systems. However, there are many systems in which GDP is not tightly bound to N and for which there is no evidence that release of GDP formed from hydrolysis of GTP is a rate-limiting step in the activation process.

Transition states

Recently, Neer & Salter (1981) have shown with solubilized N and C units that, while these units form reversible associations, activation by guanine nucleotides does not involve nucleotide-induced associations of these units. Rather, the evidence obtained suggests that the NC complex isomerizes between different states of activity and that the isomerization process is relatively slow compared to the association between N and C. Isomerization between different states of the guanine nucleotide-occupied cyclase system has been postulated (Rodbell et al 1975), based on modelling of the hepatic enzyme system in its response to Gpp(NH)p and Mg^{2+}. It was also suggested that occupation of R by glucagon increases the rate of isomerization between inactive and active states; enhanced occupancy of N by guanine nucleotides was not required to explain the actions of hormones in this model. At that time, the possibility was considered that low and high activity forms of the enzyme reflected differing affinities for inhibitory forms of ATP. However, in view of subsequent evidence that the enzyme systems contains regulatory sites for divalent cations and that these sites require the N unit for the expression of their effects (Londos & Rodbell 1975), the isomerization process more likely involves changes in the reactivity of the N unit (the 35 000 M_r protein?) with divalent cations; the latter ligands may act in concert with GTP to bring about activation of the C unit. These dual requirements for both GTP and divalent cations (Mg or Mn) could explain the long-known stimulatory effects of hormones on the ability of Mg ions to activate adenylate cyclase.

Properties of the catalytic unit

An important characteristic of the transition between inactive and active forms of C is that C preferentially utilizes MnATP as substrate when it is not activated by hormones, guanine nucleotides, and divalent cations. The physiological substrate, MgATP, is converted to cyclic AMP when the enzyme is activated by these ligands. Interestingly, even though activation of C by fluoride ion also involves the N unit, the fluoride-activated enzyme still prefers MnATP as substrate. Thus, the linkage of N with C is not necessarily the determining factor in the form of the enzyme that uses MnATP or MgATP as substrate. There must be other constraints imposed on the C unit that fluoride ion somehow releases: possibly this represents release of a regulatory subunit.

A soluble form of adenylate cyclase that uses primarily MnATP as substrate is found in the adult testis (Braun & Dods 1975). This form of the enzyme has none of the regulatory characteristics exhibited by the membrane-bound C unit. Moreover, its functional molecular weight (M_r) is about 60 000, or about half that of the functional C unit that uses MnATP as substrate in the membrane (Nielsen et al 1981). Possibly, therefore, the C unit of hormonally regulated systems exists in the form of dimers which, when linked with C, can show transitions between MnATP- and MgATP-states of the enzyme. If C is linked to N as dimers, principles of symmetry dictate that N is also structurally linked to C as dimers. As discussed previously, the functional N unit seems to be minimally composed of heterologous dimers of N. Theoretically, interactions between heterologous N units with C can give rise to a number of possible configurations having differing levels of activities. One could thus imagine that activation by such non-physiological activators as fluoride ion and Gpp(NH)p involves states normally not accessible to the enzyme system. The most obvious role for the hormone and its R unit is to ensure conversion of the NC complex to the most favourable, *reversible* activated state that uses MgATP as substrate. If NC dimers are required for the transition, then it follows that dimers of R units are also involved in the transition process.

Functional structure of receptors

Shorr et al (1981) have reported that the purified β_2-adrenergic receptor in frog erythrocytes contains a 58 000 M_r subunit; the turkey erythrocyte β_1-receptor appears to have subunits of M_r values 41 000 and 37 000 (Atlas & Levitzki 1978). From target analysis of the latter cyclase system (Nielsen et al 1981), the functional mass of the β_1-receptor is about 90 000 M_r whether measured from the binding of antagonists or by the activating effects of an agonist on cyclase activity. From this it would seem that the functional unit of the β_1-receptor is a dimer. Since antagonist binding also required a dimer of R, the differences in the binding and actions of agonists and antagonists probably reside in the structure of the dimer. Possibly the dimer can take two or more transition states, the one induced or stabilized by agonists causing NC to become active. In this case, partial agonists cannot distinguish in an all-or-none fashion between the antagonist and agonist forms of the R dimer. The glucagon receptor in liver membranes has also been tagged with a labelled marker (Johnson et al 1981) and yielded on sodium dodecyl sulphate–polyacrylamide gel electrophoresis primarily a single band with an apparent mass of 62 000. This size is significantly smaller than the target size (about 120 000 M_r) estimated for the glucagon R unit when linked to the activated form of the cyclase system (Schlegel et al 1979). It would appear, therefore, that the functional form of the glucagon receptor is also a dimer of either homologous or heterologous subunits. Different subunits may be involved, since the method of tagging the receptor involved linkage of glucagon via cross-linking agents which may selectively react with but one of two or more putative subunits. Nonetheless, it would appear from this limited number of studies that R units, for either peptide hormones or catecholamines, may require two or more subunits for their participation in the overall activation process. The question at this point is how dimers of R, N, and C units can serve to accommodate the properties of adenylate cyclase systems.

Theory

As a basic assumption, I suggest that the fundamental unit of the enzyme system that expresses activity in response to hormones, guanine nucleotides, and divalent cations is a dimer of RNC units. The R units in the dimer can be either homologous or heterologous with respect to the specificity of hormone binding. Because both R units of a homologous dimer can be occupied by the same hormone, RNC dimers containing homologous R units are more effective in activating the enzyme than RNC dimers containing heterologous units. Efficacy of hormone action in a multi-receptor-containing system is a function of the number of homologous R units present or formed during hormone action. Since it is likely that the amount of homologous R dimer is proportional to the concentrations of the various R units, it follows that the actions of a hormone with the highest concentration of R units will dominate activity when all hormones are added together at maximal stimulating concentrations. Thus, this postulate provides an adequate explanation for the non-additivity of hormone action on multi-receptor systems. An additional outcome is the possibility that binding of two different hormones to a heterologous dimer might give more activity than when the same dimeric RNC unit is occupied by a single hormone. Synergistic effects of combinations of hormones have been observed (Birnbaumer & Rodbell 1969).

The most difficult problem to solve with any of the theories advanced for hormone activation is the often-observed phenomenon in which minimal occupation of R can yield near maximal or even maximal activation of adenylate cyclase. In the 'collision-coupling' theory (Tolkovsky & Levitzki 1978), a single R unit can interact repeatedly with the same enzyme unit because R serves essentially as a catalyst in the activation process. Bergman & Hechter (1978) suggested a fixed matrix of R units arranged with respect to the enzyme components such that a single hormone molecule triggers, in ricochet fashion, a number of R units within the field with resultant activation of a number of C units in the matrix over a short span of time. In the context of the theory presented here, a similar matrix or cluster of RNC can be postulated, the difference being that the binding of a hormone to one dimeric unit in the cluster might cause neighbouring units to take the requisite transitions to more active states (occupied by GTP and Mg^{2+}). This theoretical triggering action of a hormone can be likened to a propagated change in contractility of an elastic set of intertwined proteins (muscle, for example) in response to a structural modification of only one protein in the complex. A tightly packed arrangement of clustered RNC units might satisfy this type of triggering mechanism, particularly if occupation of the N units by GTP and Mg ions is not dependent on hormone occupation of R—that is, the action of the hormone is primarily that of affecting the rate of transition to the active state rather than the number of units that can be occupied by the activating ligands, GTP and Mg ions.

The idea of a cluster of RNC units is not far-fetched. Target analysis of the hepatic cyclase system indicated that the ground-state structure (prior to activation) is at least four-fold larger in size than the final hormone-activated state of the system (Schlegel et al 1979). Included in this ground-state structure were R and N units. If the C unit is included and a dimer of RNC units represents the holoenzyme in its activated form, then it can be calculated that the ground state of the hepatic system is composed of a tetramer of dimeric RNC units.

Finally, a few comments on how this theory may relate to the phenomenon of desensitization, a process in which the actions of a hormone or a drug on a system can lead to loss of hormone or drug response. The current idea on this process with respect to adenylate cyclase systems is that loss of hormone response is due to uncoupling of the receptor from the system. Since desensitization follows activation one might consider that uncoupling reflects a change in the stability of the organized complex of regulatory and catalytic components when it is converted from a tightly packed matrix of RNC units to a less ordered, metastable structure of the activated state. Since hormones, GTP and divalent cations are required to achieve the activated state, desensitization should depend also on the actions of all these ligands. This dependency has been reported recently for desensitization of the luteinizing hormone-responsive adenylate cyclase system in isolated membranes of corpus luteum (Ezra & Salomon 1981).

Concluding comments

It is apparent from this brief review that rapid strides have been made towards an understanding of the components responsible for the regulation of adenylate cyclase systems. Purification and reconstitution of hormone receptors, GTP-regulatory proteins, the proteins that bind divalent cations, and the catalytic unit now seem feasible ventures. Such efforts should lead to a better understanding of the structure and organization of the system in its membrane environment. The theory presented here suggests that the components are assembled in a highly organized structure. This is based on rather modest evidence gleaned largely from target analysis, a relatively new procedure for assessing the structure of membrane-bound proteins. Nonetheless, the theory at least has the testable feature of predicting a relatively large structure having the specific characteristic of clustered receptors. With appropriately tagged hormones it should be possible to visualize such structures in isolated membranes or intact cells.

REFERENCES

Atlas D, Levitzki A 1978 Tentative identification of beta-adrenoreceptor subunits. Nature (Lond) 272:370-371

Bergman RN, Hechter O 1978 Neurohypophyseal hormone-responsive renal adenylate cyclase. IV. Random-hit matrix model for coupling in a hormone-sensitive adenylate cyclase system. J Biol Chem 253:3238-3250

Birnbaumer L, Rodbell M 1969 Adenyl cyclase in fat cells. II. Hormone receptors. J Biol Chem 244:3477-3482

Braun T, Dods RF 1975 Development of a Mn-sensitive 'soluble' adenylate cyclase in rat testis. Proc Natl Acad Sci USA 72:1097-1101

Cassel D, Selinger Z 1978 Mechanism of adenylate cyclase activation through the beta adrenergic receptor: catecholamine-induced displacement of bound GDP by GTP. Proc Natl Acad Sci USA 75:4155-4159

De Lean A, Stadel JM, Lefkowitz RJ 1980 A ternary complex model explains the agonist-specific binding properties of the adenylate cyclase-coupled β-adrenergic receptor. J Biol Chem 255:7108-7117

Ezra E, Salomon Y 1981 Mechanism of desensitization of adenylate cyclase by lutropin. J Biol Chem 256:5377-5382

Johnson GL, MacAndrew VI, Jr, Pilch PF 1981 Identification of the glucagon receptor in rat liver membranes by photoaffinity crosslinking. Proc Natl Acad Sci USA 78:875-878

Lad PM, Nielsen TB, Preston MS, Rodbell M 1980 The role of the guanine nucleotide exchange reaction. J Biol Chem 255:988-995

Londos C, Rodbell M 1975 Multiple inhibitory and activating effects of nucleotides and magnesium on adrenal adenylate cyclase. J Biol Chem 250:3459-3465

Neer EJ, Salter RS 1981 Modification of adenylate cyclase structure and function by ammonium sulfate. J Biol Chem 256:5497-5503

Nielsen TB, Lad PM, Preston MS, Kempner E, Schlegel W, Rodbell M 1981 Structure of the turkey erythrocyte adenylate cyclase system. Proc Natl Acad Sci USA 78:722-726

Northup JK, Sternweis PC, Smigel MD, Schleifer LS, Ross EM, Gilman AG 1980 Purification of the regulatory component of adenylate cyclase. Proc Natl Acad Sci USA 77:6516-6520

Rodbell M 1980 The role of hormone receptors and GTP-regulatory proteins in membrane transduction. Nature (Lond) 284:17-22

Rodbell M, Lin MC, Salomon Y et al 1975 Role of adenine and guanine nucleotides in the activity and response of adenylate cyclase systems to hormones: evidence for multisite transition states. Adv Cyclic Nucleotide Res 5:3-29

Schlegel W, Kempner ES, Rodbell M 1979 Activation of adenylate cyclase in hepatic membranes involves interactions of the catalytic unit with multimeric complexes of regulatory proteins. J Biol Chem 254:5168-5176

Schleifer LS, Garrison JC, Sternweis PC, Northup JK, Gilman AG 1980 The regulatory component of adenylate cyclase from uncoupled S49 lymphoma cells differs in charge from the wild type protein. J Biol Chem 255:2641-2644

Schramm M 1979 Transfer of glucagon receptor from liver membanes to a foreign adenylate cyclase by a membrane fusion procedure. Proc Natl Acad Sci USA 76:1174-1178

Shorr RGL, Lefkowitz RJ, Caron MG 1981 Purification of the beta-adrenergic receptor. J Biol Chem 256:5820-5826

Tolkovsky AM, Levitzki A 1978 Mode of coupling between the beta-adrenergic receptor and adenylate cyclase in turkey erythrocytes. Biochemistry 17:3795-3810

DISCUSSION

Kahn: Mammalian mutant cell lines have been described which lack the catalytic subunit of cyclase, or the GTP regulatory subunit, and even a few lacking the receptor unit (Haga et al 1977). One should be able to use target analysis, or other methods, to see if there are changes in the receptor aggregation as you would predict.

Rodbell: Perhaps I should first give some idea of what target analysis can do and what the limitations of this technique are. An excellent review of target analysis has been published recently by my colleagues Kempner & Schlegel (1979). In essence, the technique involves bombarding the material being examined for activity (enzyme or hormone binding, for examples) with very high energy ionizing particles (in our case, high energy electrons were generated by a linear accelerator). The energy applied is sufficient that a single 'hit' anywhere in the molecule destroys all function. Since the statistical probability of hitting a molecule is proportional to the size of the molecule, the larger it is, the less ionizing radiation is needed to cause loss of function. By plotting the exponential decay in activity against the amount of ionizing radiation impinging on the target, one obtains from the slope(s) the mass of the function being measured.

The beauty of this technique, at least in principle, is that it enables the investigator to examine the functional size of a macromolecule even when activity is dependent on the membrane environment—that is, activity would be lost or drastically altered if the macromolecule were solubilized. I should emphasize that functional mass is being measured, since the technique relies strictly on the ability to measure activity. In our studies of the target size of adenylate cyclase systems we were not particularly concerned with the size *per se.* To us, the critical question was whether the functional mass would change, depending on the state of the enzyme—whether it is activated by hormones and GTP, by non-physiological activators such as fluoride ion or Gpp(NH)p, or in its 'ground state' when it is not exposed to any ligand, including substrate and divalent cations. As I discussed, target sizes change significantly with the functional state of the enzyme. We interpreted these changes as reflecting the size of the components involved in the regulation of the enzyme. We know from independent evidence that minimally these components include R, N and C. Without such knowledge we would have predicted that either such components exist, or that perhaps the enzyme system was composed of a single macromolecule which changes its size through aggregation. The obvious point is that target analysis cannot yield information on the nature of the material being examined. This is one of its major limitations. But this limitation applies to all methods that determine the size of impure biological materials. The advantage of using target analysis to determine structure is that one can manipulate the system in numerous ways, including using ligands that promote activation or inhibition of enzyme activity (Schlegel et al 1980). Perhaps fortuitously, the results obtained with three systems (liver, adipocyte, turkey erythrocyte) are consistent with what is currently known of the functional masses of receptors and nucleotide regulatory units determined by more conventional techniques in their solubilized form.

I agree that one should take advantage of available mutants of adenylate cyclase systems such as those reported for mouse lymphoma variants (Johnson et al 1981). However, to my knowledge, the nature of the components missing or modified has not been fully established. For example, perhaps what we term the N unit is actually a complex group of regulatory units each having separate sites or subunits for regulation by divalent cations and guanine nucleotides. If we knew this to be the case, I believe we could manipulate the states of the enzyme system in a way that would permit target analysis to be interpreted in a unique manner. One hopes that such information will be available in the near future.

Kahn: The major advantage of radiation inactivation, or target size analysis, is that it can be used on molecules within the membrane. You can put a plasma membrane preparation, or even an intact cell preparation, in a high energy electron beam and measure the loss of activity of a given membrane component which will be related to its size, within its membrane environment. You and Schlegel have done that for the glucagon receptor; Joan Harmon and I did it for the insulin receptor (Harmon et al 1980). The subunit sizes can also be obtained by this means.

Rodbell: As you say, target sizes of receptors have also been measured by analysing the decay in receptor-binding activity as a function of ionizing radiation dose (Schlegel et al 1979, Nielsen et al 1981, Harmon et al 1981). Here we encounter both theoretical and practical problems. In the case of enzymes, it would appear that a single hit is sufficient to cause complete loss of activity. This is because the architecture of most enzymes is such that a disturbance in structure anywhere along the chain is sufficient to make the catalytic site less efficient or inactive. In a sense, this action of ionizing irradiation is analogous to the actions of regulatory ligands on allosteric enzymes, although the effect is considerably more drastic in consequence and, of course, is irreversible. By contrast, in the case of binding of small molecules to enzymes or to receptors, one cannot be certain that a single hit will destroy the binding regions. It is conceivable that the binding region requires less stringent organization than the catalytic site of an enzyme. In this sense, the theory may not strictly apply.

A more practical problem of examining the target sizes of receptors is that binding assays with hormones are less sensitive and reliable than the measurement of catalytic activity. The latter can be measured usually even when two orders of exponential decay in activity have occurred as a result of irradiation. The importance of this point is that one would like to know whether decay follows a single slope or multiple slopes with increasing dosage. A single slope has the virtue of suggesting a single target whereas multiple slopes, though more interesting from a mechanistic standpoint, may have multiple interpretations. In the case of target analysis of the insulin receptor (Harmon et al 1981) the slopes were minimally biphasic and were interpreted as evidence that the receptor may be attached to a 'regulatory' component that controls receptor affinity. For the glucagon receptor (Schlegel et al 1979), the target size of the receptor, determined from binding to the GTP-sensitive form of the receptor, was considerably larger than that measured by glucagon action on cyclase activity. By contrast, studies of the β-receptor linked to the cyclase system in turkey erythrocyte membranes (Nielsen et al 1981) suggested that the receptor has the same functional size whether measured from the binding of antagonists or from the actions of agonists on cyclase activity. Thus, the results of target analysis have raised some interesting questions about receptor structure and function.

Jacobs: If you have a protein with several functional domains, perhaps one required for binding and another required to anchor the protein within the cell membrane, and you hit say the anchoring domain with ionizing radiation, do you inactivate the binding domain? And, secondly, if you have an aggregate made up of several almost independent receptors, as you postulated, and you hit one receptor with radiation, would you expect to inactivate the whole aggregate? And are the effects of ionizing radiations transmitted across disulphide bonds? Are they transmitted across non-covalent bonds?

Rodbell: It would appear that ionizing radiation due to a single ionizing event on a macromolecule can spread along the backbone of the molecule for quite a distance (depending on the initial energy of the ionizing particle). You raise the interesting question of what happens if different macromolecules required for a particular activity are linked covalently or not. To our knowledge, with subunit-containing molecules that are not linked covalently, ionizing radiation does not spread between subunits. However, disulphide-linked molecules behave as if they are a single macromolecule, suggesting that ionizing radiation in this case traverses the disulphide bond.

The essential point you raise is whether a multi-functional subunit-containing system can be analysed by target analysis to give a unique interpretation. The simplest answer is: no. On the other hand, so far, this technique is uniquely capable of analysing the functional mass of a complex enzyme system in its native membrane environment. The results have allowed interesting speculations for assessment. This is precisely what we had hoped the technique would do.

Mitchison: To revert to the genetic analysis of the receptor, your theory predicts the existence of particular classes of mutants, Dr Rodbell. For example, there should be mutants where, for particular receptors, the normal agonist would be ineffective, but might synergize with another agonist. Are you in a position to screen for mutants of that sort?

Rodbell: I think we need better tools, such as labels that can select out one or other subunit in a membrane and say whether it is there or not.

Venter: Those tools are being developed. We have produced monoclonal antibodies to membrane receptors (Fraser & Venter 1980, Venter & Fraser 1981). Some of that work may support your dimerization theory, at least in terms of structural dimers. We find that the β_2-adrenergic receptor has a subunit relative molecular mass (M_r) of around 58 000 and a possible dimer size of around 100 000 (Venter & Fraser 1981), which is roughly what the molecular weights from our hydrodynamic data and your radiation inactivation study would predict. The human lung β_2-adrenergic receptor appears to exist both as a monomer, solubilized from the membrane, and also as a disulphide-cross-linked dimer. We don't know yet whether the β_2-receptor functions as a monomer, or both as a monomer and a dimer.

Another finding that argues somewhat against your proposal that receptors exist in the membrane precoupled to other membrane components is that if you solubilize α- and β-adrenergic or muscarinic receptors from a membrane they come out as the monomer or dimer but not linked to something else, whereas if you added hormone to the receptor before solubilization, you can obtain larger molecular complexes. We can obtain two to four different-sized complexes containing turkey erythrocyte β_1-receptor and some other components, presumably the GTPase and adenylate cyclase, after detergent solubilization in the presence of hormone. But the receptors appear to exist in the membrane as free units in the absence of hormone. They are probably in some sort of restricted domain in the membrane; but they must be mobile. Our study on high efficiency coupling of β-receptors to adenylate cyclase and cardiac contraction demonstrated that only a few (less than 10%) of the β-receptors in the membrane are required for complete (100%) hormone activation, yet the kinetics of this response indicate that the receptors must be in close association with all of the G proteins and adenylate cyclases to allow single receptors to activate multiple molecules of adenylate cyclase over short time periods (Venter 1979). Maybe one needs a combination of the mobile receptor hypothesis acting within restricted membrane domains?

Rodbell: I did not mean to imply that individual molecules cannot rotate with respect to one another. One function of membrane lipids may be to serve as a type of lubricant, allowing the individual components to move about and interact with one another. The theory raised in my paper provides an alternative to the mobile receptor theory which, at least in its current state of development, suggests that receptors are recruited by the hormones to their site(s) of action. Perhaps you are right that a mix of both theories is closer to the truth. Perhaps the receptors are in the same region of the membrane as all the other components required for action and loosely associated. Binding of the hormone may induce the formation of covalent linkages (disulphide bridges?) that initiate a particular chain of events culminating in action. In this manner, the hormone might cause the appearance of a larger structural unit which remains stable when solubilized. This idea, I believe, could accommodate the results you describe.

Rees Smith: Where do you envisage these interactions taking place? If you have three macromolecules (N, C and R) sitting in a membrane, the actual point of, and the nature of, the interaction is critical. How do you see this taking place in the membrane bilayer, or across the bilayer? I am wondering whether, if there is coupling between the receptor and the regulatory protein, this takes place in an aqueous environment, or in the lipid environment of the membrane.

Rodbell: I envisage all the events happening within the plane of the membrane with lipids playing structural roles, of lubricating and perhaps joining the various components, to give a coherent, relatively stable structure, at least in the ground state when it is not subjected to the forces of the various regulatory ligands.

Davies: You are also suggesting that the receptors interact with each other. How does that happen?

Rodbell: One could visualize the ground-state structure as being composed of individual 'polymers' of R, N and C units stacked perpendicularly to the plane of the surface membrane with receptors facing the exterior and held in place by the underlying N and C units. Since receptors seem in many systems to react with some type of N unit, it is possible that there are common structural regions or components of all receptors and N units that permit these materials to interact. My argument for different receptors interacting with one another is based solely on the synergism displayed when two or more hormones stimulate the same enzyme. If this actually reflects receptor contacts, I can imagine that the R units form reversible associations much like any polymer of similar units, such as tubulin or actin. Although I do not want to carry this analogy too far, reversible depolymerization of R units into effective dimers is one means of relating our data on target analysis.

As I view the problem of the assembly of the various components of the cyclase system, nature may have designed these systems to be in specialized regions of the membrane, concentrated in forms that permit ready access to external hormones. Most hormone-sensitive cells are organized as a syncytium, perhaps with only small areas of the cell membrane actually exposed to hormones from the blood circulation or to adjacent neurotransmitter-secreting cells. Accordingly, there must be some structural feature of receptor-linked systems that places them in the appropriate region of the membrane. One might speculate that cytoskeletal elements play some role in this organization process, but not necessarily in the moment-to-moment regulation of the receptor-mediated signal production.

Perhaps the point to be emphasized is that we are forced to consider the question of how receptor-mediated processes are organized in the membrane because of the relatively small concentrations of these materials in the membrane. If we are to understand receptor function we need some means of visualizing receptors in their functional mode. Obviously, target analysis cannot achieve this goal. With the advantages of specific antibodies to receptors, as will be discussed by others here, the tools may soon be at hand with which to relate structure and function more directly.

Venter: On the turkey erythrocyte there are only about 400 β_1-adrenergic receptor molecules per cell.

Rodbell: Yes; there must be very few, and probably in a very restricted part of the membrane.

Blecher: I am uneasy about the types of genetic analysis of the receptor complex currently in vogue, because one tends then to think in terms of the presence or absence of a particular component, and that doesn't seem subtle enough. I would like to think that included in the genetic aberrations would be changes in the structures of individual components of the complex (R, N or C), rather than simply their absence or presence. This would enable there to be an almost infinite variety of genetic aberrations rather than just, say, regulatory site-negative or cyclase-negative, in addition to the wild-type. And within that context, are you prepared to believe that one regulatory (N) protein serves for all hormone receptors in, for example, the fat cell system?

Rodbell: You are correct in citing the genetic approach for looking at subtle changes in structure. Variants of S49 mouse lymphoma cells have played an important role in establishing the connections between R and N, and in proving the essential role of the GTP-regulatory proteins in 'coupling' receptors to the enzyme system (Johnson et al 1981). For example, in one variant, N is modified so that it can't react with R; in another variant N reacts with R but cannot couple with C. Thus, subtle changes in structure, rather than deletion, may explain aberrant responses to hormones in certain disease states. Since this meeting deals with autoimmune diseases, one might speculate that a cause of the development of receptor antibodies is that slight changes occur in the receptor molecules so that they become 'foreign' bodies which the immune system detects and reacts to appropriately.

On your point about the possible multiplicity of N units, we know that all hormones or neurotransmitters that regulate adenylate cyclase do so through a GTP-requiring process. It is not so clear whether GTP acts through the same protein (N unit). I have speculated that N units for stimulatory and inhibitory receptors may be distinct macromolecules (Rodbell 1980).

Receptors present an even more difficult challenge. As a model, I would suggest that receptors are similar in structure to immunoglobulins, particularly in having variable and common regions. Variable regions could represent the sites of different hormone binding, whereas common regions may be regarded as those components containing the regulatory sites of guanine nucleotides, metal ions, etc. These 'common' regions may however vary, depending on the class of hormone receptors. For example, in the adipocyte several hormones activate a common cyclase unit through a GTP-requiring process (presumably the same N unit). Yet ACTH seems uniquely to require calcium at low concentrations (about 10^{-7} M) for action, whereas the other hormones do not show this requirement. Perhaps calmodulin or some other calcium-binding protein is attached to the ACTH receptor. Possibly we shall be able to group receptors into different classes, depending on their differences in requirements for divalent and monovalent cations.

Mitchison: How close are these molecules to being fully characterized?

Rodbell: At this juncture, I would say that our knowledge of receptor structure is nearly neck and neck with the N unit, at least for the β-adrenergic receptor systems. The structure of the catalytic unit, C, has proved to be the most elusive!

Venter: On the point that Mel Blecher raised, Henry Bourne showed that in pseudohypoparathyroidism (Farfel et al 1980) a 50% reduction in the amount of the N component is enough to explain a poor linkage between the parathyroid hormone receptor and adenylate cyclase, at least to the extent of correlating with the syndrome of pseudohypoparathyroidism (Farfel et al 1980). So this is an instance where a genetic alteration, resulting in perhaps only half a genetic complement of N, causes a physiological (pathological) change.

Bitensky: One shouldn't draw too firm conclusions about the molecular basis of this baffling condition. Our own and our colleagues' data on the activity of the N protein on repeat assays of the same sample, or on repeat samples from the same patient, show full activity, partial activity, and no activity. This condition may be more understandable in terms of the binding of a biologically inactive hormone to the parathyroid hormone receptor site, which partially blocks it. Our evidence (Nagant de Deuxchaisnes et al 1982) suggests that the high concentrations of parathyroid hormone circulating in this condition have very low biological activity. This less active hormone might in fact be the receptor blocker.

Crumpton: Martin Rodbell is suggesting that binding of a hormone stabilizes a pre-existing dimer. I would like to rephrase this suggestion in the form of a question, namely, what is the role of cross-linkage at the cell surface in triggering the receptor response? This is an important question in relation to the effect of antibodies on receptors; antibodies are, after all, divalent structures. If we consider the system of antibody against immunoglobulin as a growth promoter (i.e. polyclonal mitogen) of B lymphocytes, then we have good evidence that cross-linkage of the surface immunoglobulin of B cells is an essential event in the triggering process (Maino et al 1975). Similar evidence has been presented in the case of the antibody against the insulin receptor. Thus, in each case monovalent Fab fragments of the antibody molecule were inactive, whereas the bivalent antibody was an effective trigger. Furthermore, subsequent cross-linkage of the bound Fab fragments with a second bivalent antibody restored the response. There seems to be a dichotomy in that in many hormone systems, such as the catecholamines, the hormone is apparently acting as a univalent entity which should be equated with the antibody Fab fragment. Yet the Fab fragment fails to trigger, whereas the hormone stimulates its target cell. How do you view this difference? If you accept that cross-linkage by a divalent structure is an important event in triggering, then you are apparently arguing in support of the mobile receptor hypothesis, in the sense that the bivalent ligand brings receptors, which are initially apart, together. Isn't this contrary to your 'anti-mobile receptor' hypothesis?

Rodbell: I am really not against mobile receptors! I am in favour of some kind of coherent structure for receptors that accounts for their proper placement in the membrane, rapid action, amplification, and the ability of several receptors to react with a common N and C unit. Your idea that receptors are apart and must come together for binding and action to proceed is an excellent one. As you say, this idea is based on your experience and that of others with antibody–receptor interactions. The question at this point is what is meant by the term 'bivalency'. If bivalency means that molecules have regions for high affinity binding and distinct regions for action, then one can safely state that all hormones share this quality. Thus, with this definition, one can imagine that the receptor is composed of separate subunits, one involved in binding, the other with action; for physiological action both are required, although it is conceivable that at some concentration of the hormone, action might proceed without the tight-binding subunit being involved.

Given this hypothesis, my argument would be that there is an equilibrium between the two subunits prior to hormone binding and that the role of the hormone is to ensure that the equilibrium is toward the dimeric form of the receptor. In any event, a dimer of heterologous units of receptors would be compatible with the idea presented in my paper.

In sum, I don't disagree with some type of restrained, region-confined mobility of receptors in the membrane. Given the paucity of information on the actual distribution of cyclase-linked receptors, there is ample room for speculation. Nonetheless, we should be cautious in relating the actions of antibodies on receptors for hormones like insulin or EGF, which exist on some cells in large quantities (the order of 100 000 molecules per cell surface), to the actions of ligands on receptors linked to cyclase, which are present in quantities as low as 100 receptor molecules per cell. Perhaps this is the essential difference in the behaviour of the systems you are speaking about and what I am dealing with.

Crumpton: If the antibody is directed against a receptor, however, then surely you require no more molecules of antibody acting than molecules of the equivalent ligand?

Rees Smith: There is consistent evidence that in the case of antibodies to the thyrotropin (TSH) receptor, Fab fragments are as active in stimulating the thyroid as the intact IgG molecule (Rees Smith 1981). Consequently, cross-linkage does not appear to be a necessary factor in inducing a stimulatory signal in the TSH receptor. In other situations this may well not be the case.

REFERENCES

Farfel Z, Brickman AS, Kaslow HR, Brothers VM, Bourne HR 1980 Defect of receptor–cyclase coupling protein in pseudohypoparathyroidism. N Engl J Med 303:237-242

Fraser CM, Venter JC 1980 Monoclonal antibodies to β-adrenergic receptors: use in purification and molecular characterization of β-receptors. Proc Natl Acad Sci USA 77:7034-7038

Haga T, Ross EM, Anderson HJ, Gilman AG 1977 Adenylate cyclase permanently uncoupled from hormone receptors in a novel variant of S49 mouse lymphoma cells. Proc Natl Acad Sci USA 74:2016-2020

Harmon JT, Kahn CR, Kempner ES, Schlegel W 1980 Characterization of the insulin receptor in its membrane environment by radiation inactivation. J Biol Chem 255:3412-3419

Harmon JT, Kempner ES, Kahn CR 1981 Demonstration by radiation inactivation that insulin alters the structure of the insulin receptor in rat liver membranes. J Biol Chem 256:7719-7722

Johnson GL, Coffino P, Bourne HR 1981 Somatic genetic analysis of hormone action. In: Jacobs S, Cuatrecasas P (eds) Membrane receptors. Chapman & Hall, London (Receptors and recognition, Series B vol 11) p 173

Kempner ES, Schlegel W 1979 Size determination of enzymes by radiation inactivation. Anal Biochem 92:2-10

Maino VC, Hayman MJ, Crumpton MJ 1975 Relationship between enhanced turnover of phosphatidylinositol and lymphocyte activation by mitogens. Biochem J 146:247-252

Nagant de Deuxchaisnes C, Fischer JA, Dambacher KA, Devogelaer JP, Arber CE, Zanelli JM, Parsons JA, Loveridge N, Bitensky L, Chayen J 1982 Dissociation of bioactive and immunoreactive parathyroid hormone in pseudohypoparathyroidism Type I. J Clin Endocrinol Metab, in press

Nielsen TB, Lad PM, Preston MS, Kempner E, Schlegel W, Rodbell M 1981 Structure of the turkey erythrocyte adenylate cyclase system. Proc Natl Acad Sci USA 78:722-726

Rees Smith B 1981 Thyrotropin receptor antibodies. In: Lefkowitz RJ (ed) Receptor regulation. Chapman & Hall, London (Receptors and recognition, Series B vol 13) p 217

Rodbell M 1980 The role of hormone receptors and GTP-regulatory proteins in membrane transduction. Nature (Lond) 284:17-22

Schlegel W, Kempner ES, Rodbell M 1979 Activation of adenylate cyclase in hepatic membranes involves interactions of the catalytic unit with multimeric complexes of regulatory proteins. J Biol Chem 254:5168-5176

Schlegel W, Cooper DMF, Rodbell M 1980 Inhibition and activation of fat cell adenylate cyclase by GTP is mediated by structures of different size. Arch Biochem Biophys 201:678-682

Venter J C 1979 High efficiency coupling between β-adrenergic receptors and cardiac contractility: direct evidence for 'spare' β-adrenergic receptors. Mol Pharmacol 16:429-440

Venter JC, Fraser CM 1981 The development of monoclonal antibodies to β-adrenergic receptors and their use in receptor purification and characterization. In: Fellows R, Eisenbarth G (eds) Monoclonal antibodies in endocrine research. Raven Press, New York, p 119–134

The immunological basis of autoimmune disease

I. M. ROITT and L. C. DE CARVALHO

Department of Immunology, Middlesex Hospital Medical School, Arthur Stanley House, 40–50, Tottenham Street, London W1P 9PG, UK

Abstract Organ-specific diseases often involve cell surface antigens which when functionally characterized prove to have some receptor function. Certain restricted parts of the molecule are autoantigenic but the response to these epitopes is similar to that provoked by foreign antigens with respect to diversity of class, clonality and probably idiotypy. The mechanisms controlling the response to components on the surface of the body's cells are not fully understood but might be circumvented by polyclonal activators or by the development of T suppressor dysfunction. The latter could occur through a generalized defect in T suppressor cells, which would account for the association of autoimmune diseases in given individual subjects. Alternatively, or in addition (since genetic studies suggest multifactorial influences), the suppressor defect could be antigen specific. Our studies in chickens with spontaneous autoimmune thyroiditis show that normal antigen is obligatory for both the development and maintenance of autoantibody production and that it is possible that some abnormality or change in the presentation of the autoantigen (rather than its structure) is concerned in the initiation process.

The nature of the autoimmune response

We wish to address this discussion essentially to those disorders in which the pathological changes occur in a specific organ and are associated with autoantibodies whose reactivities are restricted to that particular organ. Typical diseases which come under this heading are Hashimoto's thyroiditis, primary myxoedema, Graves' disease, myasthenia gravis, Addison's disease and pernicious anaemia. As will become clear during the course of this symposium, many of them involve antibodies directed against surface molecules with receptor function.

One feature of organ-specific autoantibodies appears to be their reaction

1982 Receptors, antibodies and disease. Pitman, London (Ciba Foundation symposium 90) p 22-34

with only a limited number of epitopes or regions on the surface of the antigen. Dr Lindstrom will describe his work on myasthenia gravis later, but here we should like to refer to the specificity of the thyroglobulin autoantibodies in patients with Hashimoto's thyroiditis. Despite the fact that human thyroglobulin is a large molecule of relative molecular mass 650 K, which can bind up to 40 molecules of *rabbit* antibody to its surface, generally only four and very occasionally six molecules of the human autoantibody will bind (Roitt et al 1958, Shulman & Witebsky 1960). Since thyroglobulin is made up of two identical subunits, it seems likely that we are dealing with at the most two and sometimes three antigenically different regions. Interestingly, cross-blocking studies show that the same regions of the molecule are involved in different patients (Nye et al 1980), showing that certain restricted parts of thyroglobulin are consistently autoantigenic while the major part of the surface remains antigenically 'silent'. It may be that immunoglobulin (Ig) genes coding for antibodies to these silent epitopes are lacking in the variable region repertoire or that, as a result of chemical or physical structural characteristics, the 'silent' areas are considerably more efficient at inducing unresponsiveness.

Notwithstanding the small number of autoreactive determinants on thyroglobulin, the antibody response shows the same degree of diversity with respect to isotype (Hay & Torrigiani 1973) and spectrotype (Nye et al 1981) as would be expected with a foreign antigen; that is, once it is triggered, the nature of the response is the same irrespective of whether the inducing determinant is self or non-self.

Information on the idiotypic diversity of human autoantibody responses is sparse. We were successful in raising anti-idiotypic sera in only two out of six cases where thyroglobulin precipitins were bound from individual patient's serum onto solid-phase antigen and injected in rabbits; neither anti-idiotype cross-reacted with any of the other five patients (L. Nye & I. M. Roitt, unpublished observations).

In the majority of cases, autoimmune diseases tend to appear in middle-age and this suggests that their expression occurs as a result of some ageing process. Indeed, autoantibodies are not uncommon in the sera of clinically unaffected elderly people although it is noteworthy that they are usually of the IgM class, in contrast to the predominance of IgG autoantibodies in patients with disease.

Self-reactive lymphocytes

There is a growing body of evidence that potentially autoreactive lymphocytes are present in normal individuals. Of the order of 1×10^5 normal peripheral blood lymphocytes have been reported to bind radioactive thyro-globulin, and this binding can be inhibited by anti-immunoglobulin (Bank-hurst et al 1973). On technical grounds this finding has not been universally accepted but it is undoubtedly true that every vertebrate species so far studied can be pushed into producing autoantibodies by immunization with thyro-globulin, usually in association with an adjuvant such as complete Freund's or bacterial lipopolysaccharide, but sometimes without (ElRehewy et al 1981). In other words, all these animals are endowed with the apparatus required to make an immunological response to this autoantigen. Furthermore, the ability of spleen cells from animals immunized with thyroglobulin or myelin basic protein to transfer autoallergic disease to syngeneic recipients could be abrogated by 'suicidal' contact with highly radioactive antigen *in vitro*, indicating that the cells binding antigen were those able to transfer the autoimmune response (Ortiz-Ortiz & Weigle 1976). Autoreactive T cells can play a role in autoallergic thyroiditis induced in 'good responder' mice (Vladutiu & Rose 1975) and are effectors in experimental autoallergic encephalomyelitis (Ortiz-Ortiz et al 1976). T helper lymphocytes are also needed for expression of the spontaneous thyroid autoimmunity which is a feature of Obese strain chickens (de Carvalho et al 1981).

Self reactivity may also develop under quite different circumstances. Unexpectedly, lymphocytes cultured with syngeneic fibroblasts become cyto-toxic and can induce a graft-versus-host reaction when reinjected into mice of the same strain (Cohen & Feldmann 1971). These studies have been extended to show that T cells reacting with autologous brain (Orgad & Cohen 1974), testis (Wekerle & Begemann 1976) and thyroid (Charreire & Yeni 1980) can all be generated by co-culture with the appropriate organ. Lastly, one should mention the idiotype–anti-idiotype interactions of the immune network envisaged by Jerne (1974) as further examples of self reactivity.

The role of antigen

Autoimmunity could arise by antigen-independent mechanisms such as a spontaneous perturbation of the idiotype network or polyclonal activation. The Obese strain chicken provides a convenient model with which to test whether the presence of antigen is obligatory for the development of autoimmunity, since the thyroid gland can be removed *in toto* with relative ease. Of 32 chickens subjected to thyroidectomy at hatching, only four had circulating anti-thyroglobulin at 7 to 10 weeks of age and two of these had detectable thyroid remnants: in contrast, 47 of 95 controls, most of them sham-thyroidectomized, were positive for thyroid autoantibodies (L. C. de Carvalho et al, unpublished). Thyroidectomy carried out in birds with established disease produced a dramatic fall in antibody titre, often to zero, showing that the thyroid gland is also necessary for the maintenance of autoimmunity.

It has frequently been suggested that some structural abnormality in the antigen is required for the induction of autoimmunity. However, our finding (L. C. de Carvalho et al, unpublished) that an aqueous solution of thyroglobulin from the normal White Leghorn strain, without adjuvants, stimulates autoantibody production in seronegative neonatally thyroidectomized Obese strain chickens, shows that this is not the case. Furthermore, Obese strain and normal White Leghorn thyroglobulin could not be distinguished by sensitive immunoassays using either Obese strain autoantibodies or rabbit heteroantisera.

Factors affecting the generation of organ-specific autoimmunity

A picture is forming in which the normal individual would appear to have self-reactive T and B cells that can be triggered by unaltered antigens. In the case of surface receptors, these must be accessible to the circulating lymphocytes, and even thyroglobulin, which was originally thought to be confined within the thyroid follicle, is known to circulate in the blood (Roitt & Torrigiani 1967). Thus all the components needed for an autoimmune response are present normally and some controlling mechanism should be postulated that restrains these autoreactive cells. For the past few years it has been fashionable to envisage this control in terms of suppressor cells (Allison et al 1971), although even this concept may have many ramifications in view of the complex nature of the T suppression system (Germain & Benacerraf 1981); antigen stimulates antigen-specific suppressors (Ts_1) which in turn activate Ts_2 idiotype-specific suppressors directed against the receptors for antigen on the inducer cells, while finally the Ts_2 cells are thought to generate non-specific T suppressor signals from the Ts_3 population. In order to facilitate discussion, we have set out a possible scheme for the cellular interactions which could influence the development of autoimmune disease, accepting that it is simplified in some ways, and that other models could be presented, but that the general principles are likely to be valid (Fig. 1). Information on the experimental production of autoimmunity has been accommodated using a bypass concept similar to that of Allison (1971) and Weigle (1971), with the slight modification that the inducer T cells rather than the T helpers are considered to be normally unresponsive, although even this state may be spontaneously reversible.

Genetic analysis of autoimmune disease in experimental animals and in man (Rose et al 1981, Ghaffar & Playfair 1971) points strongly to multifac-

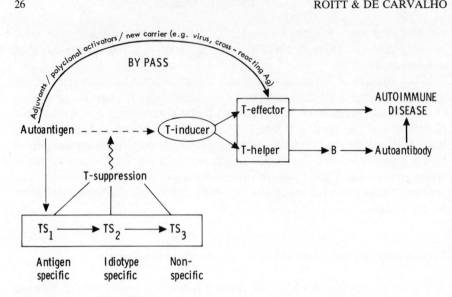

FIG. 1. Possible cell interactions involved in an immune response to self. Other schemes are of course possible and, for example, no account has been taken of the role of contrasuppressor cells (Durum et al 1980).

torial pathogenesis and one must not expect to find that these phenomena are explicable by any single defect.

It is worth drawing attention to a distinctive feature of organ-specific autoimmune diseases, namely their tendency to be associated in individual patients. Thus patients with thyrotoxicosis have a far greater chance of developing pernicious anaemia than do subjects without thyroid autoimmunity, while thyroid autoantibodies and disease are found with an uncommonly high frequency in patients with pernicious anaemia. Likewise, the first-degree relatives of these latter patients reveal a striking incidence of autoantibodies directed to both stomach and thyroid. These findings imply that some common feature underlies the overlap between organ-specific disorders, be it concerned with immunoregulation, antigen presentation or, as Knight & Adams postulate (this volume), an as yet undiscovered cross-reaction at the antigenic or idiotypic level. Additionally, there must be a factor(?s) which tends to focus the disease process more on one organ than another; one example is the greater incidence of gastric autoantibodies in the close relatives of pernicious anaemia than of Hashimoto's thyroiditis patients (Doniach & Roitt 1966). Bearing these considerations in mind, we may now explore different circumstances which might provoke autoimmunity.

(i) Defect in suppressor cells

The antigens implicated in organ-specific autoimmunity circulate at very low concentrations, oscillating about a mean value which could be set by the genetic make-up of the individual. Conceivably, in susceptible individuals, the mean concentration of a given organ-specific autoantigen may be set at a level which only marginally establishes antigen-specific Ts_1 suppressors—let us call them 'shaky' Ts_1 cells. Early in life, the Ts_2 and Ts_3 cells may adequately compensate for the marginally effective Ts_1 and unresponsiveness will be maintained, but any subsequent reduction in the performance of any of the T suppressors, as a result of an ageing process, would lead to the triggering of autoimmunity. The fact that neonatal thymectomy accelerates the onset of the spontaneous thyroid autoimmunity seen in both Obese strain chickens (Wick et al 1981) and BUF rats (Rose et al 1976) is testament to some regulatory control of the aberrant immune response by the thymus; likewise, selected strains of mice develop thyroiditis as a consequence of removal of the thymus several days after birth and the disease can be prevented by injecting young thymocytes (Kojima et al 1976).

The preference for a given organ in human disease could be attributed to differences in the genetic setting of the circulating concentrations of different antigens with corresponding selectivity in the antigen-specific Ts, which become 'shaky'.

(ii) Change in antigen concentration

Ageing of an organ, infection by a non-pathogenic organotropic virus, or perhaps the expression of some retrovirus, could influence the rate of synthesis or release of an organ-specific antigen, so affecting the balance between the T inducers and suppressors differentially. For example, depending upon the injection regimen, soluble thyroglobulin can either increase antigen-specific suppressors or actually induce autoantibodies in mice (Rose et al 1981).

From another standpoint, if one views the inhibition of autosensitization in culture by autologous serum in the experiments of Cohen and of Wekerle (see p 24) as representing blockade of lymphocyte receptors by soluble antigen in some form or other, a fall in the amount of circulating autoantigen might be expected to release the lymphocytes from suppression. Not everyone would accept the basic premise, however. Nonetheless, this does raise the question of whether some organ-specific molecules such as surface receptors do circulate at all and, if so, at what concentration.

The concentration of receptors on the cell surface as sensed by an immunocompetent lymphocyte might be important, since in most instances there are so few molecules per cell that it seems likely that they are present at subimmunogenic levels; changes in the organ which increased the surface expression of receptor could breach the threshold of immunogenicity, provided the antigen can supply an inducing signal. This brings us to the next possibility.

(iii) Change in presentation of antigen

The organ-specific surface receptors are normally associated with so-called Type I major histocompatibility molecules (H-2D/K in the mouse; HLA–A, B and C in man) and Mitchison will argue in a later chapter that unless they can be seen by a T lymphocyte on an antigen-presenting cell linked with Type II, 'Ia' molecules, they will not induce a response (see p 59). It would certainly be of interest to know the mechanism by which influenza virus infection increases the immunogenicity of a weak tumour-associated antigen (Lindenmann & Klein 1967), since this might be relevant to the development of autoimmunity to surface receptors. The virus may act as an associative 'carrier' generating the appropriate T cell help, or it might bud off as a vesicle containing the antigen and be taken up by an antigen-presenting cell. Whatever the change in presentation envisaged, it would have to be long-lived since, as shown by our studies above, the presence of antigen is still necessary to maintain a spontaneous autoimmune response.

(iv) Escape from suppression

This could occur through some mutation (? ageing) in the T inducers, resulting either in the formation of a high affinity-antigen-reactive cell, or in a general change in the responsiveness to T suppressors. The increasing resistance of T cells from New Zealand Black mice to protein-induced tolerance with age may be an example of the latter, but the genetic contribution of this mouse strain to the development of the murine systemic lupus erythematosus seen in the (NZB × NZW)F_1 suggests that this might be a feature more profitably sought at the non-organ-specific end of the autoimmune spectrum (Hijmans et al 1961).

Pathogenesis

The transient disease seen in neonates with circulating IgG autoantibodies to thyrotropin (TSH) or acetylcholine receptors (Scott 1976) acquired by transplacental passage is compelling as evidence that these antibodies play a direct pathogenetic role.

Conclusion

It is likely that autoimmune diseases have a multifactorial basis and possibly several defects, not necessarily uncommon ones, will be shown to be present before disease becomes apparent. Evidence for the individual factors is best sought in the unaffected close relatives of autoallergic patients. It must be said, however, that progress in the understanding of human autoimmune disorders is largely limited to the pace at which advances can be made in our techniques for studying antigen-specific interactions of cells in culture, particularly those involving self reactivity.

REFERENCES

Allison AC 1971 Unresponsiveness to self-antigens. Lancet 2:1401-1403

Allison AC, Denman AM, Barnes RD 1971 Cooperating and controlling functions of thymus-derived lymphocytes in relation to autoimmunity. Lancet 2:135-140

Bankhurst AD, Torrigiani G, Allison AC 1973 Lymphocytes binding human thyroglobulin in healthy people and its relevance to tolerance for autoantigens. Lancet 1:226-230

Charreire J, Yeni GP 1980 Primary sensitization of mouse lymphocytes on syngeneic monolayers of thyroid epithelial cells. Abstracts 4th International Congress of Immunology (abstr 14.3.14)

Cohen IR, Feldmann M 1971 The lysis of fibroblasts by lymphocytes sensitized in vitro: specific antigen activates a nonspecific effect. Cell Immunol 1:521-535

de Carvalho LCP, Wick G, Roitt IM 1981 Requirements of T cells for the development of spontaneous autoimmune thyroiditis in Obese strain (OS) chickens. J Immunol 126:750-753

Doniach D, Roitt IM 1966 Family studies on gastric autoimmunity. Proc R Soc Med 59:691-694

Durum SK, Eardley DD, Green DR, Yamauchi K, Murphy DB, Cantor H, Gershon RK 1980 Contrasuppression, a newly characterized immunoregulatory circuit: the inducer and acceptor. Fed Proc 39:353 (abstr 441)

ElRehewy M, Kong Y-CM, Giraldo AA, Rose NR 1981 Syngeneic thyroglobulin is immunogenic in good responder mice. Eur J Immunol 11:146-151

Germain RN, Benacerraf B 1981 Hypothesis. A single major pathway of T-lymphocyte interactions in antigen-specific immune suppression. Scand J Immunol 13:1-10

Ghaffar A, Playfair JHL 1971 The genetic basis of autoimmunity in NZB mice studied by progeny testing. Clin Exp Immunol 8:479-490

Hay FC, Torrigiani G 1973 The distribution of anti-thyroglobulin antibodies in the immuno-globulin G subclasses. Clin Exp Immunol 15:517-521

Hijmans W, Doniach D, Roitt IM, Holborow EJ 1961 Serological overlap between lupus erythematosus, rheumatoid arthritis and thyroid autoimmune disease. Br Med J 2:909-914

Jerne NK 1974 Towards a network theory of the immune system. Ann Immunol 125C:373-389

Knight JG, Adams DD 1982 The genetic basis of autoimmune disease. This volume, p 35-51

Kojima A, Tanaka-Kojima Y, Sakakura T, Nishizuka Y 1976 Prevention of post thymectomy autoimmune thyroiditis in mice. Lab Invest 34:601-605

Lindenmann J, Klein PA 1967 Viral oncolysis: increased immunogenicity of host cell antigen associated with influenza virus. J Exp Med 126:93-108

Lindstrom JM 1982 Structure of the acetylcholine receptor and specificities of antibodies to it in myasthenia gravis. This volume, p 178-191

Mitchison NA 1982 T cell recognition and interaction in the immune system. This volume, p 57-69

Nye L, Pontes de Carvalho LC, Roitt IM 1980 Restrictions in the response to autologous thyroglobulin in the human. Clin Exp Immunol 41:252-263

Nye L, de Carvalho LP, Roitt IM 1981 An investigation of the clonality of human autoimmune thyroglobulin antibodies and their light chains. Clin Exp Immunol 46:161-170

Orgad S, Cohen IR 1974 Autoimmune encephalomyelitis. Activation of thymus lymphocytes against syngeneic brain antigens in vitro. Science (Wash DC) 183:1083-1085

Ortiz-Ortiz L, Weigle WO 1976 Cellular events in the induction of experimental allergic encephalomyelitis in rats. J Exp Med 144:604-616

Ortiz-Ortiz L, Nakamura RM, Weigle WO 1976 T cell requirement for experimental allergic encephalomyelitis induction in the rat. J Immunol 117:576-579

Roitt IM, Torrigiani G 1967 Identification and estimation of undegraded thyroglobulin in human serum. Endocrinology 81:421-429

Roitt IM, Campbell PN, Doniach D 1958 The nature of thyroid auto-antibodies present in patients with Hashimoto's thyroiditis (lymphadenoid goitre). Biochem J 69:248-256

Rose NR, Bigazzi PE, Noble B 1976 Spontaneous autoimmune thyroiditis in the BUF rat. In: Friedman H et al (eds) The reticuloendothelial system in health and disease: immunologic and pathologic aspects. Plenum Publishing Corporation, New York, p 209–215

Rose NR, Kong Y-CM, Okayasu I, Giraldo AA, Beisel K, Sundick RS 1981 T-cell regulation in autoimmune thyroiditis. Immunol Rev 55:229-314

Scott JS 1976 Pregnancy: nature's experimental system. Lancet 1:78-80

Shulman S, Witebsky E 1960 Studies on organ specificity. IX. Biophysical and immunochemical studies on human thyroid autoantibody. J Immunol 85:559-567

Vladutiu AO, Rose NR 1975 Cellular basis of the genetic control of immune responsiveness to murine thyroglobulin in mice. Cell Immunol 17:106-113

Wekerle H, Begemann M 1976 Experimental autoimmune orchitis: in vitro induction of an autoimmune disease. J Immunol 116:159-161

Weigle WO 1971 Recent observations and concepts in immunological unresponsiveness and autoimmunity. Clin Exp Immunol 9:437-447

Wick G, Boyd R, Hala K, de Carvalho L, Kofler R, Muller PU, Cole RK 1981 The Obese strain (OS) of chickens with spontaneous autoimmune thyroiditis: review of recent data. Curr Top Microbiol Immunol 91:109-128

DISCUSSION

Knight: You suggested that a generalized defect in suppressor cells could account for the association of multiple autoimmune diseases in one individual. If that were so, one would not expect to see the discordance in the time of onset of the diseases which is commonly seen, as for instance in patients with both Addison's disease and diabetes mellitus. Solomon et al

(1965) found that in only 10% of 113 patients with both, did the two diseases appear simultaneously; the average interval in the remainder was six years.

Roitt: It might depend how 'shaky' the Ts_1 cells (T suppressor cells, type 1) were to the two different antigens. One might have a more shaky Ts_1 system for the thyroid autoantigens and a less shaky system for gastric antigens. One would have to postulate a continuing decline of the non-specific T suppressor cells (Ts_3) until the defects in the antigen-specific Ts_1 cells became apparent. I don't know whether that is correct; but it would be a possible way of explaining the time discordance.

Harrison: I am interested in the implications of your comments in relation to the ability to make autoantibodies. Do you think that the autoantibodies to thyroglobulin and DNA are just the tip of the iceberg and that we see them because of the high circulating concentration of autoantigens? In other words, getting back to the concept of forbidden clones, are there clonal deletions that we cannot ever compensate for in adult life? *Are* we able to make antibodies to the total repertoire of antigens that we are exposed to in, say, neonatal life? Is there such a thing as a forbidden clone, in fact?

Roitt: I think that autoreactive cells, that are precursors of so-called 'forbidden clones', *are* present for many antigens. However, where there are very high concentrations of a molecule, like serum albumin, one is presumably more likely to delete or blockade the responding clones or in some way make them unavailable. The person to disagree with that might be Göran Möller, who has evidence that lymphocytes treated with polyclonal activators produce anti-albumin antibody (Primi et al 1977), but I have not seen confirmation of this finding. I think there are some clones that are deleted. When Nicole Le Douarin manages to get chicken embryos to survive after removal of the thyroid, we hope to challenge the adult animals with thyroglobulin plus complete Freund's adjuvant, to see whether absence of the thyroid gland throughout the development of the lymphocyte system leads to the generation of a wider antibody repertoire—with more epitopes on the thyroglobulin molecule being recognized—than if the thyroid were there all the time. That sort of experiment should answer your question.

Harrison: You said that there was no evidence for common antigens between different organs at the B cell level. What did you mean by that?

Roitt: I meant that if you take say thyroglobulin antibodies and intrinsic factor antibodies, or parietal cell antibodies and thyroid microsomal antibodies, you can't detect cross-reactivity between the individual antibody specificities. However, for the anti-thyrotropin receptor antibody there is evidence that you can stimulate the adrenal gland with some sera, suggesting that they do cross-react.

Crumpton: You suggested that the potential for cross-reactivity in the immune system is greater than we have been led to believe from previous studies. There is support for this suggestion from results of E. Harlow and L. V. Crawford (Lincoln's Inn Fields Laboratories, I.C.R.F.), who have been raising monoclonal antibodies against the 'large T' antigen of SV40 virus (Crawford et al 1982). They have a spectrum of about 30 monoclonal antibodies and have been looking at their reactivity against SV40 virus-infected as well as uninfected cells. It is striking that these antibodies recognize not only the large T antigen but also a spectrum of normal cell components, with different antibodies recognizing different components within the cell. I find this surprising, because we look on antibodies as being highly specific. The degree of cross-reactivity here is completely unexpected. If we accept that this extent of cross-reactivity is a possibility and examine other systems in this light, then I think we can see similar degrees of cross-reactivity elsewhere. Some time ago we raised antisera in rabbits against skeletal muscle actin (before the days of monoclonal antibodies) and were very surprised to find that the antibodies cross-reacted with immunoglobulin (Owen et at 1978). We didn't understand this at the time, but I now believe that such cross-reactivities may be fairly common. I would, further, suggest that this type of cross-reactivity could be a major factor in autoimmune disease.

Friesen: A cautionary note must be introduced. Monoclonal antibodies may react with very restricted chemical regions of a molecule. Thus, unexpected tissue cross-reaction may simply be a reflection of the fact that chemical elements such as two or three amino acid sequences occur quite commonly among proteins. For example, one monoclonal antibody that was generated recognized an ether linkage used to attach a hapten. Initially it was felt that the monoclonal antibody had great specificity until belatedly it was appreciated that it was the ether linkage (a common chemical bond) that was the specific antigenic determinant in this case.

Newsom-Davis: You suggested that an increase in circulating antigen might trigger an autoimmune response. In some clinical conditions, the acetylcholine receptor (which is the antigenic target in myasthenia gravis) can be very greatly increased—for example, when a limb muscle is denervated. Yet these circumstances do not seem to lead to myasthenia gravis.

Secondly, how do you view the possibility of heterogeneity within a single autoimmune disease complex? There is evidence that myasthenia gravis may encompass several different categories of the disease in terms of both the HLA associations and clinical expression, suggesting that there might be several differing causative mechanisms within the disease. Why is this particular antigen, the acetylcholine receptor, 'selected', as it were, for so many forms of breakdown in tolerance, and what does that tell us about the process of autoimmunity?

Roitt: I would agree that many different processes contribute towards the breakdown of tolerance. For example, if you take recombinant, inbred NZB mouse strains, no one abnormality found by itself seems to relate to the development of autoimmunity. Perhaps you might have, say, seven different possible defects, and any four of these in combination might change the threshold of susceptibility. The acetylcholine receptor is rather an abundant receptor, by comparison to most of the other autoimmune diseases, and that may put it into a different category.

Lindstrom: On the contrary, I would say that the acetylcholine receptor is not at all abundant. Its concentration in muscle is about 3×10^{-13} mol/g or about 4×10^{-8} g/g muscle (Lindstrom & Lambert 1978).

Roitt: Of course, because the level of antigen increases, it doesn't necessarily mean that that will change the immune response in a certain way. A recent paper by Lane et al (1981) describes the response of lymphoid cells from human subjects sensitized to keyhole limpet haemocyanin. The levels of this antigen that are normally used to stimulate mitosis in lymphoid cells are orders of magnitude too high to stimulate antibody formation; so there are very critical dose ranges.

Bottazzo: I would like to stress the point that circulating autoantibodies do not necessarily imply progression to overt disease. There may be degrees of abnormality of the regulating T cell network. In the case of insulin-dependent diabetes, genetically susceptible first-degree relatives of diabetic patients have detectable islet cell antibodies for years before the acute onset of the disease. Heredity and environmental factors will contribute to the final outcome (Gorsuch et al 1981).

Mitchison: Has anybody been able to analyse this difference in target organ susceptibility?

Bottazzo: HLA restriction may influence organ susceptibility. There is disagreement as to whether DR antigens are expressed on the surface of endocrine cells. Experiments suggest that Ia molecules might become expressed only on activated cells.

Mitchison: If you demonstrated an association between the expression of an MHC molecule, say, on islet cells, and autoimmune disease, this would be very important; but until something of that sort has been done, what you are saying is highly speculative.

Harrison: The first thing is to stop using immunofluorescence and start looking specifically at cell surface molecules. Until we discover what is going on in the thyroid, in terms of particular antigens and the functional effects of autoantibodies, we shall get nowhere with the human thyroid.

REFERENCES

Crawford LV, Leppard V, Lane D, Harlow E 1982 Cellular proteins reactive with monoclonal antibodies directed against SV40 T antigen. Virology, in press

Gorsuch AN, Spencer KM, Lister J, McNally JM, Dean BM, Bottazzo GF, Cudworth AG 1981 The natural history of Type I (insulin-dependent) diabetes mellitus: evidence for a long pre-diabetic period. Lancet 2:1363-1365

Lane HC, Volkman DJ, Whalen G, Fauci AS 1981 In vitro antigen-induced, antigen-specific antibody production in man. Specific and polyclonal components, kinetics, and cellular requirements. J Exp Med 154:1043-1057

Lindstrom JM, Lambert EH 1978 Content of acetylcholine receptors and antibodies bound to acetylcholine receptors in myasthenia gravis, experimental autoimmune myasthenia gravis and Eaton-Lambert syndrome. Neurology 28:130-138

Owen MJ, Auger J, Barber BH, Edwards AJ, Walsh FS, Crumpton MJ 1978 Actin may be present on the lymphocyte surface. Proc Natl Acad Sci USA 75:4484-4488

Primi D, Smith CI, Hammarström L, Möller G 1977 Polyclonal B-cell activators induce immunological response to autologous serum proteins. Cell Immunol 34:367-375

Solomon N, Carpenter CCJ, Bennett IL, Harvey AM 1965 Schmidt's syndrome (thyroid and adrenal insufficiency) and coexistent diabetes mellitus. Diabetes 14:300-304

The genetic basis of autoimmune disease

J. G. KNIGHT and D. D. ADAMS

MRC Autoimmunity Research Unit, Medical Research Council of New Zealand, University of Otago Medical School, P.O. Box 913, Dunedin, New Zealand

Abstract The genetic predisposition to autoimmune disease in man is largely specific for each disease, indicating that these diseases are based not on a generalized breakdown of a tolerance mechanism, but on highly specific abnormalities of immune responsiveness which are subject to genetic transmission. In the presence of particular antigens encoded in the major histocompatibility complex (MHC) the relative risk of certain autoimmune diseases is increased, or in some cases decreased, and the increased risk has been widely attributed to linkage disequilibrium with unidentified disease-causing genes. Our studies on the inheritance of spontaneous autoimmune diseases in New Zealand mice have revealed that small numbers of dominant genes, some associated with the MHC but the remainder elsewhere in the genome, determine susceptibility to these diseases. That MHC-linked genes are not of paramount importance casts doubt on the linkage disequilibrium hypothesis. An alternative possibility is that major and minor histocompatibility antigens themselves predispose to the development of autoimmune diseases by altering the immune response repertoire through the effect of their clonal deletions on the network of paratope–idiotope clonal interactions. Such alterations could influence the chances of emergence, by somatic mutation, of pathogenic forbidden clones.

Autoimmune diseases in man are weakly inherited; for example, considerably less than half of the patients presenting with thyrotoxicosis have any known family history of the disease (D. D. Adams, unpublished observation, Bartels 1941). Nevertheless, it has long been recognized that many of the diseases which are now known or suspected to have an autoimmune basis do show a familial tendency. The genetic mechanisms underlying these diseases have remained mysterious and McKusick's catalogue (McKusick 1978) provides documentation of the difficulties encountered in establishing the modes of inheritance of these diseases—information which is essential for proper understanding of the aetiology of these conditions. Our current understanding of the genetic basis of autoimmunity comes firstly from the very extensive

1982 Receptors, antibodies and disease. Pitman, London (Ciba Foundation symposium 90) p 35-56

family and population studies in man, including a wealth of information on the involvement of major histocompatibility complex (MHC) antigens, and secondly from studies on the various animal models of spontaneous auto-immune diseases.

The genetic predisposition to autoimmune diseases

Twin studies have provided evidence that the familial tendency in auto-immune diseases is based primarily on genetic rather than environmental mechanisms. Thus monozygotic twins show a five-fold higher concordance rate than do dizygotic twins in juvenile-onset diabetes (Langenbeck & Jörgensen 1976) and in thyrotoxicosis (Bartels 1941). However, the approx-imately 50% discordance observed in monozygotic twins with these condi-tions indicates that, even when there is a genetic predisposition, environmen-tal factors are crucial in the expression of these diseases.

Burnet (1959) first drew attention to the probable role of somatic mutation in generating 'forbidden clones' of immunocytes with specificity for a host antigen, a concept which readily explains the incomplete penetrance observed in monozygotic twins and also the characteristic age-specific onset rates observed in autoimmune diseases (Burch & Rowell 1963). Support for this view is provided by our own observations that autoimmune haemolytic anaemia in NZB mice and lupus nephritis in (NZB × NZW)F_1 mice show highly variable ages of onset, even though the mice are genetically homogeneous, and even when they are caged together in quite large numbers and are thereby exposed to identical environmental conditions; in fact, a small proportion of NZB mice never get haemolytic anaemia, even though they live out a normal lifespan. Equally compatible with this view is the observation that the variety of autoimmune features commonly increases with age. Patients with autoimmune thyrotoxicosis commonly present with no other symptoms; not infrequently, exophthalmos, sometimes associated with pretibial myxoedema, appears later. Also, some patients initially showing thyroid-stimulating autoantibodies (TSaab) which are specific for the human thyroid may later develop TSaab which cross-react with the mouse thyroid. These phenomena suggest diversification of the forbidden clones by somatic mutation.

An additional, but related, explanation for the reduced penetrance in some diseases could be a requirement for an environmental trigger such as infection with microbial parasites bearing suitably cross-reactive antigens (Adams 1969). Exposure to such microorganisms could well alter the probability of particular mutational changes occurring, by stimulating proliferation of appropriate clones. Differing microbial environments could explain why the mean age of onset of autoimmune haemolytic anaemia is so variable among different colonies of NZB mice around the world.

Transmission of specificity

A striking feature of human autoimmune diseases is the highly specific manner in which each disease is transmitted. This feature, which should not be confused with the genetic association between certain autoimmune diseases (discussed later), has been clearly documented for several known and suspected autoimmune diseases including: Addison's disease (Spinner et al 1968), Graves' disease (Bartels 1941, Martin & Fisher 1945), Hashimoto's disease (Hall et al 1960), pernicious anaemia (Te Velde et al 1964, Doniach et al 1965), junvenile-onset diabetes (Simpson 1964), rheumatoid arthritis (Rossen et al 1980), multiple sclerosis (Visscher et al 1979), myasthenia gravis (Namba et al 1971) and ulcerative colitis (Goodman & Sparberg 1978). For example, Fig. 1a shows a pedigree in which there is specific transmission of juvenile-onset diabetes.

Patterns of inheritance

Autoimmune diseases have been characterized by uncertainty over the mode of inheritance, with some features suggesting dominance and others suggesting recessiveness. The frequent occurrence of affected individuals in two or more successive generations (Fig. 1a) suggests dominance and this feature has been documented in Graves' disease (Bartels 1941), pernicious anaemia (Doniach et al 1965, Te Velde et al 1964), myasthenia gravis (Namba et al 1971), juvenile-onset diabetes and rheumatoid arthritis (D. D. Adams, unpublished observation). However, the incidence in the siblings of probands with these diseases has invariably been found to be greater than the incidence in the parents, a feature associated with recessive conditions such as those based on enzyme defects. In fact this feature does not necessarily indicate recessiveness, but only that multiple genes are involved, at least one from each parent (Fig. 1b) but not necessarily at the same locus. These observations fit best with the contention that the predisposition for particular autoimmune diseases is determined by combinations of codominant genes (Adams 1978). Bartels (1941) recognized that his results, based on a study of the families of 204 patients with Graves' disease, were compatible with this model; however, he was influenced towards a model of recessive inheritance with virtually complete penetrance because of the very limited monozygotic twin data (13 sets) available to him, showing 75% concordance instead of the 30–50% which is now recognized.

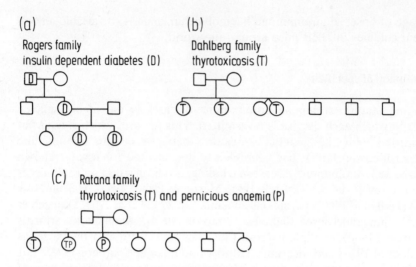

(a)
Rogers family
insulin dependent diabetes (D)

(b)
Dahlberg family
thyrotoxicosis (T)

(c) Ratana family
thyrotoxicosis (T) and pernicious anaemia (P)

FIG. 1. Some features of the inheritance of autoimmune diseases observed in family studies: (a) shows transmission of specificity through three generations; (b) shows occurrence in several offspring of unaffected parents, indicating a genetic contribution from each parent; (c) illustrates genetic association of two autoimmune diseases.

The V gene theory of inherited autoimmune disease

Adams (1978) postulated that the genetic predisposition to autoimmune disease lies in the specificity of the germline immunoglobulin variable region (V) genes, thereby explaining the genetic transmission of specificity. Germline V genes were postulated to vary in the closeness of their base sequences to those required for various autoantibodies, and so to vary in the number of sequential somatic mutations necessary to reach the autoreactive specificity. Our studies on the New Zealand mice have not substantiated this hypothesis (Knight & Adams 1981). Additionally, family studies on the inheritance of Gm allotypes in juvenile-onset diabetes suggest that there is no influence of heavy chain V genes in this condition (D. D. Adams, unpublished). However, preliminary data for Graves' disease are inconclusive and it remains possible that germline V genes influence the incidence of certain autoimmune diseases, especially as lack of allotypic markers has excluded study of the influence of V genes for λ light chains.

The genetic basis of autoimmunity in New Zealand mice

NZB mice show a high incidence of spontaneous autoimmune haemolytic anaemia, with nearly 100% incidence of anti-erythrocyte autoantibodies by

18 months. Howie & Helyer (1968) crossed NZB mice with several other strains and established that there was a strong genetic influence on development of the disease. In four of the hybrids, NZB × NZC, NZB × NZWA, NZB × NZCW and NZB × NZG, a high incidence of haemolytic anaemia, similar to that in the NZB parent, was apparent. In three of the hybrids, NZB × NZW, NZB × NZY and NZB × NZF, there was only mild or transient evidence of haemolytic disease but a very high incidence of severe renal disease resembling human lupus nephritis. These results indicate that haemolytic anaemia has a dominant mode of transmission, in that it is expressed in the heterozygous state in some strain combinations. In other strain combinations there is clearly suppression of this haemolytic anaemia phenotype by genes which also have a dominant effect. Furthermore, the lupus nephritis which occurs in three of the hybrids is clearly dependent on combinations of dominant genes because the condition is not seen in either parent.

Inheritance of lupus nephritis in (NZB × NZW)F₁ mice

Previous attempts to study the genetic basis of lupus nephritis in (NZB × NZW)F_1 mice ran into serious problems because of difficulties in distinguishing the severe, fatal renal disease characteristic of these mice from the functionally and histologically mild abnormalities found in the parental strains and in other 'normal' strains of mice. To overcome these problems we devised functional tests of renal competence which could be used to monitor the large numbers of mice required for adequate backcross studies. The onset of renal disease was monitored by fortnightly testing for proteinuria by bromophenol blue staining of urine samples on strips of chromatography paper. Detection of severe proteinuria ($> 3.3 \, \mathrm{g \, l^{-1}}$) was followed by the assessment of glomerular function using a single-injection, ^{51}Cr-EDTA clearance method (Knight et al 1977), severe renal impairment being defined by a half-value clearance time of greater than twice the normal value. Using these criteria, we observed six of 75 NZB mice (8%) and one of 40 NZW mice to have severe renal disease by 440 days, at which time 130 of 143 (NZB × NZW)F_1 mice (92%) had severe renal disease (Fig. 2).

The backcross of (NZB × NZW)F_1 mice to the NZW strain showed an incidence of renal disease which approached 50% by 440 days (Fig. 2), indicating that the NZB strain contributes a single gene, or a cluster of closely linked genes, to this condition. The backcross to the NZB strain showed an incidence of 32.7% by 440 days. As we observed a small, but significant, incidence of early severe renal disease in NZB mice we consider it more likely that this represents an over-estimate of 25% than an under-estimate of 50%

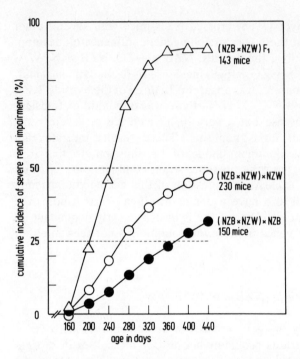

FIG. 2. The cumulative incidence of lupus nephritis in (NZB × NZW)F_1 mice and in the reciprocal backcrosses. (Reproduced from Knight & Adams 1978 by permission of the *Journal of Experimental Medicine.*)

incidence. These results are therefore compatible with the conclusion that the renal disease of the (NZB × NZW)F_1 hybrid is determined by three genes, all dominant or codominant, one contributed by the NZB strain and two, unlinked, contributed by the NZW strain (Knight & Adams 1978).

Linkage between lupus nephritis genes and the MHC

We tested for the independent segregation of histocompatibility type and renal disease in both backcrosses. In the backcross to the NZW strain, a preponderance of the mice with renal disease were heterozygous with respect to *H-2* type (the MHC in mice is termed *H-2*, and in man, *HLA*) (Table 1). This imbalance was highly significant ($\chi^2 = 26.5$, $P < 0.001$) and indicates linkage between the gene contributed by the NZB strain (*Lpn-1*) and *H-2* but with a cross-over frequency of $32.6 \pm 3.1\%$ between them. This would appear to place the *Lpn-1* locus close to the *Hh* locus which was observed by Lotzova

TABLE 1 Segregation of renal disease and *H-2* type in (NZB × NZW)F$_1$ × NZW backcross mice (Knight et al 1977)

	Histocompatibility type		Total
	$H-2^d/H-2^z$	$H-2^z/H-2^z$	
Mice with renal disease	78	36	114
Mice without renal disease	39	77	116
Total	117	113	230

& Cudkowicz (1973) to control resistance to bone marrow grafts in NZB and NZW mice, perhaps by coding for a hybrid histocompatibility antigen expressed only in heterozygotes.

In the backcross to the NZB strain, a greater preponderance of the mice with renal disease were heterozygous for *H-2* type (Table 2) ($\chi^2 = 35.2$,

TABLE 2 Segregation of renal disease and *H-2* type in (NZB × NZW)F$_1$ × NZB backcross mice (Knight & Adams 1978)

	Histocompatibility type		Total
	$H-2^d/H-2^z$	$H-2^d/H-2^d$	
Mice with renal disease	43	6	49
Mice without renal disease	35	66	101
Total	78	72	150

$P < 0.001$), indicating that one of the genes contributed by the NZW strain is tightly linked to the *H-2* complex. The occurrence of renal disease in six $H-2^d/H-2^d$ mice could indicate a cross-over frequency of approximately 8% but, as indicated earlier, a small proportion (8%) of NZB mice develop early severe renal disease indistinguishable from that of the (NZB × NZW)F$_1$ hybrid according to the diagnostic criteria used in this study.

Lupus nephritis loci are not linked to the immunoglobulin heavy chain loci

The results presented above indicate that boh *Lpn-1* and *Lpn-2* are on the 17th chromosome and therefore cannot be *Igh-V* genes (chromosome 12). The possibility of *Lpn-3* being *Igh*-linked could not be tested directly, since NZB and NZW are both *Igh-1^e*. We therefore used an appropriate outcross, as shown in Table 3, the NZC strain having the *Igh-1^a* allotype. There was no correlation between occurrence of renal disease and immunoglobulin allotype, indicating that *Lpn-3* is not an *Igh-V* gene.

TABLE 3 Lack of association between susceptibility to renal disease and immunoglobulin allotype in (NZW × NZC)F₁ × NZB outcross mice (Knight & Adams 1981) (with permission)

	Immunoglobulin allotype		Unknown	Total
	$Igh\text{-}1^{a/e}$	$Igh\text{-}1^{e/e}$		
Mice with renal disease	23	23	8	54
Mice without renal disease	84	84	18	186
Total	107	107	26	240

Inheritance of autoimmune haemolytic anaemia in NZB mice

The incidence of anti-erythrocyte autoantibodies was measured in NZB × NZC hybrids and backcrosses by the direct Coombs test (Fig. 3). The (NZB × NZC)F₁ and (NZB × NZC)F₁ × NZB backcross mice showed a similar age of onset to that observed in the NZB strain. The (NZB × NZC)F₂ mice showed a 76% incidence at 600 days, whereas 57% of the backcross to the NZC strain became Coombs-positive. These results indicate that the haemolytic anaemia is determined by a single dominant gene difference between the NZB and NZC strain.

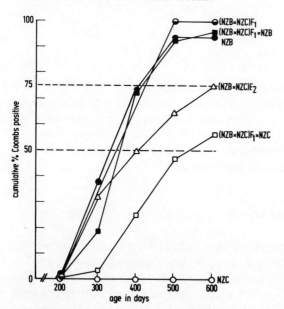

FIG. 3. The cumulative incidence of anti-erythrocyte autoantibodies in NZB and NZC mice, their F₁ and F₂ hybrids, and the reciprocal backcrosses. (Reproduced from Knight & Adams 1981 by permission of the *Journal of Clinical and Laboratory Immunology*.)

Evidence that two genes determine the occurrence of anaemia in NZB mice

The results shown in Fig. 3 suggested that the backcross to the NZC strain approached a 50% incidence more slowly than the backcross to the NZB approached a 100% incidence. In order to test this we compared the ratio:

$$\frac{\text{proportion Coombs-positive (NZB} \times \text{NZC)F}_1 \times \text{NZC}}{\text{proportion Coombs-positive (NZB} \times \text{NZC)F}_1 \times \text{NZB}}$$

at 400 days with the same ratio at 500 days by χ^2 test and found a significant difference ($\chi^2 = 5.6$; $0.01 > P < 0.025$), indicating that the time of onset of Coombs positivity in the backcross to the NZC was later than expected. One simple explanation of this difference, if it is real, is that two dominant genes determine the autoimmune haemolytic anaemia in NZB mice and that an allele of one of them, present in the NZC strain, causes a later onset of anaemia. The non-transmission of haemolytic anaemia to some hybrids suggests that some strains must have dominantly acting genes able to override the effect of the gene(s) causing autoimmunity, for example via an anti-idiotype reaction. Table 4 demonstrates that the observed results conform closely to the predictions of this model.

TABLE 4 **Comparison of observed incidence of Coombs-positive mice with predicted incidence if condition determined by two dominant genes in NZB, one also in NZC, and a dominant inhibitor in BALB/c[a] (Knight & Adams 1981) (with permission)**

	% Coombs-positive	
	Observed	Predicted
NZB (40)[b]	94	100
NZC (30)	0	0
(NZB × NZC)F$_1$ (30)	100	100
(NZB × NZC)F$_2$ (90)	75.5	75
(NZB × NZC)F$_1$ × NZB (100)	96	100
(NZB × NZC)F$_1$ × NZC (180)	57	50
(NZB × NZC)F$_1$ × (NZB × BALB/c)F$_1$ (140)	43[c]	37.5[c]

[a] Proposed genotypes of NZB, NZC and BALB/c mice:

NZB	AA	BB	ii
NZC	aa	B'B'	ii
BALB/c	aa	bb	II

Presence of both *A* and *B* and absence of *I* needed for autoantibody production.
[b] Number of mice.
[c] Data from Warner (1973).

Apparent linkage between haemolytic anaemia and the black/brown coat colour locus

Warner & Moore (1971) suggested that there was a relationship between coat colour and susceptibility to haemolytic anaemia in NZB backcrosses and intercrosses. Table 5 shows that in the backcross to the NZC strain consider-

TABLE 5 Non-independent segregation of anti-erythrocyte autoantibody production and black/ brown coat colour in (NZB × NZC)F$_1$ × NZC mice (Knight & Adams 1981) (with permission)

	Coat colour		Total
	Black	Brown	
Coombs-positive	68	35	103
Coombs-negative	31	46	77
Total	99	81	180

$\chi^2 = 10.8$, $P < 0.002$.
Cross-over frequency = $37 \pm 4\%$.

ably more of the Coombs-positive mice were black than were brown. This suggests that the NZB autoimmune anaemia gene (*Aia-1*), not represented in the NZC strain, is distantly linked to the *b* locus on chromosome 4. The observed cross-over frequency between these loci was $37 \pm 4\%$, which could place *Aia-1* in the vicinity of the minor histocompatibility locus *H-18*. We have been unable so far to find suitable genetic markers to enable a three-point test cross to be done, to position the *Aia-1* locus more accurately.

Conclusions to be drawn from genetic studies on the New Zealand mice

Table 6 summarizes the results from these genetic studies. Our studies have shown that a number of dominant genes determine the predisposition to these diseases, three genes governing the occurrence of lupus nephritis and two the occurrence of haemolytic anaemia. One of these five genes (*Lpn-2*) is closely associated with the MHC, and we have been unable to demonstrate whether or not *Aia-2* is also, but what are the others? They determine the occurrrence of specific immune responses (Knight et al 1980) and yet they are not MHC-associated immune response (Ir) genes. Having virtually excluded the possibility of these non-MHC genes being immunoglobulin V genes, we are left to consider alternative explanations. In view of the apparent proximity of *Lpn-1* and *Aia-1* to the minor histocompatibility loci *Hh* and *H-18* respectively, we have postulated that the non-MHC genes which predispose to autoimmune disease could themselves code for minor histocompatibility antigens—a theme that will be expanded upon below.

TABLE 6 Genes governing the occurrence of autoimmune disease in NZB mice and their hybrids (Knight & Adams 1981) (with permission)

Disease	Gene	Strain	Linkage	Chromosome	Cross-over	Neighbourhood
Lupus nephritis in	Lpn-1	NZB	H-2	17	33 ± 3%	Hh
(NZB × NZW)F₁	Lpn-2	NZW	H-2	17	0 or 8%[a]	H-2
	Lpn-3	NZW	Not H-2	Not 17	—	—
			Not Igh	Not 12		
Autoimmune anaemia	Aia-1	NZB	b	4	37 ± 4%	?H-18[b]
in NZB and	Aia-2	NZB	—	—	—	
(NZB × NZC)F₁		and				
		NZC				

[a] Observed cross-over was 8% but this can be accounted for by the observed incidence of renal disease in the NZB strain.
[b] Three-point cross not yet done.

Other animal models illustrating genetic determination of autoimmune disease

Since the discovery by Vladutiu & Rose (1971) that genes in the MHC govern susceptibility to adjuvant-induced thyroiditis in mice, Rose and his colleagues (1981) have made extensive observations on the genetic basis of this phenomenon and also of the spontaneous thyroiditis of Obese strain chickens. The adjuvant-induced thyroiditis appears to be principally dependent on a gene at the K end of the MHC, but a gene at the D end of the H-2 complex and genes elsewhere in the genome are also important (Rose et al 1981). In the Obese strain chicken the spontaneous development of thyroiditis is controlled not only by a gene or genes within the MHC but also by genes outside the MHC.

HLA and disease associations

The important discovery that the presence of particular MHC antigens influences the chance of developing particular diseases has resulted in a wealth of information which is of great value for analysis of the genetic basis of autoimmune disease. McDevitt & Bodmer (1972) and others have proposed that these associations in man are due not to the direct effects of the serologically determined HLA antigens, but to the effects of closely linked 'disease susceptibility' loci which are in linkage disequilibrium with the HLA-A, B, C and D loci. Linkage disequilibrium arises within populations when particular alleles at closely linked loci occur together on the same chromosome more often than would be expected by chance; this phenomenon has been well established for antigens within the HLA system

(Bodmer & Bodmer 1978), thus leading to the proposal that linkage disequilibrium is responsible for the observed disease associations.

Nevertheless, we have been influenced by our findings in the New Zealand mice, and by the results already discussed on the mode of inheritance of human autoimmune diseases, to consider an alternative explanation for the association of histocompatibility antigens with susceptibility to autoimmune diseases, namely that these antigens themselves cause alterations in the immune response repertoire through clonal deletions, as explained below.

Multiple genes acting in concert determine predisposition to autoimmune disease

The linkage disequilibrium explanation is based on the assumption that single disease-susceptibility loci, linked to or part of the MHC, are responsible for the genetic predisposition to these diseases. However, the results from our studies on New Zealand mice and the studies of Rose et al (1981) on the Obese chickens demonstrate that multiple genes determine these conditions, and that the MHC-linked genes are not more, nor less, important than the non-MHC-linked genes. As already discussed, the finding that in human autoimmune diseases the incidence in siblings of probands is higher than the incidence in parents provides evidence that, in man also, multiple genes acting together determine predisposition to autoimmunity.

Are D-locus effects pre-eminent?

The search for associations between HLA antigens and specific diseases was stimulated by the demonstration that, in the mouse, the MHC contains genes which influence specific immune responses and resistance to viral leukaemogenesis. Central to the linkage disequilibrium concept has been evidence that the *HLA-D* locus in man is equivalent to the *I* region of the mouse MHC, and that observed associations between specific diseases in man and antigens of the *A, B* or *C* loci are in fact due to *D* locus antigens with which corresponding *A, B,* or *C* locus antigens are in linkage disequilibrium. It has been proposed that the 'disease-susceptibility loci' are closely linked to the *D* locus. If this is so, then one would expect to find that *D* locus associations are considerably stronger than *A, B,* or *C* locus ones. To some extent this is borne out by available data, but there are notable exceptions in which the relative risk for particular diseases seems influenced more by *B* locus antigens than by any reported *D* locus ones (e.g. Abdel-Khalik et al 1980) (Table 7). Furthermore, there does not seem to be any consistent

TABLE 7 Some of the highest relative risks imposed by various MHC and the H-Y antigens, showing that _D_ locus antigens are not pre-eminent for autoimmune diseases

Disease	Antigen	Relative risk
Ankylosing spondylitis	B27	× 87
	H-Y	× 8
Dermatitis herpetiformis	DRW3	× 56
Reiters disease	B27	× 37
Insulin-dependent diabetes mellitus	DW2	÷ 33
	DRW3	× 5.7
Ulcerative colitis (Japanese)	AW19	÷ 25
	B5	× 3.9
Chronic active hepatitis	DRW3	× 13.9
Goodpasture's disease	DRW2	× 13.1
Systemic lupus erythematosus	H-Y	÷ 10
	B8	× 2.1
Addison's disease	DW3	× 6.3
Graves' disease	H-Y	÷ 6
	DW3	× 3.7
	B8	× 2.3
Myasthenia gravis		
females	B8	× 5.5
	DR3	× 2.9
young adults	H-Y	÷ 3

The HLA relative risks were extracted from Ryder et al (1979).

relationship between the ratios of relative risk associated with D/DR 3 and the risk associated with B8 for those diseases in which both associations have been noted (Table 8). This would imply that the disease-susceptibility loci are scattered all along the 6th chromosome, for some diseases being closer to the _B_ locus than to _D_ and for others being to the left of _D_ (the order of the MHC loci being _D-B-C-A_).

In contrast to the increase in relative risk conferred by some antigens is the protective effect conferred by others. Some of these protective effects are quite strong, as shown in Table 7. For example DW2 is associated with a 33-fold decreased risk for insulin-dependent diabetes mellitus and AW19 with a 25-fold decrease in risk for ulcerative colitis in Japanese.

There is evidence to suggest that in some diseases when certain antigens occur together, the relative risk resulting is the product of the relative risk which each confers. This has been reported in insulin-dependent diabetes for B8 and B15 occurring together (Nerup et al 1977) and for D/DR 3 and D/DR 4 occurring together (Deschamps et al 1979). This suggests either that there is a separate disease-susceptibility gene in linkage disequilibrium with each of these alleles, or that the effect is mediated by the histocompatibility antigens themselves.

TABLE 8 Are *B* locus associations attributable to linkage disequilibrium with *D* locus antigens?

Disease	Antigen	Relative risk	Ratio of risk associated with D3 or DR3 to risk associated with B8
Coeliac disease	DW3	64.5	8
	B8	8.1	
Chronic active hepatitis	DRW3	3.4	0.6
	B8	6.1	
Graves' disease	DW3	5.1	1.4
	B8	3.6	
Juvenile-onset diabetes	DRW3	1.8	0.7
	B8	2.5	
Myasthenia gravis	DRW3	2.3	0.7
	B8	3.1	
Idiopathic Addison's disease	DW3	6.3	1.6
	B8	3.9	

Data from Bodmer (1980) except for Addison's disease, for which the data came from Ryder et al (1979).

The increase or decrease in relative risk conferred by sex (Y chromosome) is as great as many of the apparent *HLA* effects (Table 7). Thus, thyrotoxicosis is about six times more common in females than in males, systemic lupus erythematosus is 5–10 times more common in females than males, myasthenia gravis in young adults is about three times commoner in females than males, and ankylosing spondylitis is about eight times commoner in males than in females. The patterns of inheritance of these disorders are not compatible with this effect being due to genes on the X chromosome.

A new explanation for the effect of histocompatibility antigens and sex on predisposition to autoimmune disease

Jerne (1974) proposed that clonal deletions by anti-idiotype reactions are a frequent happening both in fetal life, where various combinations of germline V genes will produce interacting clones, and in adult life, where new clones arise by somatic mutation. Jerne envisaged a network of paratope–idiotope reactions, influencing the immune response repertoire of each individual.

Burnet (1959) proposed that tolerance to self antigens is caused by clonal deletion by antigenic contact in fetal life, a concept for which Nossal has coined the name 'clonal abortion'. It now seems likely that this phenomenon is not restricted to the fetus but applies to immature B cells throughout life (Nossal & Pike 1975).

We consider that the influence of histocompatibility antigens and sex on predisposition to autoimmune disease can be completely explained in terms of the above concepts (Adams & Knight 1980). It is proposed that histocompatibility antigens, both major and minor and also H-Y, alter the immune response repertoire by clonal deletion and thereby influence the probability of clones with specificity for self antigens arising by somatic mutation from the clonal repertoire initially determined by germline V genes. Such clonal deletions could have both positive and negative effects, depending on whether the deleted clone is the precursor of a 'forbidden clone' or the precursor of a clone which could otherwise act as an anti-idiotype clone against a forbidden clone.

According to this hypothesis (which we have termed the H gene theory of inherited autoimmune disease) the effect of sex on the incidence of an autoimmune disease is exerted by male-specific antigens coded for by genes on the Y chromosome; these antigens would impose certain deletions, like other histocompatibility antigens, and so have positive effects (e.g. ankylosing spondylitis—deletion of clones reactive with the idiotopes of the precursors of pathogenic clones) and negative effects (e.g. thyrotoxicosis—deletion of certain potential precursors of thyroid-stimulating autoantibody clones) on the incidence of autoimmune diseases. That there may be differences in the H-Y antigens of different individuals is suggested by studies on BXSB mice, which spontaneously develop autoimmune lupus nephritis. The development of this disease is markedly accelerated in males as compared to females, and the acceleration is not hormonal (Eisenberg & Dixon 1980). Acceleration of the disease is seen in F_1 hybrid males only if the Y chromosome is derived from the BXSB strain (Murphy & Roths 1979).

The genetic association between autoimmune diseases in man

Autoimmunity affecting the thyroid, the parathyroids, the adrenals, the stomach and the pancreatic islets shows a genetic association, individuals and families with one condition having an increased incidence of the other condition (for example, see Fig. 1c). Thus in patients with Addison's disease the incidence of diabetes is increased six times and in patients with diabetes the incidence of Addison's disease is increased five times. Similarly, the incidence of diabetes in myxoedema is increased about six-fold (Adams 1978). Thyrotoxicosis shows an increased frequency in patients with pernicious anaemia (McNichol 1961) and autoantibodies to intrinsic factor are unduly common in diabetes (Irvine 1980). These data suggest pathogenic genes, perhaps coding for alloantigens, in common for these conditions. When more than one autoimmune disease occurs in the same patient, the time of onset of the two conditions is usually discordant. Thus Solomon et al (1965) found that in only 10% of 113 patients with both Addison's disease and diabetes mellitus did the two diseases appear apparently simultaneously; the average interval in the remainder was nearly six years. These observations suggest that the genetic influence operates on precursors of the pathogenic clones rather than on the clones themselves. A possible mechanism is that there are shared idiotypic determinants between precursors of the pathogenic clones in these diseases.

REFERENCES

Abdel-Khalik A, Paton L, White AG, Urbaniak SJ 1980 Human leucocyte antigens A, B, C, and DRW in idiopathic 'warm' autoimmune haemolytic anaemia. Br Med J 280:760-761

Adams DD 1969 A theory of pathogenesis of rheumatic fever, glomerulonephritis and other autoimmune diseases triggered by infection. Clin Exp Immunol 5:105-115

Adams D D 1978 The V gene theory of inherited autoimmune disease. J Clin Lab Immunol 1:17-24

Adams DD, Knight JG 1980 H gene theory of inherited autoimmune disease. Lancet 1:396-398

Bartels ED 1941 Heredity in Graves' disease. Munksgaard, Copenhagen

Bodmer WF 1980 The HLA system and disease. J R Coll Physicians Lond 14:43-50

Bodmer WF, Bodmer JG 1978 Evolution and function of the HLA system. Br Med Bull 34:309-316

Burch PRJ, Rowell NR 1963 Autoimmunity. Aetiological aspects of chronic discoid and systemic lupus erythematosus, systemic sclerosis and Hashimoto's thyroiditis. Lancet 2:507-513

Burnet FM 1959 The clonal selection theory of acquired immunity. Cambridge University Press, London

Deschamps I, Lestradet H, Marcelli-Barge A, Benajam A, Busson M, Hors J, Dausset J 1979 Properdin factor B alleles as markers for insulin-dependent diabetes. Lancet 2:793

Doniach D, Roitt IM, Taylor KB 1965 Autoimmunity in pernicious anaemia. Ann NY Acad Sci 124:605-625

Eisenberg RA, Dixon FJ 1980 Effect of castration on male-determined acceleration of autoimmune disease in BXSB mice. J Immunol 125:1959-1961

Goodman MJ, Sparberg M 1978 Ulcerative colitis. Wiley, New York

Hall R, Owen SG, Smart GA 1960 Evidence for genetic predisposition to formation of thyroid autoantibodies. Lancet 2:187-188

Howie JB, Helyer BJ 1968 The immunology and pathology of NZB mice. Adv Immunol 9:215-266

Irvine WJ 1980 Autoimmunity in endocrine disease. In: Fougereau M, Dausset J (eds) Immunology 80. Academic Press, London (Proc 4th Int Congr Immunol) p 930-958

Jerne NK 1974 Towards a network theory of the immune system. Ann Inst Pasteur (Paris) 125C:373-389

Knight JG, Adams DD 1978 Three genes for lupus nephritis in NZB × NZW mice. J Exp Med 147:1653-1660

Knight JG, Adams DD 1981 Genes determining autoimmune disease in New Zealand mice. J Clin Lab Immunol 5:165-170

Knight JG, Adams DD, Purves HD 1977 The genetic contribution of the NZB mouse to the renal disease of the NZB × NZW hybrid. Clin Exp Immunol 28:352-358

Knight JG, Knight A, Winchester G 1980 Evidence that autoimmunity in NZB mice is caused by a defect in immune specificity rather than a generalised defect in tolerance of self-antigens. Cell Immunol 56:317-322

Langenbeck U, Jörgensen G 1976 The genetics of diabetes mellitus—a review of twin studies. In: Creutzfeldt W et al (eds) The genetics of diabetes mellitus. Springer-Verlag, Berlin, p 21-25

Lotzova E, Cudkowicz G 1973 Resistance of irradiated F_1 hybrid and allogeneic mice to bone marrow grafts of NZB donors. J Immunol 110:791-800

Martin L, Fisher RA 1945 The hereditary and familial aspects of exophthalmic goitre and nodular goitre. Q J Med 56:207-219

McDevitt HO, Bodmer WF 1972 Histocompatibility antigens, immune responsiveness and susceptibility to disease. Am J Med 52:1-8

McKusick VA 1978 Mendelian inheritance in man, 5th edn. Johns Hopkins University Press, Baltimore, Md.

McNichol GP 1961 Thyrotoxicosis associated with pernicious anaemia. Am J Med Sci 241:336-342

Murphy ED, Roths JB 1979 A Y chromosome associated factor in strain BXSB producing accelerated autoimmunity and lymphoproliferation. Arthritis Rheum 22:1188-1194

Namba T, Brunner NG, Brown SB, Muguruma M, Grob D 1971 Familial myasthenia gravis. Arch Neurol 25:49-60

Nerup J, Cathelineau Cr, Seignalet J, Thomsen M 1977 HLA and endocrine diseases. In: Dausset J, Svejgaard A (eds) HLA and disease. Munksgaard, Copenhagen, p 149-167

Nossal GJV, Pike BL 1975 Evidence for the clonal abortion theory of B-lymphocyte tolerance. J Exp Med 141:904-917

Rose NR, Kong YM, Okayasu I, Giraldo AA, Beisel K, Sundick RS 1981 T-cell regulation in autoimmune thyroiditis. Immunol Rev 55:299-314

Rossen RD, Brewer EJ, Sharp RM, Ott J, Templeton JW 1980 Familial rheumatoid arthritis: linkage of HLA to disease susceptibility locus in four families where proband presented with juvenile rheumatoid arthritis. J Clin Invest 65:629-642

Ryder LP, Andersen E, Svejgaard A 1979 HLA and disease registry, third report. Munksgaard, Copenhagen

Simpson NE 1964 Multifactorial inheritance: a possible hypothesis for diabetes. Diabetes 13:462-471

Solomon N, Carpenter CCJ, Bennett IL, Harvey AM 1965 Schmidt's syndrome (thyroid and adrenal insufficiency) and coexistent diabetes mellitus. Diabetes 14:300-304

Spinner MW, Blizzard RM, Childs B 1968 Clinical and genetic heterogeneity in idiopathic Addison's disease and hypoparathyroidism. J Clin Endocrinol Metab 28:795-804

Te Velde K, Abels J, Anders GJPA, Arends A, Hoedemaeker PhJ, Nieweg HO 1964 A family study of pernicious anaemia by an immunologic method. J Lab Clin Med 64:177-187

Visscher BR, Detels R, Dudley J, Haile RW, Malmgren RW, Terasaki PI, Park MS 1979 Genetic susceptibility to multiple sclerosis. Neurology 29:1354-1360

Vladutiu AO, Rose NR 1971 Autoimmune murine thyroiditis: relation to histocompatibility (H-2) type. Science (Wash DC) 174:1137-1139

Warner NL 1973 Genetic control of spontaneous and induced anti-erythrocyte autoantibody production in mice. Clin Immunol Immunopathol 1:353-363

Warner NL, Moore MAS 1971 Defects in haemopoietic differentiation in NZB and NZC mice. J Exp Med 134:313-334

DISCUSSION

Kahn: It seems that in the immune system, as in most endocrine systems, there are mechanisms for both positive and negative feedback control. There are T helper cells and T suppressor cells, with several subtypes of each, so one could reach the same final disease state via a defect on the helper side, or a defect on the suppressor side. In any of the animal models where it would be possible to analyse this, has anyone yet dissected out the cell populations to see where the defect is?

Knight: This is a controversial field! There are good studies by De Heer & Edgington (1977) at the Scripps Institute. If they take B cells from one mouse strain (NZB) and put them into lethally irradiated mice of other, normal strains that do not normally develop autoimmune disease, the recipients will get haemolytic anaemia. If they take B cells from these other strains and transfer them to NZB mice, they won't. If they do transfers of mixtures of B cells and T cells, the essential ingredient leading to haemolytic anaemia is the B cells.

Kahn: What about measurement of helper and antigen-specific suppressor T cells in any antigen-specific autoimmune disease?

Knight: Beall & Kruger (1980) studied the production of anti-thyroglobulin antibodies by human peripheral blood lymphocytes *in vitro*. They can generate these antibodies from peripheral blood lymphocytes from Hashimoto's disease patients, providing that there are T cells present. It doesn't matter whether the T cells come from the patient or from normal subjects. You can suppress this response by putting in more T cells; again there is adequate suppression, whether the suppressor cells come from patients or from normal individuals. The implication is that production of anti-thyroglobulin antibodies is not due to a suppressor T cell defect.

Mitchison: You are seeing this as a controversy between T cells and B cells as the site of the defect, but Dr Kahn is asking how—considering just T cell regulatory defects for the moment—do you see the future of dissecting out helper and suppressor cell defects? Or, more generally, how do you see the dissection of the T cell system developing, in these human diseases? To my mind, the answer to this question is that the analysis will have to be done by cloning, and that until clones have been counted, we shall not make much progress.

Roitt: It is extremely difficult to develop an antigen-specific system for this dissection. One needs to produce T helper lines and see what cells can influence their activity.

McLachlan: Also, you will have to look at both T cell replication and antibody synthesis.

Mitchison: I am worried about something else, namely the interpretation of the linkage on chromosome 17 that you described. The evidence (Table 1, p 41) that you interpreted in terms of a locus on chromosome 17, loosely linked to H-2, could be interpreted in other ways, for instance in terms of incomplete gene penetration. Do you have further evidence for your claim of linkage between H-2 and an autoimmune disease gene on chromosome 17?

Knight: This H-2-linked gene (*Lpn-1*) is fully penetrant, because the F1 hybrids almost all develop the disease.

Mitchison: That also is interpretable in other ways; it would be important to have evidence from further backcrosses.

Knight: We haven't yet looked at other markers on chromosome 17, or on chromosome 4.

Roitt: With respect to the possible deletion of an anti-idiotype clone, to support this idea you have to suppose the existence of a common idiotype shared between say the T cells that are recognizing a whole spectrum of autoantigens in thyroid *and* those recognizing another spectrum of autoantigens in the stomach. To some extent you could simplify that by saying that once one autoimmune response has begun in one organ there is an escalation, because the microenvironment of the tissue destruction may provide cellular bypasses; but it remains a problem. In the thyroid, after all, there are possibly three different antigens, and even thyroglobulin itself bears different epitopes. So there is a problem with the idea of a common idiotype which sets off these responses.

Knight: The idiotypic cross-reactivity could occur in the precursors of forbidden clones.

Mitchison: How far do the recent results of R. Riblet's group (unpublished) using inbred recombinant NZB mice agree with your interpretation?

Knight: They find a number of genes throughout the genome which seem to be relevant to the development of autoimmunity; the problem is that when you use different strain combinations, you find that different, additional genes are important for the production of autoantibodies. This to us is the most relevant point. It could have been that the only relevant genes are MHC genes and/or immunoglobulin V genes, but that is not the way it is turning out. The extra genes could code for minor histocompatibility antigens.

Roitt: They found *no* correlation between any one parameter in their recombinant inbred mice and the development of autoimmunity.

Knight: Yes, but I am not happy about the different parameters that are claimed to be parts of the autoimmune syndrome in the NZB mouse. The production of natural thymo-cytotoxic autoantibody, for instance, may be a normal, physiological event which can be found in every strain of mouse.

Roitt: Certainly, but they failed to find an association between inherited V region genes, spontaneous production of IgM, and loss of the autologous MLR on the one hand, and the development of lymphocyte or thymus responsiveness to thymo-cytotoxic autoantibodies on the other. This is why I wonder whether having any three out of six features *is* enough to give the autoimmune response.

Mitchison: Are you implying that the minimum number of genes which John Knight spoke about may be a gross underestimate and that there may be a much larger number involved? That was certainly my impression from his results. You can't draw conclusions from a single backcross about the number of genes involved, without isolating the genes by further backcrosses.

Knight: I think you can; we have the NZB strain which does get haemolytic anaemia, and these other New Zealand strains, which have a large part of their genome in common with NZB and do not develop haemolytic anaemia, or any other autoimmune disease. What makes the NZB strain different from these other strains? I think you can analyse that, as we have tried to do. As soon as you bring in genes from a completely unrelated genome the pictures become much more complicated and, probably, unanalysable.

Kahn: If you consider all the potential steps that could be under genetic control, until you segregate each step you don't know where in the autoimmune mouse the genetic defect is. There could be as many as 10 different defects that could lead to the same final autoimmune syndrome, and each one would have a different genetic locus. You could have a defect in Ts_1, Ts_2 or Ts_3 cells in the helper side of the immune network, or in the B cells. All of these might present as a clinically significant, or non-clinical, autoimmune disease. Thus, when you say there are multiple genes involved, they may not be multiple genes acting at the same locus; rather, there may be multiple *defects* producing the same phenotype. In man, that is more likely to be the case than in genetically inbred strains of animals.

Hall: I am worried about extrapolating from the non-organ-specific to the organ-specific autoimmune diseases. Your study of NZB mice is most relevant to conditions like systemic lupus erythematosus. We should remember that these are two different groups of diseases, with very little overlap— that is, few patients suffer from both an organ-specific and a non-organ-specific disease.

Knight: I am not impressed by this distinction between organ-specific and non-organ-specific autoimmune disease. Graves' disease is regarded as a classic example of an organ-specific disease, yet there is involvement of an antigen in the orbit and an antigen in the shins!

Bottazzo: We agree that there is an overlap with the non-organ-specific diseases in thyroid autoimmunity, in that anti-nuclear antibodies are frequently found. However, SLE patients very rarely possess thyroid or gastric antibodies. We still believe that the genetic background and the immunological responses are quite distinct in these two groups of diseases.

Knight: One could regard intracellular antigens as representing an organ;

one could then say that systemic lupus erythematosus invariably involves two processes, first, the destruction of cells, which makes a large amount of intracellular antigen available; and second, the ability to mount an immune response against intracellular components. The distinction that you draw is not valid. It is an over-simplification.

Newsom-Davis: It should also be pointed out that organ-specific and non-organ-specific autoimmune diseases can sometimes associate, as for example lupus and myasthenia gravis. Myasthenia is an excellent example of an organ-specific autoimmune disease, whereas systemic lupus erythematosus clearly is not.

Mitchison: It is my impression that two kinds of analysis which have been applied in the mouse argue against the linkage disequilibrium theory. One is mutational analysis, where individual mutations have been found to affect immune response functions and antigen functions at the same time, whereas the linkage disequilibrium hypothesis would predict mutations that affect one and not the other. And it has been repeatedly shown that a single monoclonal antibody will react both with the antigen and with the immune response-controlling element, which again is not in line with the hypothesis. Both lines of evidence argue that the IR gene product and the alloantigen are identical, or at least that they are part of the same protein.

Roitt: It is certainly odd that with HLA-B27, when you find 80 or 100 times the risk factor for ankylosing spondylitis, some still maintain that because a few B27-negative subjects get this disease, it must be due to another gene close to it.

Unfortunately, we have not yet been able to produce experimental systems with which to study the interactions occurring in human autoimmune conditions, particularly with diseases like thyroiditis where most of the cells committed to the thyroid antigens are drawn in to an 'antigen sink' within the thyroid itself. When one looks at the peripheral blood, therefore, one examines a pale reflection of the real situation. That makes analysis difficult. But I agree with Av Mitchison that as one develops lines of cells one will be able to ask specific questions about different cellular types. At the moment we have only this 'catalogue' of possibilities. We have many model systems, but in the final analysis we may be remote from the thing we are trying to model.

Hall: There are models in man. Just considering antigen concentration, if you give radioactive iodine to a patient with a toxic multinodular goitre, there is no increase in receptor antibodies, whereas the majority of patients with Graves' disease given 15 mCi of ^{131}I show a rise in receptor antibody titre. So release of antigen does not necessarily produce an antibody response. You can produce models in man to answer certain of these problems in a restricted way.

Mitchison: John Knight's theory (the H theory) for the association of particular MHC antigens with autoimmune diseases would predict that minor antigens (non-MHC) should serve as specific immune response genes. There are an increasing number of animal systems in which the immunogenetics of the immune response has been looked at and where there are well-defined contributions from genes outside the MHC to immune responsiveness. These antigens are also being studied in their own right. Are you aware of any instance in which an H gene has been shown to function as an immune response gene in an experimental system?

Knight: There is one example of a minor histocompatibility antigen, H-Y, seemingly having an effect on an autoimmune disease, in the BXSB mice (see my paper, p 49). The autoimmune lupus nephritis to which this strain is prone is much more rapid in onset in males than in females. Hybridization studies show that the Y chromosome has to come from the BXSB strain to have this effect. Castration makes no difference at all, so it is not a hormonally determined acceleration.

Roitt: Alan Ebringer was one of the first to propose the idea of cross-tolerance as the basis for high and low response linked to the MHC. He and Davies looked for cross-reactivity between antibodies to the synthetic polymer TGAL and to the MHC alloantigens of CBA mice which give a poor response to TGAL (Ebringer & Davies 1973). There was a suggestion of cross-reactivity. However, Ebringer was not looking at the most appropriate parameter, since a (responder × non-responder)F_1 tends to show dominance of the responder genes and the results cannot be explained in terms of tolerance of the major histocompatibility antigens themselves. Rather, it would now be postulated that cross-reaction should be sought with (MHC + minor) antigens. It might be interesting to look at those results again.

REFERENCES

Beall GN, Kruger SR 1980 Production of human antithyroglobulin in vitro. II. Regulation by T cells. Clin Immunol Immunopathol 16:498-503
De Heer DH, Edgington TS 1977 Evidence for a B lymphocyte defect underlying the anti-X-erythrocyte autoantibody response of NZB mice. J Immunol 118:1858-1863
Ebringer A, Davies DAL 1973 Cross reactivity between synthetic T,GA-L and transplantation antigens in CBA mice. Nat New Biol 241:144-147

T cell recognition and interaction in the immune system

N. A. MITCHISON

Imperial Cancer Research Fund Tumour Immunology Unit, Department of Zoology, University College London, Gower Street, London WC1E 6BT, UK

Abstract This paper discusses mechanisms of regulation within the immune system. The only cells known to be specialized for regulatory activity within this system are helper and suppressor T cells. Like other T cells, most of these cells recognize antigen only in association with products of the major histocompatibility complex. This is a mechanism which ensures that these cells function appropriately, by being activated by and exerting their effects upon their proper cellular targets. It is likely but not certain that this mechanism of dual recognition is involved in the acquisition of self tolerance, and that inappropriate associations may be a factor in the induction of autoimmunity. There is extensive but circumstantial evidence that regulatory T cells govern to a large extent not only the induction but also the course (relapse and remission) of autoimmunity.

An understanding of the mechanisms involved in activating suppressor T cells is of special importance for the treatment and prevention of autoimmune disease. A variety of factors which favour activation of suppression have been identified in experimental studies. These include the nature of the antigen, the way in which it reaches the immune system, antigenic dosage, and the involvement of antigen-presenting cells. It is proposed that certain cells within the suppressor cell circuit (suppressor-effector cells) do not operate dual recognition, and that this may explain the factors which favour suppression.

The high incidence of sex-linked immunodeficiency diseases is discussed. It is proposed that this can be accounted for, at least in part, by the preferential elimination of autosomal deleterious genes in heterozygotes. This emphasizes the importance of measuring the fitness of carriers of these diseases.

This discussion is divided into three parts. In the first, I review the special importance of T cells as distinct from B cells in understanding and controlling autoimmunity. In the second, I review some of the circumstances in which cell surface antigens generate immunosuppression. The third part contains a discussion of sex linkage and sex limitation in relation to immunological

1982 Receptors, antibodies and disease. Pitman, London (Ciba Foundation symposium 90) p 57-81

diseases; this is a separate section which is not closely related to the rest, and is meant only for those who like solving genetical puzzles.

Three features of the T cell system are of special importance in understanding and attempting to control autoimmunity. These are (i) dual recognition, (ii) the low threshold of response of T cells, and (iii) the emphasis within the system on regulatory rather than effector functions. I shall discuss these in detail.

Dual recognition by T cells

The only receptors possessed by B cells which are known to play a part in the immune response are surface-bound immunoglobulin molecules (SIg) which recognize antigens. This is a slightly qualified generalization, for B cells do have other receptors which may possibly play a part, but which are not known to do so, although investigators are trying hard to find a functional role for them. These include complement (C) receptors and immunoglobulin Fc receptors. Since no role for them has yet been established, there is little more to say about them at the present time. Perhaps one should also add that other, less well-defined receptors have been postulated, such as those which may enable the B cell to find its way across heightened endothelial cells and others which may enable the specialized B cell of the gut to find its way into the lamina propria of the intestine. While C and Fc receptors are structures in search of a function, these others are essentially functions in search of a structure. At any rate, what matters is the SIg receptor for antigen.

For T cells the situation is different (for a general review of T cell reactivity, see Mitchison 1981). T cells recognize antigens in association with products of the major histocompatibility complex (MHC). It is generally believed that they do so in one of two possible ways, either by possessing two receptors, or by possessing one receptor which recognizes a conformational change in an MHC molecule imposed by binding antigen (there are various intermediate possibilities which need not detain us here). If the first possibility is correct, the difference between T and B cells lies principally in the number of receptors. If the second, the difference lies in their receptor repertoires. For a cogent statement of the arguments in favour of the second alternative, see Matzinger (1981)—although that review omits consideration of idiotype sharing between T and B cells, which is the strongest argument in favour of the two-receptor possibility.

Although the mechanism of dual recognition is thus unclear, its purpose is well understood. It performs two functions. Firstly, it ensures that T cells are triggered only when they are in contact with other cells, and not when they are free in body fluids. This is important because they, unlike B cells, act through products which either are not secreted at all (their antigen receptors) or are secreted but act locally (lymphokines). Secondly, dual recognition enables T cells of different subsets (cytotoxic, helper, suppressor) to be guided to their appropriate sites of action by means of the different components within the MHC. Cytotoxic T cells are guided by class I molecules (in the mouse, products of the K, D and L loci), helper T cells by certain class II molecules (products of the A and E loci), and suppressor T cells by another partially overlapping set of class II molecules (product of the J locus, but also of E). The J locus is of uncertain status because it has not yet been characterized by immuno-precipitation, and the whole question of dual recognition by suppressor cells is poorly understood.

This state of affairs has two major consequences for autoimmunity (Mitchison 1978). First, normal self tolerance probably results in part from a failure of self molecules to associate with class II MHC molecules. The argument runs as follows. No doubt there are many ways in which immunological tolerance of self is brought about. These include clone elimination and suppression mediated by T suppressor cells. Obviously, the immune system is under severe constraint in this way, and it is likely that any mechanism which could potentially prevent responses to self will in practice be selected by evolution to do so. One obvious possibility is to keep potentially dangerous antigens apart from class II MHC molecules, and thus ensure that they do not activate T helper cells. The problem is that the antigen-presenting part of the immune system has no obvious way of distinguishing self from non-self molecules and it certainly cannot afford indiscriminately to keep antigens apart from class II molecules—for this association is part of the normal working of the system. Indeed, we now have formal proof that antigen-presenting cells cannot discriminate between self and non-self (Sunshine et al 1982). This still leaves the possibility that the immune system may discriminate according to type of antigen during the MHC-association step. For example, membrane-bound antigens might constitute a special class for purposes of presentation. Foreign antigens bound to cell membranes are not the kind of thing which the immune system has much experience of in the course of its normal working, and one could imagine that it might pay the system to strike a balance such that this type of antigen would be poorly processed at the association step. This would have the consequence that such antigens would be poorly immunogenic, and thus would relieve the immune system of some of its burden of discriminating between self and non-self. While there is no direct evidence that the immune system works in this way, the possibility that it may do so provides an incentive for further study of antigen processing. And a fascinating and somewhat contradictory body of evidence exists on the question of how membrane-bound antigens are processed (Bevan 1976, Gordon et al 1976).

We are ourselves investigating this question at present, by exploring a system in which minor alloantigens are presented *in vivo* to MHC-heterozygous responding T helper cells in association with a parental MHC product (Bromberg et al 1979). In such a system the responding cells divide into two sets of clones, each restricted to one of the parental sets of MHC products; we can find out whether the minor alloantigens are processed in the sense defined above by determining whether both sets of clones respond. In practice we have been using B10 × B10.D2(H-$2^{b/d}$) T helper cells responding to BALB.B (H-2^b) or BALB.C(H-2^d) non-MHC (minor) alloantigens; we find that the BALB minor antigens appear to enter the responding immune system through the indirect route (i.e. in association with both responder MHC products), involving processing by responder antigen-presenting cells, and not to a detectable extent through the direct route, in association with stimulator MHC products. Our evidence, which is still incomplete, suggests thus far that in their preference for the indirect route antigens associated with class II MHC molecules behave very differently from antigens associated with class I molecules as described by Gordon et al (1976).

The second major consequence of dual recognition for autoimmunity is that it accounts for MHC-linked immune response (Ir) effects. It is now generally agreed that Ir genes are not a special category of MHC genes, but rather that the class I and II products of the MHC themselves control Ir functions (Klein et al 1981). They can do so in principle in two quite different ways, either by making or failing to make a physical association with a particular antigen, or by controlling the T cell receptor repertoire (probably by means of selection within the thymus) so that the antigen is or is not recognized. Both possibilities may operate in practice, and although a lot of effort has been devoted to resolving this question there are few clear answers. The human disease associations include many autoimmune diseases, and indeed it has long been known that the effects of the MHC are characteristically stronger in immunological diseases than in infectious ones.

The low threshold of response of T cells

It has long been known that T cells are more sensitive to low doses of soluble antigens than are B cells. This point was first demonstrated using foreign serum proteins such as albumin and immunoglobulin (Howard & Mitchison 1975). It has been further verified in a comprehensive study which colleagues of mine have made of the response of mice to the alloantigen F (Czitrom et al 1981). This is a protein which is present in normal serum at a concentration in the range of 10^{-8}–10^{-9} M. This concentration is sufficient to induce tolerance in T but not B cells (the question whether B cells become at all tolerant of F has not yet been answered). The system provides a clear-cut example of what is likely to be a general rule, that tolerance of self is determined mainly by T rather than B cells.

It is questionable whether this generalization applies to membrane-bound antigens of the type important in clinical autoimmunity. One obvious difficulty is that concentration, as applied to this type of antigen, does not have the same simple meaning that it does when applied to soluble antigens. The subject has not been studied systematically, and one cannot reach firm conclusions. The following points are worth making. (i) There are definite antigen dosage effects in the induction of tolerance by membrane-bound antigens. Thus, for example, classical neonatal tolerance is critically dependent on the number of cells inoculated, and the mechanisms which mediate tolerance vary with this number: at high doses, clone elimination predominates over suppression, while at lower doses this is reversed (Brent & Hutchinson 1981). (ii) There are dosage effects also in the induction of T suppressor cells, and membrane-bound antigens seem particularly to favour the induction of suppression. Both these effects are discussed further below. (iii) The location in which lymphocytes first see antigen is critically important. Exposure in the thymus is often crucial and when circumstances are arranged experimentally in such a way that an alloantigen is first encountered outside the thymus, abnormal tolerance may result (Waterfield et al 1981). (iv) B cells are known to pass through a developmental phase in which they are particularly susceptible to tolerance induction ('clonal abortion'). Whether this applies to T cells is not known. (v) Prolonged exposure of B cells to membrane-bound alloantigens in the absence of a T cell response often leads to clone elimination (Knight et al 1979).

In summary, we may conclude that in some way which is not fully understood T cells can detect the concentration of cell-bound antigens, and that they are probably more sensitive in this respect then B cells.

These conclusions have important implications for autoimmunity. They suggest that as a rule autoimmune responses are likely to be controlled primarily by T rather than B cells. For some antigens it is likely that only the T cell compartment ever becomes fully tolerant, and that departures from tolerance reflect T cell activation which may subsequently lead to B cell activation. For others the normal condition may be tolerance in both compartments. In that case, perturbations of tolerance may well be more likely to affect T cells, because of their greater sensitivity. Yet another possibility is that antigenic sequestration occurs in a way which may normally be sufficiently complete to prevent self-immunization. In that case one could imagine that the odd 'trickle through' of antigen in quantities sufficient to stimulate only T cells might generate autoimmunity. One way or another, their lower threshold of response would seem to make T cells more dangerous than B cells in the development of autoimmune disease.

T cells as regulatory cells

The third major difference between T and B cells lies in the amount of effort which they devote to regulating other cells. No compartment of the B cell population is known to be devoted solely to regulation. Admittedly, B cell products can and do exert immunoregulatory effects. The best known such effect is antibody-mediated feedback-inhibition of the immune response, and there is no doubt that this plays an important part in controlling the number of lymphocytes triggered in the response, the shut-off of the response, and maturation of the quality of antibody produced. Antibodies are also known to be capable of modulating the response through the idiotype network, although the extent to which they do so in clinically important situations is still uncertain. Yet another immunoregulatory effect, also of uncertain importance, is elimination of antigen via the liver, mediated by polymeric IgA. No doubt these and other antibody-mediated effects should be borne in mind when thinking about autoimmunity. But there are two considerations which tend to diminish their interest. First, so far as is known, these effects are all mediated by antibodies which primarily have protective functions. Therefore any defect in them should expose the body to infective rather than regulatory disease. Second, no autoimmune disease, whether naturally occurring or experimentally induced, has yet been shown to be associated with a defect in B cell regulatory function.

The situation with T cells is different. T helper and suppressor subsets are mainly regulatory in function, particularly if one includes in this category the control of other bone marrow-derived cells (macrophages, granulocytes, possibly also erythroid stem cells) as well as other lymphocytes. Indeed, the only known strict effectors among T cells—cytotoxic T cells—comprise a minor population. It is not surprising, therefore, that autoimmune disease has repeatedly been found to be associated with a defect in these regulatory cell populations. If we look at the history of the subject, when T cell subset markers were discovered in the mouse it took several years for them to reach general acceptance and even longer for subset deficiencies to be associated with particular autoimmune diseases. When similar T cell subset markers were eventually found in men, it took only a few months to find associations with autoimmune disease (Reinherz & Schlossman 1980).

Just how far need the regulatory T cell sets be subdivided? This is a 'question of the day' in cellular immunology which has attracted much discussion. Opinion divides broadly between the splitters and the lumpers. One point of view, adopted by Gershon, Tada and others, enthusiastically embraces the idea that the immune system operates through complex regulatory circuits involving at least a dozen distinct cell types: suppressor-inducers, contrasuppressors, ThAg cells, ThId cells, and so on (Tada &

Okumura 1979, Gershon et al 1981). The other viewpoint is more sceptical: it questions whether all the functions that can be distinguished *in vitro* are actually performed *in vivo*; it emphasizes the importance of repopulation experiments in which the stability of lymphocyte phenotypes or functional subsets is tested under prolonged *in vivo* 'parking' conditions; it is inclined to wait for the verification of postulated subsets by cloning methods. I am on the whole a sceptic, as I have indicated on several recent occasions (Mitchison 1981, 1982).

The generation of suppressor cells by membrane-bound antigens

This topic is worth discussing here because the antigens which matter most in clinical autoimmunity are mainly membrane-bound. Furthermore, suppression is important not only as a major natural cause of remission, but also as a principal aim of therapeutic intervention.

It has long been known that antigens presented on cell membranes tend to generate suppressor T cells. This principle applies to haptens and proteins (Battisto & Bloom 1966), alloantigens (Lake 1976), and idiotypes (Sy et al 1979). Lake's work (1976) with Thy 1, a non-MHC membrane-bound antigen, is particularly pertinent: Thy 1, as released by cultured cells into supernatants, generates an excellent *in vitro* suppressor response, which can be completely inhibited by Thy 1 as presented on intact cells.

Evidence that membrane-bound antigens tend to induce suppression can be found further afield. For example, mice exposed to ultraviolet light generate suppressor cells specific for u.v.-induced tumour cells. This phenomenon is central to any up-to-date discussion of the immune surveillance of cancer, and may be interpreted in terms of Sercarz's concept of determinants uniquely adapted to triggering Ts cells (Mitchison & Kinlen 1980). Another interesting group of examples are the glycoproteins of retroviruses which under certain circumstances confront the immune system with very large amounts of membrane-bound antigen. This is a situation which in some cases clearly (Yefenof et al 1980) and in others less clearly (Myburgh & Mitchison 1976) leads to the production of suppressor T cells.

Yet it cannot be true that membrane-bound antigens always generate suppression. After all, allografts are normally rejected; or, to take a particular example, membrane-bound Thy 1, as just mentioned, is suppressive *in vitro* but an excellent immunogen *in vivo* (Lake 1976). There must therefore be rules about when and where this type of antigen generates suppression; or, to put it a little differently, there must be rules about the balance of activation between T cell subsets. We can, I believe, define some empirical rules.

Firstly, the nature of the antigen may favour activation of one type of T cell rather than another. Perhaps the clearest examples of this are given by the alloantigens of the MHC. Those MHC products whose normal function is to guide a particular subset of self T cells—for example, the class I products which guide cytotoxic T cells—tend preferentially to provoke a response in the same subset when serving as allogens. This is a tendency rather than an absolute rule, although there is some evidence that the exceptions tend to involve T cells with abnormal phenotypes. Circumstantial evidence suggests that certain non-MHC membrane alloantigens may be particularly active in stimulating particular T cell subsets. Thus just two to three such antigens, among the many segregating in a backcross between two inbred strains of mouse, are responsible for all the stimulation of T helper cells detectable in a system investigated by Lake & Douglas (1978).

A second rule is that the mixed lymphocyte reaction *in vitro* can be manipulated to favour activation of one T cell subset or another, and in particular that it can be used to favour the induction of suppressor cells. Short-term anti-HLA-D mixed lymphocyte reactions tend to generate cytotoxic T cells (discussed in Mitchison 1981), while longer-term cultures generate helper cells (C. Mawas, personal communication). The anti-H-2D MLR easily generates suppressor T cells (Holan et al 1980).

Thirdly, small doses of antigen *in vivo* tend preferentially to activate helper cells, while large doses preferentially activate suppressor cells. This activation of suppressor cells by large doses has been clearly demonstrated by Brondz and his colleagues using various MHC alloantigens in the mouse (Brondz et al 1981). In their system, suppressor T cells are assayed by their capacity to suppress a mixed lymphocyte reaction. I have examined a similar point with panels of non-MHC alloantigens, using for assay an adoptive transfer system in which the helper and suppressor T cells regulate B cells producing anti-Thy 1 antibody. The results so far may be summarized as follows. The activation of helper T cells by a single dose of allogeneic spleen cells can be detected after injecting as few as 10^4 cells, and increases regularly with doses up to 10^7 cells. To detect this helper cell activation, we deplete the activated spleen lymphocytes of T suppressor cells at the time of adoptive transfer by treating them with rat monoclonal anti-Lyt 2,3 antibody without C or anti-Ig. Lymphocytes activated by a dose of 10^7 allogeneic cells shows an 18–52% (in three experiments) increase in activity after depletion, while lymphocytes activated by a 10^8 cell dose show a larger, 49–166% increase.

Fourthly, impairing the function of antigen-presenting cells (or avoiding them altogether) favours the development of suppression and tolerance. The older literature contains numerous instances where freeing protein antigens of aggregates tends to favour tolerance induction (Howard & Mitchison 1975), and the selective removal of adherent cells was a feature of the first successful attempt to generate T suppressor cells *in vitro* (Feldmann 1974). The effect of exposing mice to u.v. radiation, which, as has been mentioned, favours the generation of suppressor cells to tumour-specific antigens, has been interpreted in terms of impaired dendritic cell function.

What is the mechanism which underlies these empirical rules? A long time ago, before we knew anything about dual recognition, I proposed that direct access of antigens to lymphocytes, as distinct from access via macrophages, favoured the induction of tolerance. This simple theory is not compatible with what we now know about dual recognition, but perhaps it can be resurrected in modern guise. Suppressor T cells are of two kinds, suppressor-effectors and suppressor-inducers. Of these, suppressor-effector cells have been found not to be MHC-restricted, and they are indeed the only T cells which are at all securely known not to operate dual recognition. True, suppressor-inducer cells are absolutely required for their activation and these cells do operate dual recognition (Gershon et al 1981). Nevertheless, one could well suppose that suppressor-effector cells might bind non-MHC-associated antigen and then subsequently use it to interact with their suppressor-inducers. The point is that in their capacity as the only, or at least the principal regulatory cells able to bind antigen directly, their activation might well be favoured by non-processed or abnormally processed antigen.

Sex-linked immunodeficiency: the importance of measuring the fitness of carriers

The sex linkage and sex incidence of immunological diseases is a fascinating subject. An intriguing hypothesis of a general character has recently been introduced by Purtilo (1979; see also Purtilo & Sullivan 1979), which was instigated by the discovery, made by Purtilo and his colleagues, of a new form of X-linked immunodeficiency. I was at first inclined to accept this hypothesis, not only because of its intrinsic elegance but also because it offered an explanation for the relatively high incidence of skin cancer among northern Australian immunosuppressed men, as distinct from women (Mitchison & Kinlen 1980). The high incidence of skin cancer under these circumstances provides, in turn, one of the few sets of data which are encouraging for the theory of the immunological surveillance of cancer. At any rate, the hypothesis of Purtilo now seems to me mistaken, at least in part, for the reason explained below. The matter is of some importance to this symposium, because the hypothesis purports to explain the relatively high incidence of autoimmune disease among females. Even if it is mistaken, Purtilo & Sullivan have assembled a mass of interesting information about sex linkage and incidence which will have to be explained one way or another.

The main facts that Purtilo & Sullivan assemble can be grouped as follows:
(i) Recessive mutations on the X chromosome account for five immunodeficiency syndromes in man, and this degree of sex linkage is far greater than would be expected at random. These syndromes include Bruton's agammaglobulinaemia, Wiskott-Aldrich syndrome, and Purtilo's own discovery, Duncan's syndrome. All are immunologically crippling diseases which gravely impair fitness. At least one comparable sex-linked immunoregulatory disease occurs in the mouse in the CBA/N strain, again caused by a recessive mutation.

(ii) Human males are systematically hyporeactive immunologically, and females hyperreactive. Again, comparable data are available from animals.

(iii) Males are systematically more susceptible than females to a variety of infections, and to many cancers.

(iv) Females, on the other hand, are more susceptible to autoimmune diseases. Data in support of this contention come from systemic lupus erythematosus, Graves' disease, thyroiditis, and myasthenia gravis. Similar sex ratios exist for autoimmune disease in NZB and B/W mice.

Purtilo's hypothesis to explain these facts comes in two parts. In the first, it proposes that these gross deficiencies occur in males rather than females because the female is protected by having two X chromosomes. The minor, qualitative deficiencies of males reflect at least in part the action of other X-linked genes with similar but smaller effect (the argument becomes complex here, because sex limitation is more important than sex linkage at this point), while the hyperreactivity of females represents an evolutionarily balancing effect. That females are protected against these gross deficiencies by the possession of two X chromosomes is of course true; the question is why the deficiency genes occur preferentially on the X chromosome. The second part of the hypothesis attempts to answer this question, and it is here that the difficulties lie. The suggestion is made that two copies of the genes in the X chromosome may have evolved as an adaptive response to protect the female from the deleterious immunosuppressive effects of pregnancy. This does not mean that duplication of the X chromosome occurred as an evolutionary adaptation to pregnancy, for of course the XX–XY mechanism long antedates pregnancy, but means rather that immunoregulatory genes will tend to accumulate on the X chromosome. For an alternative suggestion, which raises the same objections in its population genetics as does Purtilo's, see Gatti et al (1979).

The idea of compensation for pregnancy-associated immunosuppression may or may not be correct, but let us for a moment explore another way of looking at the frequent sex linkage of immunologically crippling diseases. My first reaction to Purtilo's paper was to think as follows. Of course one should observe a preponderance of sex-linked immunologically crippling disease, not because regulatory genes occur preferentially on the X chromosome, but rather because recessive mutations occurring in these X chromosomes will be *expressed* more often than those occurring on autosomes: haploidy of the X chromosome would ensure this. This argument, though superficially attractive, is on second thoughts specious for the following reason. At equilibrium, deleterious genes must leave the gene pool at the same rate as they enter it, and therefore a sex-linked and an autosomal disease with the same impact on fitness, caused by recessive mutation occurring at the same rate, will occur at the same frequency (give or take a factor of two to allow for the fact that a lethal autosomal disease disposes of two genes while a sex-linked disease disposes of only one). However, the gene frequencies in the two cases will be very different: for an autosomal gene the number of carriers will greatly exceed the number of overt immunological cripples, but this will not be so for a sex-linked gene.

At this point we can formulate an alternative to Purtilo's pregnancy-compensation hypothesis. One possibility is that rare diseases will be identified as heritable more frequently if they are sex-linked, because of their incidence among a kindred. An effect of this sort may operate, and will do so to an extent that reflects the notoriously difficult problem of ascertainment. I prefer another possibility, which is that these crippling diseases are not fully recessive. In that case selection would operate to a minor extent against carriers, and to that extent would diminish the frequency of the full disease. If the carrier frequency is much higher than the disease frequency, as is the case for autosomal genes, this effect would be large. The net effect would be to diminish the frequency of the autosomally determined group of diseases, in comparison with the sex-linked group. This effect, it seems to me, could well account for the preponderance of sex linkage among severe immunodeficiencies noted by Purtilo.

It will not, however, account for the other three groups of facts that he noted. Autosomal immunoregulatory genes, in contrast to sex-linked ones, will, according to this hypothesis, tend to have their impact on immunocompetence more as high frequency minor-regulators than as low frequency major-regulators. The *net* impact of a deleterious mutation will in either case be the same, although autosomal mutations will be more spread out in their effect than sex-linked ones. This means that we cannot along this line of argument link the preponderance of sex-linked crippling diseases to the sex-limited incidence of hyper- and hyporesponsiveness. Perhaps the attempt to link something which is sex linked to something which is sex limited was in any case misconceived.

I do not see how we can tell at present whether Purtilo's hypothesis is correct. What is clear is that to the extent that selection of the proposed type does operate on carriers, Purtilo's hypothesis in its original form is weakened.

It so happens that the best evidence known to me of immunoregulatory defects in carriers actually comes from Purtilo's group. Their careful recent work discloses a significant defect among T cell subpopulations in female carriers of the Duncan's syndrome X-linked gene (Purtilo et al 1982). We do not yet know just what impact this has on fitness; information of this kind is critical for understanding what is really going on.

REFERENCES

Battisto JR, Bloom BR 1966 Dual immunological unresponsiveness induced by cell membrane coupled haptens or antigen. Nature (Lond) 212:156

Bevan MJ 1976 Cytotoxic T cell response to histocompatibility antigens: the role of H-2. Cold Spring Harbor Symp Quant Biol 41:519-528

Brent L, Hutchinson V 1981 Specific immunosuppression and graft survival. Transplant Proc 13:541-546

Bromberg J, Brenan M, Clark EA, Lake P, Mitchison NA, Nakashima I, Sainis KB 1979 Associative recognition in the response to alloantigens (and xenogenisation of alloantigens). In: Kobayashi H (ed) Immunological xenogenisation of tumor cells. Japan Scientific Societies Press, Tokyo. (GANN Monograph on Cancer Research) vol 23:185-192

Brondz BD, Karavlov V, Abronina IF, Blandova ZK 1981 Requirements for induction of specific suppressor T cells and detection of their H-2 antigen-binding receptors by fractionation on target monolayers. Scand J Immunol 13:517-534

Czitrom AA, Mitchison NA, Sunshine GH 1981 I-J, F, and hapten-conjugates: canalization by suppression. In: Zaleski MB et al (eds) Immunology of the major histocompatibility complex. Karger, Basel, (7th Int Convoc on Immunology) p 243-253

Feldmann M 1974 T cell suppression in vitro. I. Role in regulation of antibody responses. Eur J Immunol 4:660-666

Gatti RA, Kempner DH, Leibold W 1979 The role of the MHC antigens in the mature and immature host. Pediatrics (Suppl) 64:803-813

Gershon RK, Eardley DD, Durum S, Green DR, Shen F-W, Yamauchi K, Cantor H, Murphy DB 1981 Contrasuppression. A novel immunoregulatory activity. J Exp Med 153:1533-1546

Gordon RD, Mathieson BJ, Samelson LE, Boyse EA, Simpson E 1976 The effect of allogeneic presensitization on H-Y graft survival and in vitro cell-mediated responses to H-Y antigen. J Exp Med 144:810-820

Holan V, Hasek M, Chutna J 1980 Skin allograft tolerance induced by in vitro educated suppressor cells. Immunol Lett 1:265-267

Howard JG, Mitchison NA 1975 Immunological tolerance. Progr Allergy 18:43-96

Klein J, Juretic A, Baxevanis CN, Nagy ZA 1981 The traditional and a new version of the mouse H-2 complex. Nature (Lond) 291:455-460

Knight J, Knight A, Mitchison NA 1979 The kinetics and consequences of latent help to murine alloantigens. In: Kaplan JG (ed) The molecular basis of immune cell function. Elsevier/North-Holland Biomedical Press, Amsterdam, pp 139-146

Lake P 1976 Antibody response induced in vitro to the cell surface alloantigen Thy-1. Nature (Lond) 262:297-298

Lake P, Douglas TC 1978 Recognition and genetic control of helper determinants for cell surface antigen Thy-1. Nature (Lond) 275:220-222

Matzinger P 1981 A one-receptor view of T-cell behaviour. Nature (Lond) 292:497-501

Mitchison NA 1978 New ideas about self-tolerance and auto-immunity. Clin Rheum Dis 4:539-548
Mitchison NA 1981 Allospecific T cells. Cellular Immunol 62:258-263
Mitchison NA 1982 Differentiation within the immune system: the importance of cloning. In: Fitch F, Fathman CG (eds) Isolation, characterization, and utilization of T lymphocytes. Academic Press, New York, in press
Mitchison NA, Kinlen L 1980 Present concepts in immune surveillance. In: Fougereau M, Dausset J (eds) Immunology 80. Academic Press, London (Proc 4th Int Congr Immunol) pp 641-650
Myburgh JA, Mitchison NA 1976 Suppressor mechanisms in neonatally acquired tolerance to a Gross virus induced lymphoma in rats. Transplantation 22:236-244
Purtilo D 1979 X-Associated immunocompetence. Lancet 1:327
Purtilo D, Sullivan JL 1979 Immunological basis for superior survival of females. Am J Dis Child 133:1251-1253
Purtilo D, Sakamoto K, Barnabei V, Seeley J 1982 Clues to pathogenesis of Epstein-Barr virus-induced diseases from analysis of 100 cases of X-linked lymphoproliferative syndrome (XLP). In: Yohn DS, Blakeslee JR (eds) Comparative research on leukemia and related diseases. Elsevier/North-Holland Biomedical Press, Amsterdam, in press
Reinherz L, Schlossman SF 1980 The differentation and function of human lymphocytes. Cell 19:821-827
Sunshine GH, Cyrus M, Winchester G 1982 In vitro responses to the auto-antigen F. Immunology 45:357-363
Sy M-S, Bach BA, Brown A, Nisonoff A, Benacerraf B, Greene MI 1979 Antigen- and receptor-driven regulatory mechanisms. II. Induction of suppressor T cells with idiotype-coupled syngeneic spleen cells. J Exp Med 150:1229-1240
Tada T, Okumura K 1979 The role of antigen-specific T cell factors in the immune response. Adv Immunol 28:1-87
Waterfield JD, Nixon DF, Mair MG 1981 Lymphocyte-mediated cytotoxicity against allogeneic tumour cells. IV. Fine specificity mapping and characterization of concanavalin A-activated cytotoxic effector lymphocytes. Immunology 44:685-693
Yefenof E, Meidav A, Kedar E 1980 In vitro generation of cytotoxic lymphocytes against radiation- and radiation leukemia virus-induced tumors. III. Suppression of anti-tumor immunity in vitro by lymphocytes of mice undergoing radiation leukemia virus-induced leukemogenesis. J Exp Med 152:1473-1483

DISCUSSION

Knight: Why do you think immune responses to weak alloantigens are an appropriate model of autoimmunity? To my knowledge, autoimmune diseases are never directed against alloantigens, but against antigens common to all members of a species. Ronald Kahn has evidence for this in his system. Certainly with thyroid-stimulating antibody, there is no special affinity of one person's antibodies for his or her own thyroid antigen compared to thyroid antigen from other subjects (A. Knight, unpublished results).

Mitchison: The reason for choosing to study alloantigens is that you can take a row of *minor* alloantigens and put them in some kind of rank order both for skin graft rejection, and as helper cells in the transfer system that I described. Our ability to rank them in this way makes these antigens attractive as subjects for the study of immunoregulation. Some of them are defined membrane molecules, others as yet have been defined only from their genetics. They are not a *direct* model for autoimmunity, certainly, but I hope that they are a relevant model.

Davies: I am interested in the role of membrane-bound antigens, as opposed to soluble antigens, in autoimmunity. Can you say more about the necessity for antigen to be membrane-bound in order to trigger an immune response in T cells?

Mitchison: This is thought to be because T cells don't release long-range products; B cells do, namely antibodies. T cells may release lymphokines but these seem to be essentially short-range products. So the immune system had to adopt a mechanism for triggering T cells *only* in the vicinity of antigen which is membrane-bound. Dual recognition seems to be a mechanism for doing that.

Davies: And a soluble antigen would be expected to stimulate a B cell directly? It is not membrane-bound when it is presented to the cell.

Mitchison: Yes.

Rees Smith: In your hypothesis it looks as though you are postulating that four macromolecules are specifically interacting simultaneously for dual recognition. This seems to be an unlikely event, in physicochemical terms; one can't easily conceive that four independent molecules (MHC product, MHC receptor, antigen, and T cell receptor) come together in a multimolecular interaction. So how does dual recognition work at the level of protein–protein interactions?

Mitchison: I am not the first person here to talk about four molecules interacting! Dr Rodbell discussed precisely that, in the binding of glucagon to the three-component adenylate cyclase system (R, N and C).

Crumpton: In the 'one-receptor' model of the recognition of complexes of major histocompatibility antigen with foreign antigen, there is an apparent requirement for a specific interaction between the antigens. I find this concept difficult to accept, because it apparently requires the class I and class II histocompatibility antigens to have the capacity to recognize a large spectrum of molecular structures—that is, a similar range of specificities to that of antibodies. It seems to me that a related problem may exist in respect of the suggestion that a collection of different hormonal receptors interact with the same GTP regulatory protein of the adenylate cyclase system. One would have to say that all these different hormonal receptors have some common site with which the GTP protein interacts. This is perhaps no different from saying that class I or class II histocompatibility antigens have to interact with a variety of different molecules.

Roitt: There is a difference between the probability of three or more molecules meeting in three dimensions and the probability of interactions of molecules moving in the two-dimensional planes of two cell surfaces in contact.

Rees Smith: I am quite happy for you to say that initially there is an interaction between two cell surface molecules, and then *subsequently* there is interaction between another set of molecules. That was the type of comment I was hoping for. *Is* that what actually goes on? The probability of a simultaneous interaction between four independent macromolecules must be very low.

Mitchison: I think that when we have the T cell receptor molecules expressed in plasmids, we should be better able to decide between these possibilities. This is just what Dr S. Tonegawa is trying to do at present.

Bottazzo: Do you think that the full complement of receptors is present on the cells at all times or do you envisage a progressive expression of receptors in response to an initial signal?

Mitchison: The failure of MHC product alone or specific antigen alone to compete out the binding of MHC plus antigen complexes argues against either receptor being able to work on its own.

Roitt: You can absorb cytotoxic T cells out on the right target fibroblasts in the cold without them reacting.

Kahn: Dr Mitchison is saying that for T cell proliferation—that is, DNA synthesis—the two molecules (MHC product and antigen) have to be present at the same time. But it seems to me that that event—namely, stimulation of DNA synthesis—requires a chain of events to be triggered which may have to occur simultaneously in the same cells, and yet could be independently triggered.

Mitchison: If that were the case I would still have expected one or other molecule on its own to be able to compete.

Harrison: How is that blocking experiment done?

Mitchison: You can use cytotoxic T cells that kill target cells which carry BGG plus MHC. No matter how much free BGG is put into the system, that cytotoxicity is not blocked.

Vincent: What is known about the nature of the antigen on the antigen-presenting cell? Is there a complete antigen on the surface of that cell, or is it an epitope only?

Mitchison: That is debatable. How would one answer that question? Since one can't block the T cell receptor with antigen alone, one can't answer that question in any simple way.

Vincent: Is it possible, therefore, that some MHC-restricted T cells are being stimulated by epitopes on antigen-presenting cells which are quite different antigenically from those on the soluble antigens which the suppressor cells respond to?

Mitchison: That is a most interesting idea. It is akin to the hypothesis which Eli Sercarz has advanced, that certain determinants on an antigen such as lysozyme are uniquely suppressive.

Roitt: Dr J. Charreire cultures mouse thyroid cells with syngeneic lymphocytes and claims to generate a *de novo* priming of the T cells which will subsequently give a mitogenic response to thyroglobulin (Yeni & Charreire 1982). Anti-thyroglobulin and H-2D/K prevents that induction, but anti-Ia does not block. She can't detect Ia on the upper surface of the thyroid cells. Is that relevant?

Mitchison: That is part of my argument. When people have looked for T cells that can be stimulated by antigen in the absence of MHC molecules, or that will adsorb to solid-phase antigen without MHC molecules, or release factors that bind to antigen alone without these MHC molecules, they always end up with suppressor cells with Lyt 2,3 markers. I therefore imagine that she is looking at the hypothetical *unrestricted* suppressor cells.

Roitt: But she transfers these cells to syngeneic mice and anti-thyroglobulin antibodies are detected.

McLachlan: She is able to generate a helper T cell for autoantibody synthesis.

Roitt: What is the current thinking about the type of helper cell required for making T cells cytotoxic to a virally infected, Ia-negative cell? Are you convinced that there has to be some macrophage processing, or can the help be direct? In other words, are we prejudiced by the response to allogeneic antigens where we see anti-Ia recognition giving a mixed lymphocyte response, which helps the generation of cytotoxic T cells? Perhaps we should allow that the class I MLC molecules (D and K) might 'help' as well. There might in fact be helper cells that recognize H-2D *plus* thyroglobulin. If Dr Charreire's results are correct and if people were to dissect the helper response to virally infected cells, they might find class I help. If this is true, it is difficult to sustain your thesis that Ia presentation is the major source of autoimmunity. So this is a critical piece of information that we need.

Mitchison: I quite agree that we need to know more about these apparent exceptions, where helper cells seem to recognize antigen in association with class I MHC molecules, rather than class II, as expected.

Kahn: Also on dual recognition, do we know that the MHC protein and the antigen-presenting site are physically adjacent on the cell? Do the antigens co-cap with H-2 markers, or are they at opposite ends of the cell? And do we know anything about the affinity of each of these binding sites? In a dual recognition hypothesis, if there were a totally unrestricted system the predicted affinity would be the multiple of the individual affinities. With affinities of 10^6 for each site, the affinity of the dual recognition would be 10^{12}; for 10^8, it would be 10^{16}, and so on. Eventually you would reach such a high affinity that the two cells in contact would never separate! In other words, I am trying to imagine how this takes place at a molecular level.

Mitchison: One other difficulty is that a virus, say, needs to be recognized in association with, say, a class II MHC molecule. There are all the other non-MHC molecules on that antigen-presenting cell, which, when they function as alloantigens, are apparently 'seen' in association with the Ia molecule. So an incoming virus has to 'compete out' H-Y and all the other non-MHC products on the cell membrane (Bubbers et al 1978).

On the affinities, Frank Lilly's group has studied this for viral proteins and has found roughly the kinds of associations that one would want (e.g., a leukaemia virus associates physically with the very MHC molecules which act as restriction elements). So there seems to be some physical interaction of the kind that one would predict. These results have been extended to other viruses and to bacteria and have run into trouble: in certain cases the organism does display preference among MHC molecules, but not for those that act as restriction elements. In other words, viruses associate with an MHC product which is not the one coded by the immune response gene for that virus. This tells us that the physical association can mislead.

Rees Smith: The point should be made that one cannot usually just multiply up affinities in that way. The free energy of binding is proportional to the log of the equilibrium constant and with multiples of completely independent binding sites, multiplication would be justified. However, for linked sites, such as the two binding sites on an IgG molecule, the probability of interaction with one site changes when the other is bound by a large ligand. Consequently, multiple binding sites do not always lead to large increases in affinity. This is certainly evident in the case of IgG antibodies, where Fab fragments usually have similar affinities for antigen as the intact molecule (Mason & Williams 1980).

Kahn: Although it may be a dual site recognition system, this may be much more like the interaction of a cell with an affinity column with multiple antigens on it, in the sense that there are two *classes* of sites with many copies of each. So even if the affinity of each class is very small, you have to multiply that by the few hundred or thousand molecules that might be interacting simultaneously as the two cell surfaces come together.

Venter: Would one expect that there would be more suppressor cells to integral membrane proteins in existence than to other cellular proteins and, therefore, by loss of suppressor function, one would expect an increased chance of autoimmune reactions developing to such proteins?

Mitchison: Yes. I don't think that it is so much a matter of membrane-bound proteins associating with MHC molecules directly. It is rather that membrane-bound molecules are somehow more difficult for the antigen-processing cells to process and to associate with self Ia.

Venter: So you wouldn't be surprised if humans carried suppressor cells to β-adrenergic or glucagon or insulin receptors in their normal suppressor cell repertoire?

Mitchison: That's exactly what one would expect. Suppression, in my view, is likely to be more important as a second line of defence than as a first one. The main reasons we don't make antibodies to glucagon receptors or other hormone receptors is to do with the first line of defence, which relates to failures of antigen processing, and also elimination of self-reactive clones. Suppression is probably more important as a second line. I like to think of potential self antigens such as hormone receptors as a volcanic magma which is constrained by geological strata of clonal elimination and presentation mechanisms. These normally keep the magma safely underground, but every now and then it erupts as a volcano. But this doesn't mean complete disaster, because the system can still use suppressor cells to plug the volcano. That is my reading of experimental autoimmune diseases, such as experimental allergic encephalitis, where, if you paralyse a rat's hind legs by giving it emulsified spinal cord in Feund's adjuvant, and keep it alive for a few days, it recovers movement in its legs and is, then, full of suppressor cells (Welch & Swanborg 1976). It has enough such cells to stop another rat being paralysed.

Roitt: However, insulin receptors are present on macrophages, which also bear plenty of Ia molecules. Perhaps, Dr Kahn, you would then argue that that is not related to conventional organ-specific autoimmune disease, because your studies with Franco Bottazzo show that patients with autoantibodies to insulin receptors don't have organ-specific antibodies of other kinds, whereas in organ-specific diseases in general there tends to be an association with other organ-specific antibodies.

McLachlan: There has been a report of acetylcholine receptors on human monocytes (Whaley et al 1981); it would be of great interest if this can be confirmed.

Vincent: I thought the evidence looked very good. Complement synthesis by human monocytes was stimulated by cholinergic agonists and inhibited by cholinergic antagonists, including α-bungarotoxin. The 'receptor' was also antigenically related to *Torpedo* and human acetylcholine receptor.

Harrison: There are TSH receptors on macrophages. In fact, all the receptors involved in endocrine autoimmunity are probably present on thymic lymphocytes.

Venter: We are interested in the antigenicity of receptor molecules like the β-adrenergic receptor, which exist in very low concentrations on cell membranes. Using the turkey erythrocyte β-receptor as the antigen, Dr Claire Fraser has raised a number of monoclonal antibodies to the β-receptor (Fraser & Venter 1980, Venter & Fraser 1981). Some of these monoclonal antibodies have very interesting properties. For example, as with the autoantibodies to the β-receptor (Venter et al 1980), a major antigenic determinant is the adrenergic ligand-binding site. Our studies so far with monoclonal antibodies indicate that there are at least three major determinants on the turkey erythrocyte β-receptors (C. M. Fraser & J. C. Venter, abstract, ICN-UCLA Symposia, Squaw Valley, 1982). One monoclonal antibody (FV-104) acts like an antagonist, competing directly with adrenergic ligands for the ligand-binding site on the receptor. The ligands block antibody binding and the antibody blocks ligand binding. Even though there are at least two molecular forms of the β-receptor (one in heart, the β_1-receptor, and one in lung and liver, the β_2-receptor, differing in structure and molecular size) (Table 1), antibody FV-104 cross-reacts with every β-receptor we have studied, whether from mammalian or non-mammalian tissues, β_1 or β_2. So there appears to be at least one determinant in the ligand-binding site in common among all β-receptors.

We have used this antibody (FV-104) as an affinity probe to immunopurify the turkey erythrocyte β-adrenergic receptor. The basic receptor subunit

TABLE 1 (Venter) Molecular properties of β-adrenergic receptors

Property	β_1-adrenergic receptor	β_2-adrenergic receptor
Stokes radius (nm)	Dog heart: 4.2 Rat heart: 4.8 Turkey erythrocytes: 4.3	Dog lung: 5.8 Dog liver: 5.8 Calf lung: 5.8 Frog erythrocytes: 5.8 Human lung: 5.8
Relative molecular mass (M_r) (hydrodynamic)	Dog heart: 65 000 Turkey erythrocytes: 62 000	Dog lung: 91 000 Dog liver: 90 000
M_r (SDS-polyacrylamide gel electrophoresis)	Turkey erythrocytes: 70 000 Pigeon erythrocytes: 70 000	Calf lung: 59 000 (114 000 dimer) Human lung: 50 000 (88 000 dimer)
M_r (target size analysis (see Rodbell, this volume)	Turkey erythrocytes: 90 000	Liver: 100 000
Cross-reactivity with autoantibodies to β_2 adrenergic receptors	Dog heart: 0%	Calf lung: 100% Dog lung: 77% Human placenta: 58%
Cross-reactivity with monoclonal antibody FV-104	Calf heart: 100% Turkey erythrocytes: 100%	Calf lung: 100% Calf liver: 100%

(Venter et al 1981.)

seems to have an M_r value of 70 000. We occasionally find a 30 000 subunit which does not derive from the 70 000 peptide by disulphide reduction and therefore could be a proteolytic fragment of the receptor. In the pigeon erythrocyte we find the same basic receptor size (70 000). The β_1-receptor appears to be a monomer and the β_2-receptor appears to be a dimer. Our studies indicate that the human β_2-receptor has a basic subunit size of approximately M_r 50 000 that appears quantitatively by disulphide reduction from an 88 000–90 000 peak (Venter & Fraser 1981). The canine and bovine lung β_2-receptors appear to be slightly larger than the human lung β_2-receptors (J. C. Venter, unpublished), but all these M_r values are in good agreement with the M_r values from target size analysis of liver β_2-receptors (see Rodbell, this volume).

So we have antibodies that distinguish clearly between β_1- and β_2-receptors with no cross-reactivity (Venter et al 1980), yet we have this one monoclonal antibody (FV-104) that cross-reacts with all β-receptors studied. There appears to be a tremendous degree of conservation of the ligand-binding site from the invertebrates up to mammals and all through the mammalian tissues. An additional point of interest is that the β-adrenergic receptors are among the lowest density membrane proteins we know of, yet from these very small amounts of material we seem to be able to generate good antibodies.

Mitchison: There is evidently no question of self tolerance here; presumably an antibody to mouse receptor could be raised in the mouse too, since you have cross-reactivity between mouse and *rat* tissues. This tells us that there are reactive B cells in mice; mice evidently have B cells which are able to react with their own receptors.

Knight: That surely is just analogous to the rat cell-induced haemolytic anaemia in the mouse; these clones are not the same ones that cause spontaneous autoimmunity.

Kahn: That raises the question of whether your animals in which antibodies are raised have any manifestation of the antibodies which they possess.

Venter: The mice appear to have some manifestation of the presence of antibodies to the β-receptor; however, we have not attempted to document the effects. BALB/c mice in which we grow our control ascites tumours remain alive for weeks, even when their abdomens become so enlarged from the tumours that they cannot easily walk. In contrast, the mice with, for example hybridoma FV-104, which produces the monoclonal antibody to the ligand-binding site of the β-receptor, do not live long enough to develop full ascites tumours. They become emaciated, extremely weak and are unable to respond to even strong stimuli.

Crumpton: What about the mice that were immunized with the receptor preparation in order to obtain the spleen cells for the cell fusion?

Venter: In general they have received one immunization followed by a boost four weeks later, with the fusion four days subsequent to the booster. There was no apparent effect of immunization with the isolated receptor in terms of obvious pathological changes. It may be important to keep in mind the normal physiological roles of the β-receptor. Blocking the β-adrenergic receptors by antibody in the mouse or human won't necessarily produce a pathological state. We have stressed this point in our studies on the possible role of autoantibodies to β-receptors in allergic disease (Venter et al 1980, Fraser et al 1981). β-Receptors have important roles in the regulation of such parameters as the heart beat and normal cardiac rhythm (Venter 1981) and in the control of blood vessel and airway diameter, as other examples. β-Adrenergic receptors are physiological modulators of numerous functions, but do not appear to be required for life in the absolute sense. For example, in order for the diaphragm to function in its role of promoting respiration, intact functional nicotinic acetylcholine receptors are required. Skeletal muscle contraction requires these receptors in an absolute manner.

Mitchison: Why don't these mice go into cardiac arrest?

Venter: This has to do with the role of adrenergic control of the heart. You can completely denervate the heart, as with heart transplants, and the heart still responds to stress, by the action of adrenal catecholamines. If the heart has its normal innervation, very high concentrations of β-blockers are required to completely suppress nerve activation of the heart. The heart during rest can function normally with complete denervation and β-blockers.

Kahn: If you give pharmacological β-adrenergic blocking agents you slow the heart rate, so an antibody that acts like a β-blocking agent and has a certain pharmacological potency would be expected to slow heart rate, and an antibody mimicking β-agonists would be expected to speed it up.

Venter: Yes. One would expect to see physiological modulation but not a life-threatening situation.

Bitensky: If the β-adrenergic receptor sites were blocked, you would only be able to detect the consequences of that blockage either if you stressed the animal and forced it into a maximal physiological state, or if you gave pharmacological agents that either accelerated or blocked that response. One would not expect to see *clinical* responses in the mouse to the antibody.

Venter: Exactly. We didn't expect to see any obvious effects of the antibody in the mice. However, it would be interesting to test these mice under stressful conditions and assess physiological function. Clearly the monoclonal antibodies have an effect on the longevity of the mice, and the depressed activity of the mice with the anti-β-receptor antibodies is consistent with extensive β-receptor blockade.

Jacobs: You said that the antibody competes with adrenergic agonists and antagonists. Was this competition specific for, say, antagonists which selectively bind to the β_1-receptor?

Venter: Antibody FV-104 competes directly with the non-selective β-adrenergic antagonists, such as propranolol, which bind with equal affinity to β_1 and β_2 receptors. Propranolol competes very well with both forms of β-receptor; so does hydroxybenzylpindolol. There is no apparent receptor selectivity in terms of these ligands or antibody FV-104. We haven't investigated antibody competition with agonists to the same extent, but it appears that the determinant in the receptor recognized by monoclonal antibody FV-104 is that part of the ligand-binding site of the receptor that determines the specificity for the non-β-receptor-selective antagonists. Two other monoclonal antibodies that we have made to the β-receptor are to different determinants from the one recognized by FV-104. One has no effect on ligand binding but only immunoprecipitates the receptor, whereas the other monoclonal antibody non-competitively modulates ligand binding, perhaps only by steric hindrance.

Engel: What proportion of patients with chronic asthma have such antibodies?

Venter: The incidence we find with immunoprecipitation appears to be around 10-15% of our patients.

Harrison: The β-receptor is a big molecule and only a small part of it is the ligand-binding site. There are therefore many ways in which you could modulate the receptor's function. Using the binding assay to screen asthmatics you may get 10–15% with β-receptor autoantibodies, but using another assay, say of biological function, you might get a higher frequency of positives. We need to use as many parameters as possible to qualify our conclusions. Talking about effects on binding is not enough.

Mitchison: Nevertheless, one important application of such a monoclonal antibody is to assay for antibodies in patients that will block binding of the monoclonal.

Venter: That is the direction in which we are moving. The assays we have now for autoantibodies are tedious and involve methodology that requires experience to obtain good results. We are trying to set up a competitive binding assay using the monoclonal antibodies; however, we do not know whether or not we have monoclonals to all of the determinants on the receptor, at this point.

Dr Harrison's point about the actual concentrations of autoantibodies is an important one. I worry when I hear people say that a given patient has *no* autoantibody to a given antigen. The detection of autoantibodies very much depends on the sensitivity of the assay used. With our various receptor assays we can easily detect femtomoles (10^{-15} moles) or less of the receptor molecule, but in work on autoantibodies to the β-adrenergic receptor we have screened at relatively low serum concentrations, compared for example to the insulin receptor autoantibody data. We screen at a 1:100 dilution of patient serum and therefore would not find a patient with an antibody titre of 1:3.

Davies: We have been analysing a type of idiotypic antibody raised by Dr Nadir Farid in rabbits against anti-human TSH. This anti-anti-TSH inhibited the binding of radioiodinated TSH to human thyroid membrane. We have studied the activity of this IgG preparation in a human thyroid cell bioassay system which measures the accumulation of cyclic AMP as an end point and has a sensitivity of 10–20 μU/ml. The idiotypic antibody caused almost total suppression of TSH stimulation in a dose-related manner (Fig. 1). Furthermore, there was no anti-TSH activity in the preparation. Hence, an anti-anti-TSH antibody both inhibited the binding of TSH and actually blocked the biological action of TSH without causing stimulation of the TSH receptor itself. Hence, there appears to be an IgG molecule which has determinants consistent with a mirror image of the TSH receptor.

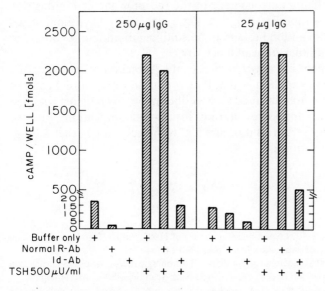

FIG. 1 (Davies). Antibody to anti-human TSH inhibits human thyroid cell bioassay. Normal human thyroid cells (30 000/well) were incubated with or without normal rabbit IgG (R-Ab) or IgG from rabbit immunized with anti-hTSH (Id-Ab), for 2 h in the presence or absence of bTSH (500 μU/ml) in a final incubation volume of 250 μl. Intracellular cyclic AMP was measured by radioimmunoassay after ether extraction.

Fuchs: So it might therefore be expected to act like the stimulatory anti-receptor antibodies?

Davies: Yes!

Mitchison: How often do you raise that particular kind of antibody?

Davies: So far, I understand Dr Farid has raised it in only one rabbit out of 12.

Mitchison: How much of the anti-idiotype antibody in such a rabbit has this biological activity?

Davies: I don't know. It's a relatively sensitive assay system, where gross suppression is produced by 25 µg of IgG.

Kahn: One point about this type of experimental design is that frequently the antibodies that are formed to the hormone ligand, in this case the anti-TSH antibody (and this is true for anti-insulin antibodies), are not directed at the biologically active site of the hormone molecule (Karlsson et al 1982). So even if an animal develops an anti-idiotype antibody to the first antibody molecule, it would not have anything to do with the bioactive surface.

Fuchs: Antibodies to insulin, which are found in patients with insulin resistance, may look like a mirror image of the receptor and can in this way trigger anti-receptor antibodies. Sege & Peterson (1978) have immunized rabbits with anti-insulin antibodies and the resulting anti-antibodies bound to insulin receptor and mimicked insulin activity.

Kahn: This experiment has never been repeated successfully by that or any other group, because the antibodies that they produced were transient and of very low titre. We have not observed such antibodies in any patients who had developed anti-insulin antibodies during insulin administration, but we haven't looked at every serum. If it occurs it must be very rare in that setting. It may occur in other settings.

REFERENCES

Bubbers JE, Chen S, Lilly F 1978 Nonrandom inclusion of H-2K and H-2D antigens in Friend virus particles from mice of various strains. J Exp Med 147:340-351

Fraser CM, Venter JC 1980 Monoclonal antibodies to β-adrenergic receptors: use in purification and molecular characterization of β-receptors. Proc Natl Acad Sci USA 77:7034-7038

Fraser CM, Venter JC, Kaliner M 1981 Autonomic abnormalities and autoantibodies to β-adrenergic receptors. N Engl J Med 205:1165-1170

Karlsson FA, Harrison LC, Kahn CR, Itin A, Roth J 1982 Subpopulation of antibodies directed against evolutionarily conserved regions of the insulin molecule in insulin-treated patients. Submitted for publication

Mason DW, Williams AF 1980 The kinetics of antibody binding to membrane antigens in solution and at the cell surface. Biochem J 187:1-20

Rodbell M 1982 Structure–function relationships in adenylate cyclase systems. This volume, p 3-11

Sege K, Peterson PA 1978 Use of anti-idiotypic antibodies as cell-surface receptor probes. Proc Natl Acad Sci USA 75:2443-2447

Welch AM, Swanborg RH 1976 Characterization of suppressor cells involved in regulation of experimental allergic encephalomyelitis. Eur J Immunol 6:910-912

Whaley K, Lappin D, Barkas J 1981 C2 synthesis by human monocytes is modulated by a nicotinic cholinergic receptor. Nature (Lond) 293:580-583

Venter JC 1981 β-Adrenoceptors, adenylate cyclase and the adrenergic control of cardiac contractility. In: Kunos G (ed) Adrenoceptors and catecholamine action. Wiley, New York, vol 1:213-245

Venter JC, Fraser CM 1981 The development of monoclonal antibodies to β-adrenergic receptors and their use in receptor purification and characterization. In: Fellows R, Eisenbarth G (eds) Monoclonal antibodies in endocrine research. Raven Press, New York, p 119-134

Venter JC, Fraser CM, Harrison LC 1980 Autoantibodies to β₂-adrenergic receptors: a possible cause of adrenergic hyporesponsiveness in allergic rhinitis and asthma. Science (Wash DC) 207:1361-1363

Venter JC, Fraser CM, Soiefer AI, Jeffrey DR, Strauss WL, Charlton RR, Greguski R 1981 Autoantibodies and monoclonal antibodies to β-adrenergic receptors: their use in receptor purification and characterization. Adv Cyclic Nucleotide Res 14:135-144

Yeni GP, Charreire J 1982 Eur J Immunol, in press

Insulin receptors and insulin receptor antibodies: structure–function relationships

STEVEN JACOBS and PEDRO CUATRECASAS

Wellcome Research Laboratories, Research Triangle Park, North Carolina 27709, USA

Abstract The insulin receptor has been purified by affinity chromatography and studied by affinity-labelling techniques. It appears to be a disulphide-linked heterotetramer, $(\alpha\,\beta)_2$, composed of two copies of a 135 000 M_r subunit (α), and two copies of a 90 000 M_r subunit (β). β is readily proteolysed to generate a 45 000 M_r fragment (β_1). α, β and β_1 all contain sialic acid and are, therefore, probably all exposed on the external surface of the membrane. Although α is predominantly labelled in affinity-labelling studies, β and β_1 can also be labelled. Therefore, α, β and β_1 are all in proximity to the insulin-binding site and may contain part of the binding site.

Antibodies have been prepared against the intact, purified receptor and against the isolated α subunit. Both antibodies directly interact with the insulin receptor as indicated by their ability to immunoprecipitate the receptor. Neither antibody, however, directly competes with insulin binding. Therefore, they are probably directed against regions of the receptor distinct from the insulin-binding site. In spite of this, these antibodies have a wide range of insulin-like activities.

Several methods have been used to assess the structure of the insulin receptor. These include purification by affinity chromatography with insulin–Sepharose (Cuatrecasas 1972a, Jacobs et al 1977), or with insulin receptor antibodies (Harrison & Itin 1980), photoaffinity labelling with aryl azide derivatives of insulin (Yip et al 1978, 1980, Jacobs et al 1979, Wisher et al 1980), and by affinity cross-linking insulin to its receptor with bifunctional reagents (Pilch & Czech 1979, 1980, Massague & Czech 1980). It is gratifying that these diverse methods have produced similar results.

1982 Receptors, antibodies and disease. Pitman, London (Ciba Foundation symposium 90) p 82-90

Receptor purification

The major approach of our laboratory has been to purify the insulin receptor using insulin–Sepharose affinity chromatography (Cuatrecasas 1972a, Jacobs et al 1977). Rat liver membranes are solubilized with Triton X-100 and purified by DEAE–cellulose chromatography followed by insulin–Sepharose affinity chromatography and concanavalin A–Sepharose affinity chromatography. After concanavalin A–Sepharose, three main Coomassie blue-stained bands that have approximate relative molecular masses (M_r) of 135 000, 90 000 and 45 000 (these have been designated α, β and $β_1$ respectively, by Massague & Czech (1980)) are visible on sodium dodecyl sulphate (SDS)–polyacrylamide gels of the reduced receptor. The 90 000 and 45 000 M_r bands are visualized more clearly if the receptor is iodinated, and bands on the gel are detected by radioautography.

There is considerable evidence to indicate that these three bands are components of the receptor: they migrate with the peak of insulin-binding activity when the purified receptor is analysed by gel filtration (Stokes radius, 72 Å) and isoelectric focusing (pI, 4.0) (Jacobs et al 1977). The photoaffinity label, 4-azido-2-nitrophenyl insulin, labels a protein with identical mobility to the α band of the purified receptor (Jacobs et al 1979). This labelling is specific since it can be inhibited by physiological concentrations of insulin and proinsulin, but not by peptides that do not bind to the insulin receptor. Not only does the photoaffinity-labelled band have the same mobility as the 135 000 M_r band present in preparations of the purified receptor, but treatment with proteolytic and glycosidic enzymes results in the production of several similar products, clearly establishing their identity (Jacobs et al 1980b). Although by using 4-azido-2-nitrophenyl insulin we have not been able to identify photoaffinity-labelled bands corresponding to the β and $β_1$ components of the purified receptor, bands in this region have been identified by Yip et al (1980) using $N^{εβ29}$-(azidobenzoyl)insulin, and by Massague & Czech (1980) and Massague et al (1980, 1981) using disuccinimidyl suberate to affinity cross-link insulin to its receptor.

Further evidence that these three bands are components of the receptor is provided by antibodies prepared against the isolated α subunit excised from an SDS–polyacrylamide gel of the purified receptor (Jacobs et al 1980b). These antibodies immunoprecipitate solubilized insulin-binding activity and mimic many of the biological effects of insulin, thus associating this protein with the two expected functions of a true biological receptor for insulin; namely, binding, and triggering a biological response. Further support for α, β and $β_1$ being components of the insulin receptor is the presence of similar components when the receptor is purified from human placenta with spontaneously occurring anti-insulin receptor autoantibodies from sera of patients with insulin-resistant diabetes (Harrison & Itin 1980, Van Obberghen et al 1981). While both insulin and anti-insulin receptor antibodies would be expected to have high affinity and selectivity for insulin receptors, it is unlikely that they would cross-react with the same contaminating proteins; therefore, the similar results obtained with these two methods are reassuring.

Subunit structure

Massague & Czech (1980) and Massague et al (1980, 1981) have used the affinity-labelling technique to provide evidence that the β_1 subunit is a proteolytic fragment of β. We have reached similar conclusions from studies with purified receptor. The relative amounts of α, β and β_1 varies considerably in different preparations of purified receptor (Jacobs et al 1979). Modification of the original purification scheme to minimize proteolysis by including the protease inhibitors, phenylmethylsulphonyl fluoride, EDTA, and leupepsin in the buffers, and by eliminating overnight dialysis steps early in the procedure, results in an increase in the relative amount of β at the expense of β_1. This suggests that β_1 is a proteolytic fragment of β. Peptide maps of the three subunits are consistent with this. Most of the peptide fragments produced from β_1 are also produced from β. There also appears to be some similarity between many of the fragments produced from α and β. Whether this is merely a coincidence or whether it represents some degree of homology between the subunits is not clear. However, it is interesting to note that the distinct subunits of the nicotinic acetylcholine receptor do share a considerable degree of homology (Raftery et al 1980).

Under non-denaturing conditions, solubilized insulin receptor has a Stokes radius of about 70 Å and a sedimentation coefficient of about 11 S, from which a relative molecular mass (M_r) of about 300 000 to 360 000 can be calculated (Cuatrecasas 1972b, Siegel et al 1981) (Fig. 1). Even after the receptor is denatured by boiling in 2% SDS, and analysed by SDS–polyacrylamide gel electrophoresis, it remains as an intact entity with a molecular weight of approximately 360 000 (Jacobs et al 1979, 1980a, b, Pilch & Czech 1979). The denatured receptor dissociates into isolated α, β and β_1 components only after it is reduced with dithiothreitol. Two-dimensional SDS–polyacrylamide gel electrophoresis (first dimension run without reduction of the receptor; second dimension run after reduction with dithiothreitol) indicates that the unreduced receptor is a disulphide-linked complex composed of two copies of the α subunits, and two copies of the β subunits, or, when partially proteolysed, two copies of the α subunits, and two copies of the β_1 subunits (Jacobs et al 1980, Massague & Czech 1980).

There is considerable evidence that the insulin receptor is a glycoprotein.

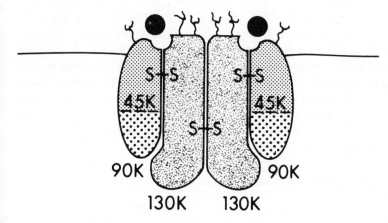

FIG. 1. Schematic model illustrating several structural aspects of the insulin receptor.

Glycosidic enzymes alter insulin binding and the biological response (Cuatrecasas & Illiano 1971). Lectins such as wheat germ agglutinin and concanavalin A modulate insulin binding and have insulin-like activity (Cuatrecasas 1973, Cuatrecasas & Tell 1973). Furthermore, solubilized insulin receptor is adsorbed to lectin affinity columns and can be eluted with the appropriate sugar (Cuatrecasas & Tell 1973). In addition, tunicamycin inhibits the synthesis of insulin receptors (Rosen et al 1979, Ronnett & Lane 1981). It is now clear that both subunits of the receptor are glycoproteins. Neuraminidase alters the mobility of α, β and β_1, indicating that these components contain sialic acid (Jacobs et al 1980b, Van Obberghen et al 1981). Recently, it has been shown that both α and β are biosynthetically labelled with tritiated sugars (Hedo et al 1981). Since the carbohydrate portions of cell membrane glycoproteins are located exclusively on the external part of the cell membrane, these results indicate that both the α and β subunits of the receptor as well as the β_1 fragment are exposed on the external surface of the cell membrane. This is supported by the fact that α, β and β_1 are labelled in affinity-labelling studies in intact cells where, presumably, the affinity label would have access only to the external surface of the cell membrane.

Anti-receptor antibodies

We have produced two types of antibodies to the insulin receptor. The first was prepared by immunizing a rabbit with non-denatured purified insulin receptor (Jacobs et al 1978); the second by immunizing with reduced and denatured α subunit isolated from the purified receptor by SDS-polyacrylamide gel electrophoresis. The two antibodies have several properties in common. Both immunoprecipitate solubilized insulin receptor (this can be demonstrated either by labelling the receptor with ^{125}I-labelled insulin or by directly iodinating the purified receptor), yet neither inhibits insulin binding. Thus, both antibodies appear to recognize regions of the insulin receptor which are distinct from the insulin-binding site, but which must be on the external surface of the cell, since both antibodies recognize the receptor in intact cells, as indicated by their ability to mimic several of the biological activities of insulin (Table 1).

TABLE 1 Insulin-like effects of anti-insulin receptor antibodies

System tested	Reference
Stimulation of glucose transport	Jacobs et al 1978
and glucose oxidation	Rosen et al 1979
Anti-lipolytic effects	Jacobs et al 1978
Stimulation of lipogenesis	Caro & Amatruda 1981
Stimulation of H_2O_2 production	Mukherjee et al 1982
Stimulation of pyruvate dehydrogenase	Seals & Jarrett 1980
Phosphorylation of ribosomal S6 protein	Smith et al 1980
Down regulation of insulin receptors	Caro & Amatruda 1980
Production of a putative insulin mediator	Seals & Jarett 1980
	Rosen et al 1981
Induction of tyrosine aminotransferase	J. W. Koontz, unpublished results 1981
Stimulation of [^{3}H]thymidine incorporation	J. W. Koontz, unpublished results 1981

It is further possible to demonstrate that the antibody prepared using the isolated α subunit recognizes only this subunit. These antibodies will immunoprecipitate both the α and β subunits and the β_1 fragment of the native receptor, and of receptor that has been denatured with SDS or reduced with dithiothreitol; however, when the receptor is both denatured and reduced, only the α subunit is immunoprecipitated. These results indicate that the antibody recognizes only the α subunit, and that precipitation of β and β_1 occurs only because of their association with α by both inter-chain disulphide bonds and non-covalent interactions.

Antibodies to the purified insulin receptor have been shown to mimic the biological effects of insulin on all systems in which they have been tested. These are listed in Table 1. It can be seen that the antibody affects processes that occur intracellularly, such as lipolysis, phosphorylation of the ribosomal protein, S6, and stimulation of pyruvate dehydrogenase, as well as processes that occur at the cell membrane. It is not clear whether the antibody must be internalized to regulate at least some of these intracellular processes. Both insulin and anti-receptor antibody are internalized (see Kahn et al 1981, Posner et al 1981 for recent reviews), and we have found that our antibodies cross-react with intracellular Golgi binding sites (unpublished observations). On the other hand, interaction of both insulin and anti-receptor antibody with plasma membrane receptors has been shown to lead to the production of a substance(s) capable of mediating several of the intracellular effects of insulin (Seals & Jarrett 1980, Rosen et al 1981). This provides a mechanism by which interaction with receptors at the cell surface could indirectly modulate intracellular events.

In many tissue culture cell lines, insulin is mitogenic, but only at supraphysiological concentrations. In cultured human fibroblasts, King et al (1980) have shown that these mitogenic effects, which require micromolar concentrations of insulin, result from insulin acting not at its own receptor, but cross-reacting with receptors for insulin-like growth factors. Recently, Koontz & Iwahashi (1981) have described a rat hepatoma cell line in which 1 nM-insulin, well within the physiological range, maximally stimulated mitogenesis. In these cells, anti-receptor IgG was also able to stimulate mitogenesis (J. W. Koontz, personal communication). These results indicate that in some cells activation of the insulin receptor can stimulate mitogenesis, and this process can be triggered by anti-receptor antibodies.

REFERENCES

Caro JF, Amatruda JM 1980 Insulin receptors in hepatocytes: post receptor events mediate down regulation. Science (Wash DC) 210:1029-1031

Caro JF, Amatruda JM 1981 Evidence for modulation of insulin action and degradation independently of insulin-binding. Am J Physiol 240:E325

Cuatrecasas P 1972a Affinity chromatography and purification of the insulin receptor of liver cell membranes. Proc Natl Acad Sci USA 69:1277-1281

Cuatrecasas P 1972b Properties of the insulin receptor isolated from liver and fat cell membranes. J Biol Chem 247:1980-1991

Cuatrecasas P 1973 Interaction of wheat germ agglutinin and concanavalin A with the insulin receptor of fat cells and liver. J Biol Chem 248:3528-3534

Cuatrecasas P, Illiano G 1971 Membrane sialic acid and the mechanism of insulin action in adipose tissue cells: effects of digestion with neuraminidase. J Biol Chem 246:4938-4946

Cuatrecasas P, Tell GPE 1973 Insulin-like activity of concanavalin A and wheat germ agglutinin—direct interactions with insulin receptors. Proc Natl Acad Sci USA 70:485-489

Harrison LC, Itin A 1980 Purification of the insulin receptor from human placenta by chromatography on immobilized wheat germ lectin and receptor antibody. J Biol Chem 255:12066-12072

Hedo JA, Kasuga M, Van Obberghen E, Roth J, Kahn CR 1981 Direct demonstration of the glycosylation of insulin receptor subunits by biosynthetic and external labeling. 63rd Annual Meeting of the Endocrine Society, Cincinnati, p 626 (abstr)

Jacobs S, Shechter Y, Bissel, K, Cuatrecasas P 1977 Purification and properties of insulin receptors from rat liver membranes. Biochem Biophys Res Commun 77:981-988

Jacobs S, Chang K-J, Cuatrecasas P 1978 Antibodies to purified insulin receptor have insulin-like activity. Science (Wash DC) 200:1283-1284

Jacobs S, Hazum E, Shechter Y, Cuatrecasas P 1979 Insulin receptor: covalent labeling and identification of subunits. Proc Natl Acad Sci USA 76:4918-4921

Jacobs S, Hazum E, Cuatrecasas P 1980a The subunit structure of rat liver insulin receptor. J Biol Chem 255:6937-6940

Jacobs S, Hazum E, Cuatrecasas P 1980b Digestion of insulin receptors with proteolytic and glycosidic enzymes—effects of purified and membrane-associated receptor subunits. Biochem Biophys Res Commun 94:1066-1073

Kahn CR, Baird KL, Flier JS, Grunfeld C, Harmon JT, Harrison LC, Karlsson FA, Kasuga M, King GL, Lang UC, Podskalny JM, Van Obberghen E 1981 Insulin receptors, receptor antibodies, and the mechanism of insulin action. Recent Prog Horm Res 37:477-538

King GL, Kahn CR, Rechler MM, Nissley SP 1980 Direct demonstration of separate receptors for growth and metabolic activities of insulin and multiplication-stimulating activity (an insulin-like growth factor) using antibodies to the insulin receptor. J Clin Invest 66:130-140

Koontz JW, Iwahashi M 1981 Insulin as a potent, specific growth factor in a rat hepatoma cell line. Science (Wash DC) 211:947-949

Massague J, Czech MP 1980 Multiple redox forms of the insulin receptor in native liver membranes. Diabetes 29:945-947

Massague J, Pilch PF, Czech MP 1980 Electrophoretic resolution of three major insulin receptor structures with unique subunit stoichiometries. Proc Natl Acad Sci USA 77:7137-7141

Massague J, Pilch PF, Czech MP 1981 A unique proteolytic cleavage site on the β subunit of the insulin receptor. J Biol Chem 256:3182-3190

Mukherjee SP, Attaway EJ, Mukherjee C 1982 Insulin-like stimulation of hydrogen peroxide production in adipocytes by insulin receptor antiserum. Submitted

Pilch PF, Czech MP 1979 Interaction of cross-linking agents with the insulin effector system of isolated fat cells. J Biol Chem 254:3375-3381

Pilch PF, Czech MP 1980 The subunit structure of the high affinity insulin receptor. J Biol Chem 255:1722-1731

Posner BI, Bergeron JJM, Josefsberg Z, Khan MN, Khan RJ, Patel BA, Sikstrom RA, Verma AK 1981 Peptide hormones: intracellular receptors and internalization. Recent Prog Horm Res 37:539-582

Raftery MA, Hunkapiller MW, Strader CD, Hood LE 1980 Acetylcholine receptor: complex of homologous subunits. Science (Wash DC) 208:1454-1456

Ronnett GV, Lane MD 1981 Post-translational glycosylation-induced activation of aglycoinsulin receptor accumulated during tunicamycin treatment. J Biol Chem 256:4704-4707

Rosen OM, Chia GH, Fung C, Rubin CS 1979 Tunicamycin-mediated depletion of insulin receptors in 3T3-L1 adipocytes. J Cell Physiol 99:37-42

Rosen OM, Rubin CS, Cobb MH, Smith CJ 1981 Insulin stimulates the phosphorylation of ribosomal protein S6 in a cell-free system derived from 3T3-L1 adipocytes. J Biol Chem 256:3630-3633

Seals JR, Jarett L 1980 Activation of pyruvate dehydrogenase by direct addition of insulin to an isolated plasma membrane/mitochondria mixture: evidence for generation of insulin's second messenger in a subcellular system. Proc Natl Acad Sci USA 77:77-81

Siegel TW, Ganguly S, Jacobs S, Rosen OM, Rubin CS 1981 Purification and properties of the human placental insulin receptor. J Biol Chem 256:9266-9273

Smith CJ, Rubin CS, Rosen OM 1980 Insulin-treated 3T3-L1 adipocytes and cell-free extracts derived from them incorporate ^{32}P into ribosomal protein S6. Proc Natl Acad Sci USA 77:2641-2645

Van Obberghen E, Kasuga M, LeCam A, Hedo JA, Itin A, Harrison LC 1981 Biosynthetic labeling of insulin receptor: studies of subunits in cultured IM-9 lymphocytes. Proc Natl Acad Sci USA 78:1052-1056

Wisher MH, Baron MD, Jones RH, Sönksen PH, Saunders DJ, Thamm P, Brandenburg D 1980 Photoreactive insulin analogues used to characterise the insulin receptor. Biochem Biophys Res Commun 92:492-498

Yip CC, Yeung CWT, Moule ML 1978 Photoaffinity labeling of insulin receptor of rat adipocyte plasma membrane. J Biol Chem 253:1743-1745

Yip CC, Yeung CWT, Moule ML 1980 Photoaffinity labeling of insulin receptor proteins of liver plasma membrane preparations. Biochemistry 19:70-76

DISCUSSION

Hall: I gather that you did not produce any blocking antibodies when you immunized rabbits against the purified receptor or the isolated α subunit?

Jacobs: No. Both these antibodies bind to the insulin receptor, yet neither of them inhibits subsequent insulin binding.

Mitchison: Do you have any evidence for patching or for capping by these antibodies and on the role of dimer formation in regulation?

Jacobs: Our antibodies have not been studied to determine this. However, Dr Kahn and his colleagues have shown that autoantibodies to insulin receptor cause either capping or patching, depending upon the cell type.

Kahn: We have found that on lymphocytes, insulin receptor antibodies form distinct caps (see my paper, this volume) and even co-cap with fluorescently labelled insulin. On 3T3-L1 cells these ligands patch when the cells are attached to the dish, but cap when put in suspension (C. Grunfeld, J. Schlessinger & C. R. Kahn, unpublished observation).

Mitchison: It seems that the common feature between hormone and regulatory antibody may be the cross-linking of sub-membrane cytoskeletal assemblies?

Jacobs: Insulin may cause capping or patching of receptors by causing them to interact with the cytoskeleton or other membrane proteins. In a way, this would result in indirect cross-linking of receptors. There is no evidence that insulin cross-links receptors directly.

Harrison: We have some unpublished results supporting the possibility that when insulin binds to its receptor there is a process of disulphide exchange, whereby the disulphide bonds of a small fraction of the bound insulin molecules exchange with thiol groups on receptor subunits, forming a covalent hormone–receptor complex. This could provide a mechanism for cross-linking by insulin—'insulin bridging'—and may be related to the insulin-like effects of known cross-linkers, like receptor antibodies and lectins, as well as oxidants.

Rees Smith: Is the process reversible or irreversible?

Harrison: Disulphide exchange occurs rapidly at 37 °C, reaching a steady state in 10–15 minutes. We haven't yet looked at the 'turnover' of the covalent hormone–receptor complex. It is resistant to denaturants and can be degraded only by reducing agents when extracted from cells in Triton X-100.

Jacobs: In what you are describing, insulin is being cross-linked to a single receptor. Insulin is not serving as a cross-bridge between adjacent receptors.

Drachman: Does the Fab fragment of anti-insulin receptor antibody affect the turnover of the receptor? We found that divalent antibodies against the acetylcholine receptor accelerate the turnover of this receptor, while the monovalent Fab fragments do not (Drachman et al 1978). Secondly, do Fab fragments mimic the *physiological effects* of insulin, as the intact antibodies do?

Jacobs: We haven't yet looked at the effects of isolated Fab fragments on the receptor. However, Dr Kahn has shown that Fab fragments lose the agonist properties.

Kahn: The Fab fragment does lose its agonist properties, but we have some preliminary evidence that it may still accelerate receptor turnover.

Drachman: Have you used a 'piggy-back' technique to determine whether cross-linking of Fab fragments bound to insulin receptor would produce physiological effects or accelerated degradation of the receptor? To test this, you would first bind the Fab fragment to the insulin receptor, and then add a second antibody to cross-link the Fab fragments.

Kahn: No, we haven't done this.

Mitchison: Finally, Dr Jacbos, may one ask how you are getting on with cloning the genes for the receptor?

Jacobs: At present we are not undertaking that task. However, other groups with considerable experience are interested in cloning insulin receptors. I think, with a little luck, they will be successful.

REFERENCES

Drachman DB, Angus CW, Adams RM, Michelson JD, Hoffman GJ 1978. Myasthenic antibodies cross-link acetylcholine receptors to accelerate degradation. N Engl J Med 298:1116-1122

Kahn CR, Kasuga M, King GL, Grunfeld C 1982 Autoantibodies to insulin receptors in man: immunological determinants and mechanisms of action. This volume, p 91-105

Autoantibodies to insulin receptors in man: immunological determinants and mechanism of action

C. RONALD KAHN, MASATO KASUGA, GEORGE L. KING and
CARL GRUNFELD*

*Elliott P. Joslin Research Laboratory and Department of Medicine, Brigham and Women's Hospital, Harvard Medical School, Boston, Massachusetts 02215 and *Veterans Administration Hospital, University of California, San Francisco, California 94121, USA*

Abstract The insulin receptor is a membrane glycoprotein of high M_r which binds insulin with high affinity and specificity and transmits some intracellular signal(s) that initiate(s) insulin action. Antibodies to the receptor have been identified in patients with a syndrome characterized by severe resistance to endogenous and exogenous insulin, varying degrees of glucose intolerance, and the skin lesion acanthosis nigricans. The syndrome is most common in non-Caucasian, middle-aged women, but occurs in patients of all races, both sexes, and spanning the ages of 12–62. Most patients have evidence of other autoimmune disease with increased erythrocyte sedimentation rate and gamma globulins, anti-DNA and anti-nuclear antibodies, leucopenia, and other signs and symptoms of autoimmune disease. Antibodies to the insulin receptor are detected by their ability to inhibit ^{125}I-insulin binding or to immunoprecipitate solubilized insulin receptors. *In vitro* these antibodies acutely mimic most of insulin's metabolic effects. This insulin-like activity depends on antibody bivalence; monovalent Fab fragments block insulin binding and action but lack intrinsic activity. With prolonged exposure of cells to anti-receptor antibody the insulin-like effect is lost and a state of insulin resistance ensues. This is due to both a blockage of insulin binding and a form of post-receptor desensitization. The possible causation of anti-receptor antibodies in this condition is discussed.

Insulin-resistant diabetes due to autoantibodies to the insulin receptor is the rarest of the clinical syndromes caused by anti-receptor antibodies. Despite the infrequency of the disease, studies of these antibodies have proved extremely fertile, since they have provided many insights into the structure of the insulin receptor, the mechanism of insulin action and the mechanism by which antibodies to membrane receptors might modify cell function. In this report we shall briefly review the clinical and laboratory features of the

1982 Receptors, antibodies and disease. Pitman, London (Ciba Foundation symposium 90) p 91-113

disease caused by anti-insulin receptor antibodies and attempt to answer several critical questions concerning its pathogenesis. These questions are important since they are fundamental not only to this disease but to all the diseases being considered in this symposium. The questions include: (1) Where on the receptor do the antibodies bind? (2) What happens to the cell-bound antibody? (3) How is cellular function altered? (i.e., how do these antibodies produce insulin resistance?) (4) What factors might initiate this type of autoimmune response?

Clinical syndromes associated with antibodies to the insulin receptor

Antibodies to the insulin receptor were first discovered during the evaluation of several patients with insulin resistance (Flier et al 1975). Since that time, approximately 25 cases have been uncovered throughout the world. The general clinical features of the patients have been summarized by Kahn & Harrison (1981). Like many autoimmune disorders, there is a female predominance. In addition, there is an unusual racial distribution. Over 50% of the patients have been Blacks from North America or the Caribbean islands, although the disease has been reported in American and European Caucasians and in Japanese. The mean age of onset has been 42 years, with a range from 12 to 62 years.

The most common clinical presentation has been symptomatic diabetes, with polyuria, polydipsia, polyphagia and weight loss. Three of the patients presented primarily as autoimmune disorders, and in one case the anti-receptor antibodies were found as part of a family screening evaluation. In three patients, reactive and/or fasting hypoglycaemia has been the major presenting feature. This is not surprising, in view of the ability of the anti-receptor antibodies to mimic the action of insulin (see below), but appears to be a much less common presentation than insulin resistance.

In addition to abnormalities in carbohydrate metabolism, almost all of the patients have had the skin disease acanthosis nigricans. In some cases there has been very severe involvement of the entire trunk and face with the typical velvety lesions. Many patients also have multiple skin tags on the face and upper body. The aetiology of the acanthosis nigricans remains unknown, but appears to be related to the insulin resistance rather than the autoimmune syndrome. Acanthosis nigricans is also seen in a variety of other insulin-resistant syndromes (Wachslicht-Rodbard et al 1981), as well as other endocrine diseases. Because of this association, however, these patients have been designated as having the Type B syndrome of insulin resistance and acanthosis nigricans (Kahn et al 1976).

Many of the patients have symptoms suggestive of autoimmune disease, including alopecia, vitiligo, arthralgias and arthritis, enlarged salivary glands and/or clinical Sjögren's syndrome, splenomegaly, and Raynaud's phenomenon. In about one-third of cases these manifestations can be classified into a clinically defined generalized autoimmune disease such as Sjögren's syndrome or lupus erythematosus.

The major laboratory findings can be divided into those related to the disordered carbohydrate metabolism and those related to the autoimmune disease. Although almost all patients presented with insulin-resistant diabetes, the degree of insulin resistance and carbohydrate intolerance has varied considerably. Two of the patients had little or no abnormality in glucose tolerance testing at the time of the diagnosis despite the marked insulin resistance. On the other hand, most patients have seen glucose intolerance and in those patients in whom insulin was administered therapeutically, doses have ranged from 150 to as much as 177 500 units of insulin per day without control of blood glucose levels (Tucker et al 1964, Kahn et al 1976). We have recently given one patient up to 15 000 units of insulin per hour intravenously without normalizing the blood glucose concentration. Endogenous insulin levels when measured are always elevated and have ranged from 80 to 950 µU/ml in the basal state (normal level, 11 ± 4 µU/ml). Most patients also give exaggerated responses to insulin secretagogues such as glucose, tolbutamide and leucine (Kahn et al 1976).

In addition, all patients have laboratory findings typical of generalized autoimmunity, with an elevated erythrocyte sedimentation rate, leucopenia, proteinuria, increased gamma globulins, and positive tests for anti-nuclear and anti-DNA antibodies. Interestingly, evidence for organ-specific autoimmunity, such as anti-thyroid antibodies, is rare in these patients.

Assays of insulin receptors and receptor antibodies

The interaction of insulin with its receptor in patients with anti-receptor antibodies and other states of altered insulin action has been primarily studied using circulating mononuclear leucocytes prepared by density gradient centrifugation. Cells from these patients show a marked decrease in insulin binding (Fig. 1, left). This is due to a decrease in receptor affinity with little or no change in receptor number (Bar et al 1980). In kinetic experiments, this loss of affinity appears to be due to an increase in the spontaneous rate of dissociation. Circulating erythrocytes (Dons et al 1981) and subcutaneous adipocytes (Pedersen et al 1981) show a similar defect.

Evidence that the syndrome was due to antibodies to the insulin receptor first came when it was found that sera from these patients inhibited the binding of insulin to normal cells, thus mimicking in vitro the defect observed

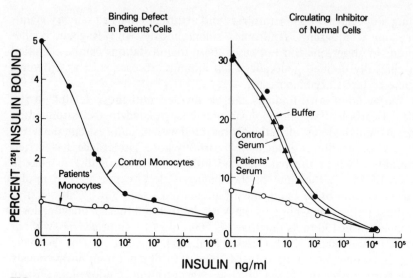

FIG. 1. Insulin receptor dysfunction in patients with anti-receptor antibodies. Left panel shows decreased binding of insulin to peripheral monocytes isolated from a patient with the type B syndrome of insulin resistance and acanthosis nigricans. Right panel shows the ability of this patient's serum to inhibit insulin binding to normal cultured human lymphocytes.

with the patient's cells *in vivo* (Fig. 1, right). Antibodies to the insulin receptor have subsequently also been detected by their ability to immunoprecipitate solubilized insulin receptors (Harrison et al 1979). Both direct and indirect studies showed that these antibodies bind to the insulin receptor with an extremely high affinity (10^9–10^{10} M^{-1}) (Flier et al 1977, Jarrett et al 1976). Evidence that these antibodies indeed bind to the insulin receptor rather than some other membrane protein is summarized in Table 1.

In most cases, the antibody activity is either exclusively or predominantly of the IgG class and is polyclonal in nature (Flier et al 1976). Naturally occurring IgM antibodies to the insulin receptor have also been found in man (Flier et al 1976, Bar et al 1978, Harrison et al 1979) and in the sera of New Zealand Obese mice (Harrison & Itin 1979).

TABLE 1 Evidence that the antibodies in patients with insulin resistance and acanthosis nigricans bind to the insulin receptor

1. They inhibit insulin binding to a wide variety of tissues from species as diverse as fish, birds, rodents and man
2. They immunoprecipitate the insulin receptor quantitatively
3. They mimic most of insulin's metabolic effects on cells
4. Labelled antibodies bind to cells in proportion to the number of insulin receptors and this binding is inhibited by insulin analogues in order of their affinity for the insulin receptor

Structure and antigenic determinants of the insulin receptor

Over the past few years great progress has been made toward elucidating the structure of the insulin receptor and toward its purification (for a review see Kahn et al 1981, Jacobs & Cuatrecasas 1982). By means of a variety of methods of labelling, followed by immunoprecipitation and sodium dodecyl-sulphate (SDS)–polyacrylamide gel electrophoresis, two major subunits of the insulin receptor have been demonstrated (Fig. 2) (Van Obberghen et al

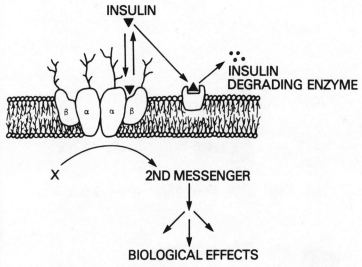

FIG. 2. Schematic model of the insulin receptor and its subunit structure.

1981, Kasuga et al 1981, Hedo et al 1981). They have relative molecular masses (M_r) of about 135 000 and 95 000 and have been referred to as the α and β subunits of the receptor, respectively (Massague et al 1980). Both subunits are glycoproteins, as demonstrated by biosynthetic labelling with ^{3}H-labelled sugars, and both are expressed on the external surface of the cell, as can be demonstrated by surface-labelling techniques. On peptide mapping the α and β subunits show marked differences, suggesting that they are structurally unrelated (M. Kasuga et al, unpublished, Jacobs & Cuatrecasas 1982). In the native receptor the two subunits appear to be held together by disulphide bonds. The exact stoichiometry of the subunits in the native receptor is uncertain, although currently an $\alpha_2 \beta_2$ model is favoured (Fig. 2). The two subunits of the receptor may serve different functional roles. The α subunit appears to contain or be nearer the insulin-binding site and is preferentially labelled by affinity labelling techniques (Wisher et al 1980, Yip et al 1978, Pilch & Czech 1979). Current studies in our own laboratory suggest that the β subunit may act as the effector limb of the system and undergo rapid phosphorylation upon insulin binding (Kasuga et al 1982).

When cells are labelled and the insulin receptors immunoprecipitated by a variety of human sera containing autoantibodies to the receptor, similar patterns are found on SDS gel electrophoresis (Fig. 3). Small pools of free receptor subunits exist in the cell, as determined by non-reduced gels, and

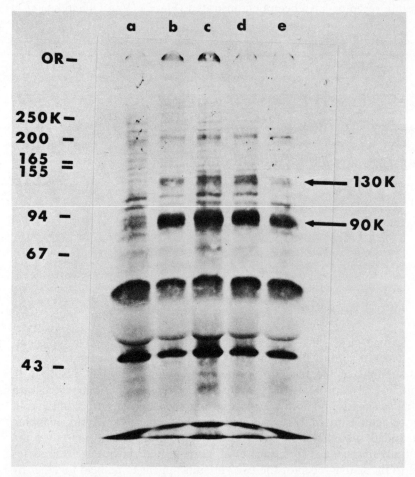

FIG. 3. Identification of the insulin receptor by [35S]methionine labelling and immunoprecipitation. Cells were labelled with [35S]methionine and solubilized in Triton X-100. The insulin receptors were partially purified and immunoprecipitated as described. The precipitate was solubilized in SDS with dithiothreitol, electrophoresed, and an autoradiogram was prepared. The lanes from left to right represent (a) normal IgG; (b–e) anti-receptor IgG (b, B-2; c, B-5; d, B-6; e, B-8). All IgGs were used at 120 μg/ml. (From Van Obberghen et al 1981.)

these are also precipitated. This suggests that autoantibodies in the sera recognize both the major subunits of the receptor, and that all sera are similar in this regard.

It is interesting to note that all the naturally occurring antibodies inhibit insulin binding to the receptor, suggesting that they bind close to the insulin-binding site. By contrast, antibodies raised by immunizing rabbits do not (Jacobs & Cuatrecasas 1982). Both naturally occurring anti-insulin receptor antibodies and antibodies raised in animals are capable of mimicking the action of insulin (Kahn et al 1977, Jacobs et al 1978). Direct binding studies with ^{125}I-labelled IgG preparations from different patients' sera have suggested that on the receptor subunits these antibodies may have somewhat different binding sites (Jarrett et al 1976). Clearly, more detailed studies of the antibody-binding domain(s) are needed.

Fate of anti-receptor antibody bound to cells

The fate of insulin bound to cells has been determined using both biochemical and morphological approaches (Fig. 4). Briefly, it appears that insulin is initially bound diffusely over the cell surface, but after short periods of time begins to form patches and, in some cases, discrete 'caps' on the surface of the cell (Schlessinger et al 1980, Barazzone et al 1980). In some, but not all, cells this receptor aggregation appears to occur preferentially over coated areas of the membrane.

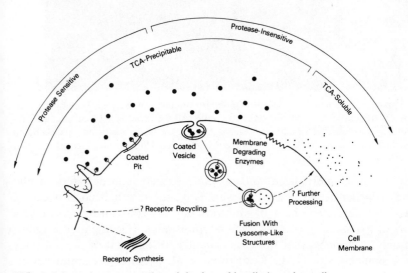

FIG. 4. Schematic representation of the fate of insulin bound to cells.

At 37 °C receptor aggregation is followed by a rapid internalization process, in which the endocytotic vesicles containing the insulin or insulin–receptor complexes fuse with lysosome-like or Golgi-like structures (Carpentier et al 1979, Posner et al 1981) and the intracellular insulin is degraded.

Cell-bound antibodies to the insulin receptor appear to follow the same course. On lymphocytes, the antibodies to the insulin receptor cap, and, indeed, co-cap with labelled insulin (Schlessinger et al 1980) (Fig. 5). The

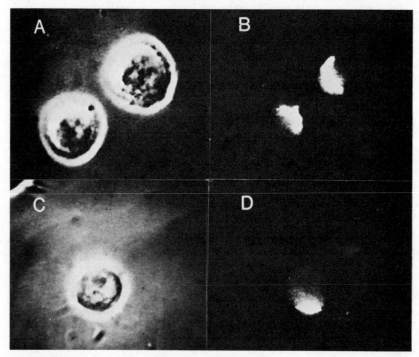

FIG. 5. Capping of insulin and anti-receptor antibody on intact lymphocytes. The upper panels show two cells treated with rhodamine-labelled insulin and the lower panel a cell treated with fluorescein-labelled anti-receptor antibody. Panels A and C use phase microscopy; panels B and D use fluorescence microscopy, both with video intensification. (From Schlessinger et al 1980.)

antibody is then internalized and is preferentially concentrated in the lysosomes (Carpentier et al 1981). Eventually, the internalized antibody is degraded and this component of antibody degradation can be blocked by inhibitors of lysosomal proteases, such as chloroquine (Grunfeld et al 1980). Interestingly, it appears that the monovalent Fab fragment of the antibody follows a similar route (J. L. Carpentier et al, personal communication), suggesting that the fate of this antibody is independent of its valence.

Mechanism of antibody effects on cell function

Antibodies which bind to membrane receptors may alter cell function by several different mechanisms (Table 2). Autoantibodies to the insulin recep-

TABLE 2 Effects of anti-receptor antibodies

1. Blockade of ligand binding/action
2. Mimic ligand action
3. Accelerate receptor degradation
   (a) Directly
   (b) Antibody-dependent, complement-mediated lysis
4. Non-competitive inhibition of receptor function
5. Post-receptor desensitization

tor appear to be able to elicit most of these. As already noted above, antibodies to the insulin receptor directly block insulin binding, and thus could produce an alteration in insulin action by acting as an inhibitor of insulin at the receptor level. Much to our surprise, however, it was found that *in vitro* the acute effect of the anti-receptor antibodies is to mimic, not block, the actions of insulin (Kahn et al 1977, Kasuga et al 1978). Antibodies to the insulin receptor mimic virtually all the metabolic effects of insulin, including those which involve glucose transport, many which are independent of glucose transport, and many which require protein synthesis. In our hands, however, the antibodies do not mimic the growth-promoting action of insulin (King et al 1980).

The biological activity of the anti-receptor antibody, in contrast to the inhibition of insulin binding, appears to require antibody bivalency (Kahn et al 1978). Purified IgG and F(ab')$_2$ inhibit insulin binding and mimic insulin's activity with equal efficacy (Fig. 6A). Monovalent Fab fragments, on the other hand, inhibit insulin binding but are without biological effect. The biological activity of the monovalent antibody fragment can be restored by adding a second antibody. This had led to the suggestion that occupancy of the insulin receptor is an insufficient signal and that cross-linking of receptors or receptor aggregation is important in both antibody and insulin action (Fig. 6B).

The apparent paradox that *in vitro* the anti-receptor antibodies are insulin-like, whereas most of the patients are insulin-resistant and suffering from apparent insulin deficiency, is explained, at least in part, by differences between the acute and more chronic effects of the antibody. Thus, when 3T3-L1 pre-adipocytes are acutely exposed to anti-receptor antibody, these cells show stimulation of biological effects similar to those seen in other cells. This insulin-like effect, however, is transient, reaching a maximum at 30 min

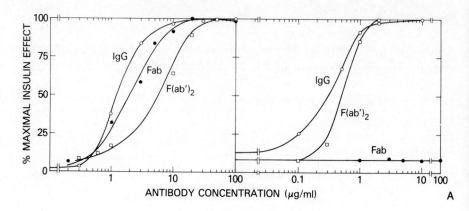

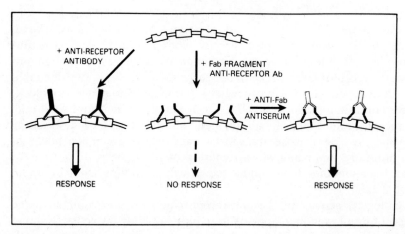

FIG. 6. A. The role of valence in the action of antibodies to the insulin receptor. Left panel shows inhibition of ^{125}I-labelled insulin binding to isolated adipocytes by anti-receptor IgG, $F(ab')_2$ and Fab. Right panel shows ability of the same preparations to stimulate glucose oxidation in these cells.
B. The role of receptor aggregation or cross-linking in the action of anti-receptor antibody.

and then decreasing, so that by 6 h of exposure the cells have returned to a normal basal activity (Karlsson et al 1979). At this time, the cells are resistant to the action of insulin (Fig. 7). This change in activity occurs without any further change in insulin binding and appears to be due to two separate mechanisms. First, since the antibody blocks insulin binding but chronically lacks insulin-like bioactivity, one would predict a shift to the right in the dose–response curve for insulin action, simply as a result of receptor blockade. In addition, there is a decrease in maximal insulin response and this latter effect has been termed 'desensitization'.

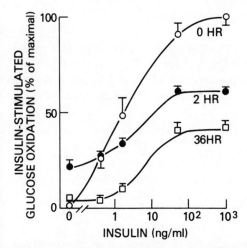

FIG. 7. Effect of prolonged exposure of 3T3-L1 cells to anti-receptor antibody. Note that after 2 and 36 hours there is a decrease in maximal insulin response and a rightward shift of the dose–response curve for insulin-stimulated glucose oxidation.

The exact site and mechanism of desensitization are not yet clear (Grunfeld et al 1980). The site appears to be at some step beyond insulin binding, but relatively early in the pathway of insulin action. The activity of spermine and vitamin K_5, two agents which produce insulin-like effects without interacting with the receptor, is unaltered. The desensitized cell will not, however, respond fully to concanavalin A or to the addition of a second aliquot of anti-receptor antibody. Like the other biological effects of the antibody, desensitization appears to require antibody bivalence. In addition, the medium must contain a source of energy such as glucose or pyruvate or a glucose derivative capable of being phosphorylated (Table 3). There is no effect of anti-microtubular, anti-microfilament, or anti-lysosomal agents on this process (Grunfeld et al 1980).

TABLE 3 Effect of medium composition on antibody-induced desensitization of 3T3-L1 cells

Medium	Desensitization
Complete culture medium	+
Glucose-free medium	−
+ glucose	+
+ pyruvate	+
+ 2-deoxyglucose	+
+ 3-O-methylglucose	−

(From data of Grunfeld et al 1980.)

Possible aetiology of antibodies to the insulin receptors

As in other autoimmune syndromes, the causation of autoantibodies to the insulin receptor in these patients remains unknown. There is much indirect evidence to suggest that the underlying receptor in these patients is normal (Table 4) (Kahn & Harrison 1981). If so, one might presume that in these

TABLE 4 Evidence that the underlying receptor is normal in patients with anti-receptor antibodies

1. Defect is reproduced by exposure of normal cells to antibody *in vitro*
2. Cultured fibroblasts and lymphocytes of patients have normal insulin binding
3. Elution of cell-bound antibodies by acid-wash or plasma exchange returns insulin binding toward normal
4. Cells from patients in remission have normal insulin binding

patients something has acted as a trigger to the production of specific receptor antibodies and/or that there is a basic defect in immunoregulation. Similar mechanisms have been postulated to be involved in the pathogenesis of a variety of autoimmune diseases (Table 5).

TABLE 5 Possible mechanisms of autoimmunity

1. Antigenic modulation with loss of tolerance (e.g. virus-induced)
2. Cross-reactivity of the autoantigen (e.g. with microbes, drugs) (may be T cell-independent)
3. Defect in suppressor T cell function
4. Intrinsic B cell abnormality
5. Non-specific (polyclonal) B cell activation (as with bacterial lipopolysaccharides)
6. Non-specific helper T cell activation (as with adjuvants, such as *Bacillus pertussis*)
7. Imbalance of the idiotypic network (e.g. the emergence of receptor antibodies as complementary anti-idiotypic antibodies—antibodies against antibodies to the natural ligand)

(Adapted from Kahn & Harrison 1981.)

In the case of the immune response to a receptor, one mechanism which is particularly attractive is the possibility that immunological tolerance is lost secondary to modulation of the antigen (i.e., receptor) by some external factor, such as a viral infection. Insulin receptors are known to be modulated in both their number and affinity by a wide variety of physiological factors (Roth et al 1975). Recently, it has been shown that cells infected with some viruses may show acute changes in the binding properties of their receptors. For example, insulin receptors decrease by more than 50% on cells infected with herpes simplex virus or vesicular stomatitis virus (Shimizu et al 1980), and epidermal growth factor (EGF) receptors are altered in cells infected with reoviruses (Maratos-Flier et al 1981). These observations provide a basis for the speculation that, in some cases, a viral disease could trigger an autoimmune response to a membrane protein as a result of antigenic modulation with a loss of immunological tolerance. Obviously, much more remains to be done before we understand the evolution and pathogenetic role of insulin receptor antibodies. Nevertheless, the direct measurement and experimental application of these antibodies illustrate that advances have been made in understanding the molecular mechanisms that mediate immune disease.

REFERENCES

Bar RS, Levis WR, Rechler MM, Harrison LC, Siebert CW, Podskalny JM, Roth J, Muggeo M 1978 Extreme insulin resistance in ataxia telangiectasia: defect in affinity of insulin receptors. N Engl J Med 298:1164-1171

Bar RS, Muggeo M, Kahn CR, Gorden P, Roth J 1980 Characterization of the insulin receptors in patients with the syndromes of insulin resistance and acanthosis nigricans. Diabetologia 18:209-216

Barazzone P, Carpentier J-L, Gorden P, Van Obberghen E, Orci L 1980 Polar redistribution of ^{125}I-labelled insulin on the plasma membrane of cultured lymphocytes. Nature (Lond) 286:401-403

Carpentier J-L, Gorden P, Freychet P, LeCam A, Orci L 1979 Lysosomal association of internalized ^{125}I-insulin in isolated rat hepatocytes. J Clin Invest 63:1249-1261

Carpentier J-L, Van Obberghen E, Gorden P, Orci L 1981 Binding, membrane redistribution, internalization and lysosomal association of [^{125}I]anti-insulin receptor antibody in IM-9 cultured human lymphocytes. Exp Cell Res 134:81-92

Dons RF, Ryan J, Gorden P, Wachslicht-Rodbard H 1981 Erythrocyte and monocyte insulin binding in man: a comparative analysis in normal and disease states. Diabetes 30:896-902

Flier JS, Kahn CR, Roth J, Bar RS 1975 Antibodies that impair insulin receptor binding in an unusual diabetic syndrome with severe insulin resistance. Science (Wash DC) 190:63-65

Flier JS, Kahn CR, Jarrett DB, Roth J 1976 Characterization of anti-insulin receptor antibodies: a cause of insulin resistant diabetes in man. J Clin Invest 58:1442-1449

Flier JS, Kahn CR, Jarrett DB, Roth J 1977 Autoantibodies to the insulin receptor: effect on the insulin-receptor interaction in IM-9 lymphocytes. J Clin Invest 60:784-794

Grunfeld C, Van Obberghen E, Karlsson FA, Kahn CR 1980 Antibody-induced desensitization of the insulin receptor: studies of the mechanism of desensitization in 3T3-L1 fatty fibroblasts. J Clin Invest 66:1124-1134

Harrison LC, Itin A 1979 A possible mechanism for insulin resistance and hyperglycaemia in NZO mice. Nature (Lond) 279:334-336

Harrison LC, Flier JS, Roth J, Karlsson FA, Kahn CR 1979 Immunoprecipitation of the insulin receptor: a sensitive assay for receptor antibodies and a specific technique for receptor purification. J Clin Endocrinol Metab 48:59-65

Hedo J, Kasuga M, Van Obberghen E, Roth J, Kahn CR 1981 Direct demonstration of the glycosylation of insulin receptor subunits by biosynthetic and external labeling: evidence for heterogeneity. Proc Natl Acad Sci USA 78:4791-4795

Jacobs S, Chang K-J, Cuatrecasas P 1978 Antibodies to purified insulin receptor have insulin-like activity. Science (Wash DC) 200:1283-1284

Jacobs S, Cuatrecasas P 1982 Insulin receptors and insulin receptor antibodies: structure–function relationships. This volume, p 82-89

Jarrett DB, Roth J, Kahn CR, Flier JS 1976 Direct method for detection and characterization of cell surface receptors for insulin by means of ^{125}I-anti-receptor autoantibodies. Proc Natl Acad Sci USA 73:4115-4119

Kahn CR, Harrison LC 1981 Insulin receptor autoantibodies. In: Randle PJ et al (eds) Carbohydrate metabolism and its disorders, vol 3. Academic Press, London, p 279-330

Kahn CR, Flier JS, Bar RS, Archer JA, Gorden P, Martin MM, Roth J 1976 The syndromes of insulin resistance and acanthosis nigricans: insulin receptor disorders in man. N Engl J Med 294:739-845

Kahn CR, Baird KL, Flier JS, Jarrett DB 1977 Effect of autoantibodies to the insulin receptor on isolated adipocytes: studies of insulin binding and insulin action. J Clin Invest 60:1094-1106

Kahn CR, Baird KL, Jarrett DB, Flier JS 1978 Direct demonstration that receptor cross-linking or aggregation is important in insulin action. Proc Natl Acad Sci USA 75:4209

Kahn CR, Baird KL, Flier JS, Grunfeld C, Harmon JT, Harrison LC, Karlsson FA, Kasuga M, King GL, Lang UC, Podskalny JM, Van Obberghen E 1981 Insulin receptors, receptor antibodies, and the mechanism of insulin action. Recent Prog Horm Res 37:477-538

Karlsson FA, Van Obberghen E, Grunfeld C, Kahn CR 1979 Desensitization of the insulin receptor at an early post-receptor step by prolonged exposure to anti-receptor antibody. Proc Natl Acad Sci USA 76:809-913

Kasuga M, Akanuma Y, Tsushima T, Suzuk K, Kosaka K, Kibata M 1978 Effects of anti-insulin receptor autoantibody on the metabolism of rat adipocytes. J Clin Endocrinol Metab 47:66-77

Kasuga M, Kahn CR, Hedo JA, Van Obberghen E, Yamada KM 1981 Insulin-induced receptor loss in cultured human lymphocytes is due to accelerated receptor degradation. Proc Natl Acad Sci USA 78:6917-6921

Kasuga M, Karlsson FA, Kahn CR 1982 Insulin stimulates the phosphorylation of the 95K subunit of its own receptor. Science (Wash DC) 215:185-187

King GL, Kahn CR, Rechler MM, Nissley SP 1980 Direct demonstration of separate receptors for growth and metabolic activities of insulin and multiplication stimulating activity (an insulin-like growth factor) using antibodies to the insulin receptor. J Clin Invest 66:130-140

Maratos-Flier E, Rubin D, Field B, Tashjian AH Jr 1981 Reovirus infection causes a decrease in EGF binding to rat pituitary cells. Program 63rd Annual Meeting Endocrine Society, June 17–19, Cincinnati, Ohio, p 237

Massague J, Pilch PF, Czech MP 1980 Electrophoretic resolution of three major insulin receptor structures with unique subunit stoichiometries. Proc Natl Acad Sci USA 77:7137-7141

Pedersen O, Hjøllund E, Beck-Nielsen H, Kromann H 1981 Diabetes mellitus caused by insulin-receptor blockade and impaired sensitivity to insulin. N Engl J Med 304:1085-1088

Pilch PF, Czech M 1979 Interaction of cross-linking agents with the insulin effector system of isolated fat cells. J Biol Chem 254:3375-3381

Posner BI, Bergeron JJM, Josefsberg Z, Khan MN, Khan RJ, Patel BA, Sikstrom RA, Verma AK 1981 Polypeptide hormones: intracellular receptors and internalization. Recent Prog Horm Res 37:539-582

Roth J, Kahn CR, Lesniak MA, Gorden P, De Meyts P, Megyesi K, Neville DM Jr, Gavin JR III, Soll AH, Freychet P, Goldfine ID, Bar RS, Archer JA 1975 Receptors for insulin, NSILA-s, and growth hormone: applications to disease states in man. Recent Prog Horm Res 31:95-139

Schlessinger J, Van Obberghen E, Kahn CR 1980 Insulin and antibodies against the insulin receptor cap on the membrane of cultured human lymphocytes. Nature (Lond) 286:729-731

Shimizu F, Hooks JJ, Kahn CR, Notkins AL 1980 Virus-induced decrease of insulin receptors. J Clin Invest 66:1144-1151

Tucker WR, Klink D, Goetz F, Knowles H 1964 Insulin resistance and acanthosis nigricans. Diabetes 13:395-399

Van Obberghen E, Kasuga M, LeCam A, Itin A, Hedo JA, Harrison LC 1981 Biosynthetic labeling of the insulin receptor: studies of subunits in cultured human IM-9 lymphocytes. Proc Natl Acad Sci USA 78:1052-1056
Wachslicht-Rodbard H, Muggeo M, Kahn CR, Saviolakis GA, Harrison LC, Flier JS 1981 Heterogeneity of the insulin-receptor interaction in lipoatrophic diabetes. J Clin Endocrinol Metab 52:416-425
Wisher MH, Baron MD, Jones RH, Sönksen PH, Saunders DJ, Thamm P, Brandenburg D 1980 Photoreactive insulin analogues used to characterise the insulin receptor. Biochem Biophys Res Commun 92:492-498
Yip CC, Yeung CWT, Moule ML 1978 Photoaffinity labeling of insulin receptor of rat adipocyte plasma membrane. J Biol Chem 253:1743-1745

DISCUSSION

Friesen: Dr Harrison suggested earlier (p 89) that there is a small fraction of the total amount of tissue insulin binding which is irreversible, and implied that it was that small proportion of irreversibly bound hormone that was mediating the biological effects of insulin. How would that affect the interpretation of conventional insulin-binding studies?

Harrison: Our suggestion helps to explain the fact that any cross-linking reagent—whether antibody or lectin, or oxidants such as H_2O_2, spermine, diamide, vitamin K_5, etc.—which encourages disulphide-bond formation, will mimic insulin. This hypothesis of natural cross-linking unifies all this information. It is only a small fraction of the specifically bound hormone that is irreversible; and I don't know whether all insulin receptors are capable of undergoing this reaction, or only a subpopulation.

Kahn: All that one can say is that there is a correlation between the amount of insulin bound (or the concentration range where binding occurs) and a biological effect. This suggests biological relevance, but you don't know that the observed binding is to the biologically relevant fraction of receptors.

Friesen: I feel just as threatened as you do by Dr Harrison's suggestion! However, there is another example suggesting that a small subpopulation of epidermal growth factor (EGF) receptors are the biologically relevant ones, and that most of the specific binding to EGF receptors is probably functionally not significant (Shechter et al 1978).

Rees Smith: Were you suggesting that the antibody to the insulin receptor undergoes some form of disulphide interchange as well?

Harrison: No. The antibody is already in a conformation which would link receptor subunits, at the microscopic level. Whether it needs to undergo disulphide exchange or not, I don't know. We haven't done that experiment.

Jacobs: There seem to be two possibilities, as you suggest: (1) that before insulin binds to the receptor, the receptors are all the same and a small fraction of them undergo this covalent disulphide interaction; or (2) a small fraction of the total receptor population is different even before insulin is present, and only this fraction interacts by covalent disulphide interchange. I don't think you were trying to choose one or the other model?

Harrison: No. I don't know which of those two possibilities it is.

Kahn: One should not give the impression here that this is the proved mechanism by which the insulin receptor is stimulated. So far, it is only a correlation.

Harrison: Yes. The experiments originated by asking the question that Dr Crumpton asked earlier, of how would insulin cross-link. Since the receptor has so many thiol groups on it, and insulin is a disulphide-bonded molecule, I wondered if the hormone could split and link up the receptor subunits. In a very simple experiment we found that if we blocked the disulphide exchange, we also blocked insulin's action, at least on glucose transport: the dose–response curves are superimposable. It is not direct evidence but it is very suggestive, to us.

Engel: How rapidly does the insulin receptor disappear after it has been bound by antibody?

Kahn: The internalization process is fairly rapid. There is some internalization of antibody, or insulin, within 10–15 minutes, increasing up to a steady-state level at about 60 minutes, at 37 °C. However, we don't know that the receptor is necessarily going into the cell at the same time. We presume it is, but we lack direct proof, because our labels are on the antibody or on insulin, and not on the receptor. Fehlmann et al (1982), using a photoaffinity-labelled insulin that covalently links with the receptor, find that the covalently labelled receptor is also internalized, so in that case one presumes that the normally occupied receptor is also going in. We don't know if that's always true.

Engel: If the insulin receptor is rapidly internalized after it is bound by antibody, this might explain why complement fixation or activation of the lytic complement pathway do not take place after the antibody binds to the receptor. Since those cells that harbour insulin receptors are not structurally damaged, one may also infer that rapid internalization of the antibody-bound receptor does not in or of itself injure the cell surface membrane.

Bottazzo: You claim immunofluorescent capping by insulin receptor antibodies using lymphocytes. Several groups, including ours, tried unsuccessfully to demonstrate fluorescence with anti-TSH receptor antibodies of Graves' disease.

You also showed that rhodamine-labelled insulin co-caps with anti-insulin receptor antibodies. If these antibodies are directed against the same antigen, would you not expect blocking rather than a two-colour fluorescent image?

Kahn: This type of experiment has to be done using a special fluorescence microscope connected to a camera designed to detect very low levels of light. With the normal fluorescence microscope you cannot see insulin or anti-receptor antibody immunofluorescence because there are not enough receptors on the surface of the cell. This is a much more sensitive technique, so the apparent strength of the fluorescence is an artifact of the fact that it is an electronically amplified signal.

In the co-capping experiment you are correct, in that if you used a fully saturating amount of insulin or of anti-receptor antibody, you would expect one to inhibit the other. We did this with radioactive label and showed this to be true. In the fluorescence experiment we chose subsaturating concentrations of antibody and insulin, and this allows us to co-label the receptors. The interpretation of that experiment is difficult, because it could mean that the two binding sites co-cap, or it could mean that the receptor is naturally multivalent, and statistically they are all brought together because half of all the sites are occupied on individual dimers or tetramers, or something like that.

Drachman: You found that the affinities of anti-insulin receptor antibodies were extremely high. However, you were testing their binding to a cell surface, so that you were in fact dealing with binding to a solid substrate. The 'avidity' of a divalent antibody binding to solid substrate is probably two or three orders of magnitude higher than the affinity that you would be able to measure in solution.

Kahn: We tried to do that experiment. The monovalent Fab fragment has a slightly lower affinity than the bivalent fragment but, as Dr Rees Smith pointed out earlier, it isn't as much lower as one might have expected if one assumed bivalent binding with no steric inhibition or other factors. It binds more tightly, but not by the addition of the exponents.

Drachman: What is the affinity of the Fab fragment?

Kahn: I can't say. I would guess that it is one or two orders of magnitude less potent than bivalent antibody, but I have no direct measurement of that in a homologous system.

Drachman: I am interested in this point, because we have measured the affinity of anti-acetylcholine (ACh) receptor antibody in a series of myasthenic patients (Bray & Drachman 1982). We found that anti-ACh receptor antibodies have extremely high affinities, of the order of $10^{10}M^{-1}$, so they bind very tightly to the ACh receptors.

Knight: You said that you found raised ESR and gamma globulin levels, and anti-DNA antibodies, in the insulin-resistant patients. That sounds like an anti-viral response to me, not an autoimmune response. You can induce anti-DNA antibodies with viruses: it has been done with polyoma virus in mice. Anti-DNA antibodies are seldom measured using human antigen, i.e. human DNA; what substrate are you using?

Kahn: Antibodies to both double-stranded and single-stranded DNA can be detected, as well as antibodies to ribonucleoprotein.

Engel: You mentioned the decrease in insulin receptors induced by herpes simplex virus. Could one do the converse experiment and try to block viral infection with the antibody?

Kahn: The results suggest that the virus does not directly compete with the insulin receptor: rather, it causes a change in the number of available receptors. It does not appear to do this by inhibiting protein synthesis, because if you inhibit protein synthesis the reduction in receptors is not as rapid as with the virus. The virus seems to be accelerating receptor degradation, although the exact mechanism is still uncertain.

Crumpton: Does treatment with interferon reproduce the effect of the virus?

Kahn: Interferon itself has no direct effect on insulin receptors, on either their binding or their expression, in the long term.

Rodbell: Dr M. C. Lin in my laboratory studied a MDCK kidney cell line which contains glucagon, vasopressin, prostaglandin and catecholamine receptors. He treated the cells with a retrovirus (Moloney sarcoma virus). The glucagon and vasopressin receptors disappeared very rapidly. If he added prostaglandins, they reappeared. The virus had evidently inhibited prostaglandin synthesis. The receptor for prostaglandin remained, and when prostaglandin was added it was able to bring about the reappearance of the vasopressin and glucagon receptors. In blocking the synthesis of prostaglandin the virus had evidently cut off the signal(s) which regulate(s) the production of the glucagon and vasopressin receptors.

Prostaglandins are local hormones; they are produced by the cell itself to regulate, apparently, receptors for other hormones. Perhaps in your particular autoimmune disease—insulin resistance with receptor antibodies—there was a virally induced change, with something like prostaglandin (it needn't be prostaglandin) synthesis being abolished, resulting in a change in the ability of these cells to make the insulin receptor. Perhaps in this way the response to insulin is lost.

Kahn: The viruses used in the study that I mentioned were non-transforming viruses, as opposed to a transforming virus such as a retrovirus. We know that cellular transformation, whether virally induced or radiation-induced or spontaneous, causes a change in the expression of many membrane proteins, including receptors (Thomopoulos et al 1976). In the study I described there was an acute viral infection which presumably, in an intact animal, would be reversible.

Mitchison: A student working in Dr Askonas's group has shown that after infection with influenza virus A, the expression of an HLA molecule (as judged by binding of a monoclonal antibody) falls dramatically in a few hours.

Later, however, the HLA molecule expression returns to normal. The cell still has plenty of viral antigen on its surface and is still a good target for cytotoxic T cells. So there is an early drastic change induced by the virus and a late recovery, which may be associated with the persistence of virus. Your experiment with the virus went on to eight hours. Have you looked at the receptors 24 hours later?

Kahn: Yes. As long as the cells remain alive (i.e., for 24 hours) the loss of insulin binding persists. It is a cytotoxic virus and eventually the cells cannot adhere; thus no recovery is observed.

Bottazzo: I also believe that the presence of anti-nuclear antibodies in patients with insulin receptor disease suggests a possible viral aetiology. What I find difficult to understand is why this disorder is so rare in comparison with Graves' thyrotoxicosis or myasthenia gravis.

Another puzzle is why spontaneous insulin antibodies are relatively common in Japan and very rarely observed in all other countries. Their appearance is transient and they were found mainly in thyrotoxic patients treated with methimazole. This is a good example of drug-induced autoantibody production (Hirata 1977).

Friesen: If one took all the untreated diabetics who have basal fasting insulin levels greater than 100 µU/ml, how many of them would have autoantibodies to the insulin receptor? My guess is that there would be rather few.

Kahn: The subclass of diabetics who have extreme insulin resistance, as shown by their high endogenous levels of insulin, must be very small, because this is not the common situation. I think the Type A patients are probably not so rare as the Type B subgroup. Many patients are referred to us with high levels of insulin resistance and, of these, only about 20% have anti-receptor antibodies as a cause. Maybe 80% have some other cause of extreme insulin resistance, like lipoatrophic diabetes, or the Type A syndrome of insulin resistance and acanthosis nigricans; ataxia telangiectasia is a subgroup of Type B insulin resistance, in that these patients also have anti-receptor antibody as a cause of their condition.

Friesen: We have examined five patients with insulin-resistant diabetes (basal insulin > 100 µU/ml) and none had any antibodies to the insulin receptor.

Hall: George Alberti in Newcastle upon Tyne examined their insulin-resistant patients and did not find any anti-receptor antibodies. This may reflect the fact that his patients were largely Caucasian. Perhaps your findings reflect your higher black population in the US.

Mitchison: How much selection is there in the antibodies that you choose to look at? Is it possible that you may be missing many anti-receptor antibodies which don't inhibit insulin binding, but turn on the insulin receptor, or antibodies which don't do either? You wouldn't pick those up in the assay.

Kahn: In the past few years all our sera have been screened using both an immunoprecipitation assay and a binding-inhibition assay. The former would presumably pick up antibodies to determinants other than the insulin-binding site itself. We do not routinely screen the sera in a bioassay, because we feel that those two assays will pick up most of the antibodies.

Mitchison: Are the results of the two assays concordant?

Kahn: With maybe one exception, all patients who were positive in one assay were also positive in the other. We have mainly been screening patients with insulin resistance, so there is a marked selection; only a few patients have been screened with unexplained hypoglycaemia. There are two cases now where the major presentation of the disease was hypoglycaemia, and where the cause appears to be an anti-receptor antibody with its persistent 'insulinomimetic' effect.

Mitchison: If you used the precipitation assay to screen a normal population would you find binding but ineffective antibodies?

Kahn: One has to use sera from normal subjects as the blank of the assay, so whatever amount of immunoprecipitation occurs with normal serum, we consider to be a non-immune blank. We have no way to distinguish that from zero since we have to use a serum control. There could be low titre anti-receptor antibodies in some individuals which we lose by calling it a non-immune blank.

Mitchison: Have you ever found a high titre in the normal population?

Kahn: Not yet.

Harrison: We define diabetes in terms of blood glucose since we have that test available. It is important to stress that when antibodies are not *detected* in 'acute' assays, it does not mean that they are absent. It depends on our definition—our criteria. Maybe, if we put the appropriate cells in culture with patients' globulins for a few days, in physiological conditions, we might see an effect. Or if we look at serum at greater concentrations than 1:20, which we never do with human serum, we may find something; but we have always been reluctant to do that because of 'non-specific' serum effects! The New Zealand Obese mouse is a good example. The titre of anti-insulin receptor antibodies in this strain is very low. They are IgM antibodies, usually, so whether they have a pathogenetic role is another question.

Mitchison: Now that human monoclonal antibodies are just round the corner, won't that open up new experimental possibilities here?

Kahn: I'm not sure. We are trying to make human monoclonal antibodies using lymphocytes from these patients. We have not had much success in raising high titre anti-insulin receptor antibodies in rabbits or mice.

Mitchison: You would be in a stronger position if you had an *in vitro* anti-insulin response that you could persuade these patients' lymphocytes to make. Since you have a radioimmunoassay, you could perhaps pick it up in that way. Have you ever tried to boost antibody production, using patients' lymphocytes?

Kahn: No.

Friesen: You mentioned the switch from insulin resistance to extreme insulin sensitivity in patients with autoantibodies to the insulin receptor and suggested that there might be a shift related to the uptake of glucose, specifically the phosphorylation of glucose. Have you looked at glucose transport units using a cytochalasin assay?

Kahn: No. We have looked at various types of substrate—glucose and other sugars—that can or cannot be phosphorylated, and pyruvate as an alternative energy source. We also looked at inhibitors of microtubules and microfilament function, but they don't seem to play a role in desensitization. The only positive factor was that antibody bivalence seems to be required for desensitization, and some source of energy—preferably a sugar that can be phosphorylated.

Friesen: I wonder if this switch has a more general application, to the sudden shifts in insulin sensitivity that are so commonly encountered in diabetics, for no apparent reason. From one day to the next, two units of insulin more or less can greatly alter the control of glucose levels in the 'brittle' diabetic patient.

Drachman: Do you have any patients in other disease categories who have extreme insulin resistance (acquired, not genetic) and very low numbers of insulin receptors but no demonstrable IgG antibody?

Kahn: Some patients have very low levels of insulin receptors and are extremely obese and insulin-resistant. These are patients with syndromes like the Type A form of insulin resistance and acanthosis nigricans that occurs primarily in the teenage years. However, we believe this to be a genetic defect that isn't expressed earlier.

Drachman: Do you have any insulin-resistant patients with a serum factor *other than IgG* that lowers the numbers of insulin receptors?

Kahn: Insulin itself does this; but no other regulatory molecules have been defined apart from insulin and the anti-receptor antibody.

Drachman: We recently found that some patients with polymyositis have reduced numbers of ACh receptors. Their serum induces accelerated receptor degradation, but we cannot attribute this effect to IgG, and have not yet identified the nature of the factor.

Engel: Is there any clinical concomitant of this, such as a decremental electromyogram, or any definite myasthenic symptoms?

Drachman: Our patients with polymyositis do not show decremental responses on repetitive nerve stimulation. They have reduced numbers of ACh receptors at neuromuscular junctions, below the established normal levels, and in the upper range seen in patients with myasthenia gravis

(A. Pestronk & D. B. Drachman, unpublished).

Newsom-Davis: Is the factor another immunoglobulin?

Drachman: I don't know yet.

Hall: Were these patients with malignant disease, for example bronchogenic carcinoma?

Drachman: No.

McLachlan: Dr Kahn, do you know where the antibodies are made in your insulin-resistant patients?

Kahn: No.

Mitchison: You would like the antibodies to be made in the pancreas, presumably!

McLachlan: In our studies of autoantibody synthesis in Hashimoto's disease and myasthenia gravis we have evidence that thyroid lymphocytes are a major site of microsomal and thyroglobulin autoantibody production (McLachlan et al 1979) and that thymic lymphocytes are a major site of ACh receptor antibody synthesis (McLachlan et al 1981). Localized autoantibody synthesis may well occur in other autoimmune diseases.

Secondly, in the binding studies using serum from your patient, Dr Kahn, could you be detecting lymphocytes expressing an anti-idiotype antibody—that is, an anti-anti-insulin receptor antibody? Some studies in rabbits have shown that during the early stages of an immune response, cells with idiotype on their surface predominate, while at a later stage cells bearing anti-idiotype became detectable (Tasiaux et al 1978).

Kahn: We have not specifically looked for any anti-idiotypes to the anti-receptor antibody in these sera. The sera inhibit insulin binding not only of lymphocytes but of almost all mammalian cell types with essentially the same titre.

McLachlan: It is possible that the production of an anti-idiotype to the receptor antibody could explain the spontaneous remissions you describe.

Kahn: We have taken serum from patients in remission to see whether it would neutralize the acute-phase serum. There doesn't seem to be anything there.

REFERENCES

Bray JJ, Drachman DB 1982 Binding affinities of anti-acetylcholine receptor autoantibodies in myasthenia gravis. J Immunol 128:105-110

Fehlmann M, Carpentier J-L, Le Cam A, Thamm P, Saunders D, Brandenburg D, Orci L, Freychet P 1982 Biochemical and morphological evidence that the insulin receptor is internalized with insulin in hepatocytes. J Cell Biol, in press

Hirata Y 1977 Spontaneous insulin antibodies and hypoglycaemia. In: Bajaj JS (ed) Diabetes. Excerpta Medica, Amsterdam (International Congress Series 240) p 278-284

McLachlan SM, McGregor A, Rees Smith B, Hall R 1979 Thyroid-autoantibody synthesis by Hashimoto thyroid lymphocytes. Lancet 1:162-163

McLachlan SM, Nicholson LVB, Venables G, Mastaglia FL, Bates D, Rees Smith B, Hall R 1981 Acetylcholine receptor antibody synthesis in lymphocyte cultures. J Clin Lab Immunol 5:137-142

Shechter Y, Hernaez L, Cuatrecasas P 1978 Epidermal growth factor: biological activity requires persistent occupation of high-affinity cell surface receptors. Proc Natl Acad Sci USA 75:5788-5791

Tasiaux N, Leuwenkroon R, Bruyns C, Urbain J 1978 Possible occurrence and meaning of lymphocytes bearing autoanti-idiotypic receptors during the immune response. Eur J Immunol 8:464-468

Thomopoulos P, Roth J, Lovelace E, Pastan I 1976 Insulin receptors in normal and transformed fibroblasts: relationship to growth and transformation. Cell 8:417-423

Structure–function relations of the thyrotropin receptor

B. REES SMITH and P. R. BUCKLAND

Department of Medicine, Welsh National School of Medicine, Heath Park, Cardiff, CF4 4XN, UK

Abstract The thyrotropin (thyroid-stimulating hormone or TSH) receptor is an amphiphilic membrane component with a relative molecular mass of about 200 000 as judged by gel filtration and an isoelectric point close to pH 5. Analyses with chemical, enzymic and affinity probes indicate that the receptor is a glycoprotein containing a disulphide bridge and that the integrity of the disulphide bond is essential for maintaining the structure of the TSH-binding site.

Serum from patients with Graves' disease contains antibodies which inhibit the binding of TSH to its receptor and there is considerable evidence that this effect is due to a direct interaction between the antibodies and the receptor. The antibody–receptor interaction is probably responsible for the TSH agonist properties of Graves' serum and, similarly, the TSH antagonist properties of the sera from a small number of patients can be explained on the basis of antibody–receptor binding.

Although TSH and IgG from Graves' disease patients appear to bind to the same receptor, the relationship between the sites for the two substances is not clearly understood. However, Fab fragments of Graves' IgG are as effective as intact IgG in competing with TSH for the receptor and gel filtration and immunoprecipitation studies indicate that the binding of hormone and antibody to the receptor is mutually exclusive. Current evidence suggests therefore that the binding sites for TSH and TSH receptor antibodies are very closely related and may well be identical.

The TSH receptor

When highly purified preparations of biologically active thyrotropin (thyroid-stimulating hormone, TSH) became available in the early 1970s (particularly through the generosity of Dr J. G. Pierce) it was possible, for the first time, to study the interaction between TSH and its receptor directly. These investigations were done using isolated cells or crude or partially purified membranes

1982 Receptors, antibodies and disease. Pitman, London (Ciba Foundation symposium 90) p 114-132

from porcine (Verrier et al 1974), guinea-pig (Manley et al 1974) or human thyroid tissue (Smith & Hall 1974) and ^{125}I-labelled bovine or porcine TSH. The binding of labelled TSH to these preparations was found to be a saturable, partially reversible process. Analysis of binding data in terms of Scatchard transformation gave linear plots for guinea-pig and porcine thyroid tissue. The conventional interpretation of this data suggested association constants in the region of 10^9–10^{10} M^{-1}. Human thyroid membranes gave curved Scatchard plots. The reason for this is not clear at present but detailed studies have indicated that negative cooperativity is not involved (Rees Smith et al 1977).

Thyrotropin has been shown to stimulate lipolysis in isolated fat cells and TSH receptors are readily demonstrable in adipose tissue (Teng et al 1975). These receptors have similar TSH-binding characteristics to those in thyroid tissue.

Thyroid stimulation by TSH appears to be mediated by the adenylate cyclase–cyclic AMP system and studies with thyroid membrane preparations have demonstrated a good correlation between receptor binding and stimulation of cyclic AMP synthesis (Verrier et al 1974, Manley et al 1974). In the case of the extremely rapid effects of TSH, such as stimulation of iodine release from isolated cells, changes in cyclic AMP levels are undetectable at the time of the effect (Povey et al 1976). This could reflect limitations in the ability to detect adenylate cyclase activation rather than a non-cyclic AMP-mediated phenomenon. However, iodine release could also be stimulated by cyclase-independent events, such as ion movement across the plasma membrane.

Thyrotropin receptors can readily be extracted from thyroid tissue preparations by the use of non-ionic detergents such as Triton X-100 or Lubrol (Manley et al 1974, Petersen et al 1977, Dawes et al 1978). The detergent-solubilized receptors have similar TSH-binding characteristics to membrane-bound receptors but appear to be much less stable.

Analysis of detergent-solubilized porcine and human TSH receptors by isoelectric focusing indicates that the molecule has an isoelectric point close to pH 5.

Gel filtration of complexes of labelled TSH, TSH receptor and Lubrol micelles on Sephacryl S-300 indicate that the complex has a K_{av} of 0.25, making very approximate corrections for the size of the hormone and detergent micelles. This type of analysis suggests that the receptor itself has a relative molecular mass (M_r) in the region of 2×10^5. However, more recent studies with sucrose density gradient centrifugation have suggested a somewhat lower molecular weight (E. D. Jones & B. Rees Smith, unpublished observations).

The nature of the TSH receptor has been investigated indirectly by using a variety of chemical, enzymic and affinity probes. The thyrotropin-binding activity of thyroid membranes is readily inactivated by proteolytic enzymes such as trypsin and reducing agents such as dithiothreitol and mercaptoethanol. These effects are also observed on detergent-solubilized receptors, which suggests that the probes are acting directly on the receptor. Consequently, the TSH receptor appears to be a protein with at least one functionally important disulphide bridge. Disulphide-blocking agents such as iodoacetamide do not influence the TSH-binding properties of membrane-bound or detergent-solubilized receptors, indicating that free SH groups are not important in forming the active site.

Detergent-solubilized TSH receptors can be reversibly bound by columns of Sepharose coupled to lentil lectin or concanavalin A. As well as providing a useful means of purifying the receptor, these observations suggest that sugar groups (particularly glucosyl and mannosyl residues) are an integral part of the receptor. However, neuraminidase in amounts ranging from $10 \mu U$ to 1 unit, and phospholipases A_2, C and D in amounts up to $10 \, mU$, have no effect on detergent-solubilized TSH receptors. This suggests that sialic acid residues and phospholipids are not important components of the TSH-binding site.

Solubilized TSH receptors can also be purified about 50-fold by columns of Sepharose coupled to TSH (Rickards et al 1981). This procedure, together with lectin chromatography, is clearly a promising approach to the purification and further characterization of the receptor.

Recently, we have used a variety of cross-linking reagents to couple ^{125}I-labelled TSH covalently to its receptor. These studies included linking the heterobifunctional reagent, hydroxysuccinimidyl-4-azidobenzoate (HSAB) to TSH before labelling with ^{125}I. The ^{125}I-labelled HSAB-TSH was then reacted with affinity-purified TSH receptors and the mixture exposed to ultraviolet light. After the TSH–TSH receptor complexes had been precipitated with polyethylene glycol, the precipitates were dissolved in sodium dodecyl sulphate and run on polyacrylamide gel electrophoresis, and the gels were analysed by autoradiography. Three bands M_r 59 000, 73 000 and 120 000 were apparent in addition to bands characteristic of TSH (M_r 28 000 and 14 000). Similar bands were obtained when cross-linking was carried out by adding disuccinimidyl suberate (DSS) to preformed TSH–TSH receptor complexes. Under the conditions used, both HSAB and DSS cross-linked the two subunits of TSH. The formation of the 59 000, 73 000 and 120 000 M_r bands was completely inhibited by unlabelled TSH in both cases. These studies suggest that the TSH receptor contains two subunits of M_r 45 000 each.

An interesting and probably important feature of the TSH–TSH receptor interaction is that hormone and receptor show a reduced tendency to dissociate with increasing time of contact (Manley et al 1974, Brennan et al 1980). Similar characteristics have been observed with other systems, including the growth hormone and luteinizing hormone receptors. In the case of TSH–TSH receptor complexes, the reduction in dissociation rate with time has been studied in isolated cells, particulate membrane preparations and detergent-solubilized membranes (Brennan et al 1980). These observations suggest that the hormone–receptor complex (HR) undergoes a configurational change to a more stable form (HR)'. The rate of formation of the more stable form is slowest in isolated intact cells, more rapid in membranes and fastest in solubilized receptor preparations. This suggests that the rate of conversion of (HR) to (HR)' is influenced by the degree of disruption of membrane structure. Similar observations have been made on the rate of dissociation of labelled human chorionic gonadotropin (hCG) from rat testis membranes, detergent-solubilized testis membranes and isolated Leydig cells (Brennan et al 1980, Karem 1979).

The role of stable hormone–receptor complexes in the actions of hormones such as TSH and hCG is not clear at present. They are clearly not important in the acute actions of TSH and hCG but may be involved in events which require prolonged contact of hormone and receptor, such as internalization or shedding from the cell surface.

Autoantibodies which interact with the TSH receptor

The presence of thyroid-stimulating activity distinct from TSH in the serum of patients with Graves' disease was established by Adams and Purves in the mid 1950s (Adams & Purves 1956, Dorrington & Munro 1966). Subsequently these antibody molecules were shown to be of the IgG class with the thyroid-stimulating site being formed by the combination of heavy and light chains in the Fab part of the molecule (Dorrington & Munro 1966, Smith et al 1969, Rees Smith 1981). The effects of the thyroid-stimulating autoantibodies on the thyroid appeared to be virtually identical to those of TSH, with the principal activities of both stimulators being mediated by the adenylate cyclase–cyclic AMP system (Dorrington & Munro 1966, Kendall-Taylor 1973).

More recently, analyses have shown that IgG from patients with Graves' disease inhibits the binding of labelled TSH to the TSH receptor. This effect could result from an interaction between the IgG and TSH or an effect of the Graves' IgG on thyroid cell membranes. However, studies using gel filtration and polyethylene glycol precipitation have failed to show any interaction between TSH and Graves' disease IgG. Furthermore, when thyroid membranes are incubated with Graves' disease IgG and then washed before the addition of labelled TSH, inhibition of hormone binding is still observed.

Consequently, the IgG of Graves' disease patients must act by binding to the membrane and not by interacting with TSH.

The Graves' IgG might interact directly with the TSH receptor. Alternatively, binding to a different membrane component could occur and this process could somehow result in the transmission of a signal through the membrane which inactivated the TSH-binding site. One way of deciding between these two possibilities is to disperse the membrane components in an excess of non-ionic detergent micelles and re-examine the effects of Graves' IgG on TSH binding. When this is done, the Graves' IgG is found to inhibit TSH binding to the detergent-solubilized receptors in a very similar manner to TSH binding to membrane-bound receptors (Petersen et al 1977). Consequently, the Graves' IgG appears to interact directly with a component of the TSH receptor. It would seem, therefore, that this IgG contains antibodies to the TSH receptor. More recent studies have shown that Graves' IgG inhibits the binding of labelled TSH to TSH receptors purified by affinity chromatography on Sepharose–TSH or Sepharose–lectin columns (Rickards et al 1981).

The regions of the TSH receptor that are involved in receptor–antibody binding are unknown at present. A molecule as large as the receptor might be expected to have multiple antigenic sites and Graves' disease IgG might contain antibodies to several different antigenic determinants on the receptor. In this respect, however, it is interesting that the Fab fragments of receptor antibodies are equally effective in inhibiting TSH binding as the intact IgG (Rees Smith et al 1977). Furthermore, the binding of TSH and TSH receptor antibodies to the TSH receptor appears to be mutually exclusive, in that there is no evidence for the formation of a complex consisting of all three components (Rickards et al 1981). It would appear therefore that the antibody-binding sites are closely linked to the hormone-binding site. The inability to form a termolecular complex between TSH, the receptor and antibodies also suggests that one receptor molecule contains only one TSH-binding site.

Freezing and thawing of human thyroid particulate preparations has been shown to release a water-soluble substance which reversibly binds to and inactivates the thyroid-stimulating activity of Graves' IgG. This material has a relative molecular mass in the region of 30 000 and an isoelectric point of about 4.5 (Smith 1971). The relationship between this binding protein and the TSH receptor is not clear at present. It would seem likely that it is a hydrophilic fragment of the amphiphilic TSH receptor cleaved off by enzymes released during freezing and thawing of thyroid tissue.

Thyroid stimulation and TSH receptor antibodies

As Ig from Graves' disease patients contains antibodies to the TSH receptor, it is likely that TSH receptor binding by these antibodies is responsible for the thyroid-stimulating properties of the IgGs. This hypothesis is difficult to prove absolutely, as it is always possible to propose that the IgG preparations also contain another antibody which stimulates the thyroid cell by interacting with another receptor. If a non-TSH receptor is involved, however, this has to be a rather specialized molecule able to undergo a complex coupling reaction with adenylate cyclase, and the simplest explanation for the thyroid-stimulating properties of Graves' IgG is to attribute them to TSH receptor antibodies. Strong circumstantial support for this hypothesis is provided by the observation that both Graves' IgG and TSH interact with TSH receptors in fat and stimulate lipolysis, and also inhibit TSH binding to TSH receptors in the testis. If thyroid stimulation by Graves' IgG is due to the effects of an antibody interaction with a membrane component other than the TSH receptor, one would have to suppose that this membrane component is also present on cells in fat and testis.

Biochemical characteristics of TSH receptor antibodies

TSH receptor antibodies have been analysed biochemically, both receptor-binding and thyroid-stimulating systems being used to assess antibody activity.

Studies using the mouse bioassay demonstrated that the thyroid-stimulating activity of Graves' serum was exclusively associated with the IgG fraction. Furthermore, the activity was formed by the combination of heavy and light chains in the Fab part of the IgG molecule. Isolated heavy chains also showed a small amount of thyroid-stimulating activity. Ion exchange and isoelectric focusing studies demonstrated that the thyroid-stimulating activity of Graves' IgG had a wide range of isoelectric points, indicating that the antibodies were of polyclonal origin (Smith 1971). Studies with immunoglobulin light chain antisera have also demonstrated that the stimulating activity is distributed approximately equally between antibody molecules with $\varkappa$ and λ light chains. In addition, stimulating activity in one Graves' serum has been shown to be associated with IgG subclasses 1, 2 and 4 but not IgG3 (Ochi et al 1977).

Analyses of the properties of Graves' IgG using assay systems other than the mouse bioassay have been less extensive. Stimulation of human thyroid adenylate cyclase has been demonstrated with the Fab fragment of Graves' IgG (Rees Smith et al 1977) and the activity has been shown to be polyclonal (Zakarija & McKenzie 1978). Similarly, the ability of Graves' IgG to inhibit

TSH binding to thyroid membranes has been localized in the Fab fragment (Rees Smith et al 1977).

The capacity of antibodies to the receptor to stimulate the thyroid rather than induce cell lysis by way of the complement system is of interest. However, as the number of receptors on the surface of the thyroid cell is small (in the region of 10^3 sites per cell) and the receptor antibodies are of the IgG class, complement activation might not be expected to occur.

The binding of Graves' IgG to thyroid preparations is not readily reversible, in contrast to the easily dissociable characteristics of the TSH–TSH receptor complex. However, antibody–receptor complexes can be dissociated by treatment with the chaotropic agent, sodium thiocyanate (Smith 1971). This suggests that hydrophobic bonding is a major factor in the antibody–receptor interaction.

Thyroid function in Graves' disease and TSH receptor antibodies

In normal subjects, thyroid function is under the control of a feedback system involving pituitary TSH and thyroid hormones (Hall et al 1975). Perturbation of the system by administration of thyroid hormones or thyrotropin-releasing hormone (TRH) can be used to assess the state of the pituitary–thyroid axis and the effects of serum TSH receptor antibodies. When this is done in Graves' disease patients who have been treated, the presence of receptor antibodies correlates well with the loss of TSH control of thyroid function (Clague et al 1976), suggesting that when the antibodies are present they are involved in thyroid stimulation.

The relationship between levels of receptor antibodies and the extent of thyroid stimulation is difficult to assess, since thyroid tissue in patients with Graves' disease is usually subject to some autoimmune destruction as well as autoimmune stimulation. However, the iodine-trapping mechanism is not markedly influenced by autoimmune destruction, and consequently early ^{131}I uptake measurements are probably one of the most useful assessments of the ability of receptor antibodies to stimulate the thyroid. Indeed, in untreated Graves' disease patients (carefully selected for absence of iodine contamination in their diets), levels of receptor antibodies are found to show a significant correlation with the ^{131}I uptake (Mukhtar et al 1975).

In addition, Endo et al (1978) have shown that levels of TSH receptor antibodies correlate significantly with uptake of [99m]Tc (used in place of ^{131}I) by the thyroid in untreated Graves' disease patients. These investigators also demonstrated a good relationship between the levels of receptor antibodies and the extent of thyroid follicle hyperplasia in needle biopsy samples.

These initial observations on the relationship between receptor antibody levels and control of thyroid function suggested that when the antibodies were present, they stimulated the thyroid. Consideration of the complexity of the immune response and the heterogeneity of antibody affinity and specificity, however, suggested that some of the receptor antibodies might act as TSH antagonists rather than as TSH agonists. Subsequently, good evidence for the existence of receptor antibodies that were unable to stimulate thyroid function was obtained in a few patients with Hashimoto's thyroiditis (Clague et al 1976) and ophthalmic Graves' disease (Teng et al 1977) (eye signs of Graves' disease in the absence of hyperthyroidism or a past history of hyperthyroidism). More recently, further support for these observations has been provided by a report of a euthyroid mother with high levels of receptor antibody (which crossed the placenta) giving birth to a euthyroid child (Hales et al 1980). It is also possible that, in some circumstances, receptor antibodies acting as TSH antagonists could induce hypothyroidism. Again, there has recently been some evidence that this can happen in the neonate (Konishi et al 1980).

As mentioned earlier in this section, Graves' disease usually has the features of both autoimmune stimulation and autoimmune destruction. In hyperthyroid Graves' disease the stimulatory process is clearly predominant. In some patients with ophthalmic Graves' disease, however, there appears to be a stable balance between autoimmune stimulation and destruction (Teng et al 1977).

A further factor affecting the process of thyroid stimulation by TSH receptor antibodies is the ability of thyroid tissue to become refractory to stimulation (Shuman et al 1976). Thyroid tissue from Grave's disease patients is known to be less responsive to TSH and receptor antibody stimulation than normal thyroid tissue (Kendall-Taylor 1972).

In summary, receptor antibodies can be of both TSH agonist and TSH antagonist types, and most Graves' sera probably contain a mixture of antibodies with agonist, partial agonist and antagonist properties. In our own experience the agonist or stimulating properties virtually always predominate and induce a stimulating signal in the receptor. This stimulating signal usually leads to thyroid stimulation and hyperthyroidism. Sometimes, however, the stimulating signal is rendered ineffective or at least attenuated by auto-immune destruction and tissue refractoriness.

Synthesis of TSH receptor antibodies by lymphocytes localized in the thyroid

In this section, Hashimoto's thyroiditis as well as Graves' disease will be considered. Hashimoto's disease is characterized by serum autoantibodies to thyroglobulin and thyroid microsomes and extensive autoimmune destruction. Lymphocytic infiltration of the thyroid is a feature of both autoimmune disorders and the immune cells in thyroid tissue from the Hashimoto's disease patients show many of the organizational features of lymph nodes. In Graves' disease, lymphocytic infiltration is less extensive but aggregates of lymphoid cells are a frequent finding.

It seems quite possible that the lymphocytes localized in the thyroid synthesize the thyroid autoantibodies found in Graves' disease and Hashimoto thyroiditis. In Hashimoto's disease there is some direct evidence for this possibility (Davoli & Salabé 1974), including studies in which lymphocytes extracted from Hashimoto thyroid tissue synthesized relatively large amounts of thyroglobulin and microsomal antibodies (McLachlan et al 1979). In Graves' disease, thyroid lymphocytes may also be a major site of TSH receptor antibody production. This evidence is provided principally by studies of the effects of treatment for Graves' disease on serum levels of TSH receptor antibodies and other thyroid antibodies (about 80% of patients with Graves' disease have serum microsomal antibodies detectable by the tanned red cell haemagglutination inhibition technique).

If lymphocytes localized in the thyroid are a major site of autoantibody synthesis, anti-thyroid treatment for Graves' hyperthyroidism might be expected to influence autoantibody production by thyroid lymphocytes as well as thyroid hormone synthesis by thyroid tissue. Three types of treatment are generally used in Graves' hyperthyroidism:

(1) Anti-thyroid drugs such as carbimazole or propylthiouracil, which are concentrated by the thyroid and block iodine organification.
(2) Destructive therapy with [131]I.
(3) Removal of a large part of the thyroid by surgery (subtotal thyroidectomy). In addition, treatment directed against the effects of thyroid hormones at the tissue level is also given, in the form of the β-blocking drug, propranolol.

These different forms of therapy are followed in most, but not all patients, by characteristic changes in serum levels of microsomal and TSH receptor antibodies (for review see Rees Smith 1981).

Treatment with anti-thyroid drugs is accompanied by a marked fall in the titres of both autoantibodies and this appears to be independent of changes in thyroid status, such as serum thyroid hormone levels. By contrast, ^{131}I treatment is followed by a marked increase in thyroid autoantibody synthesis. Serum levels are maximal about three months after therapy and then fall away over the succeeding months.

The effects of surgery are more difficult to analyse because most patients are treated with anti-thyroid drugs until immediately before thyroidectomy. However, in patients who have detectable microsomal or TSH receptor antibodies, serum levels tend to fall after surgery and remain low or undetectable. Treatment of patients for short periods (two months) with propranolol, or placebo, is not accompanied by any significant change in serum autoantibody levels.

These observations indicate that:

(a) Spontaneous changes in autoantibody levels do not tend to occur, at least over short periods of time;
(b) Anti-thyroid drugs inhibit autoantibody synthesis, directly or indirectly;
(c) Irradiation of the thyroid transiently stimulates autoantibody production;
(d) Removal of a large proportion of the thyroid results in reduced thyroid autoantibody synthesis.

Studies *in vitro* have demonstrated that concentrations of anti-thyroid drugs similar to those found in the thyroid during treatment readily inhibit autoantibody synthesis by lymphocyte cultures. Furthermore, lymphocytic infiltration of the thyroid is markedly reduced during anti-thyroid drug treatment. Consequently, the anti-thyroid drugs, concentrated in the thyroid and acting directly on thyroid lymphocytes to inhibit autoantibody production, appear to be a likely explanation for the fall in serum autoantibody levels during treatment.

Similarly, irradiation of lymphocytes *in vitro* can be shown to generate a population of cells capable of stimulating autoantibody synthesis. Such a mechanism could be important in the increase in autoantibody synthesis observed after irradiation of the thyroid. With regard to surgery, the removal of a large proportion of the lymphocytes synthesizing thyroid autoantibodies would be expected to result in a marked reduction in serum antibody levels.

The effect of the antigen release which probably occurs during ^{131}I treatment and surgery on autoantibody synthesis is not clear. The two procedures (surgery and ^{131}I treatment) seem to result in similar marked elevations in serum concentrations of autoantigen, from estimations of serum thyroglobulin levels. However, the changes in serum autoantibody levels are in opposite directions after these two procedures (increase after ^{131}I treatment, decrease after surgery) and this suggests that antigen release does not have a major role in the acute changes in autoantibody levels observed after surgery or ^{131}I treatment. In addition, stimulation of autoantibody production *in vitro* by irradiated lymphocytes can be demonstrated in the absence of autoantigen.

In summary, therefore, the evidence that lymphocytes localized in the thyroid are a major site of autoantibody production is as follows:

(1) Relatively large amounts of microsomal antibodies are produced by lymphocytes isolated from Hashimoto thyroid tissue.

REES SMITH & BUCKLAND

(2) Microsomal and TSH receptor antibody synthesis in Graves' disease are influenced by anti-thyroid drug treatment in a parallel fashion.

(3) The effects of anti-thyroid drugs, ^{131}I and surgery on microsomal and TSH receptor antibody production are consistent with the autoantibodies being synthesized by thyroid lymphocytes.

REFERENCES

Adams DD, Purves HD 1956 Abnormal responses in the assay of thyrotropin. Proc Univ Otago Med Sch 34:11-12

Brennan A, Petersen VB, Petersen MM, Rees Smith B, Hall R 1980 Time-dependent stabilisation of the TSH–TSH receptor complex. FEBS (Fed Eur Biochem Soc) Lett 111:35-38

Clague R, Mukhtar ED, Pyle GA et al 1976 Thyroid stimulating immunoglobulins and the control of thyroid function. J Clin Endocrinol Metab 43:550-556

Davoli C, Salabé GB 1974 Tissue-specific gamma-globulins in human thyroid. Clin Exp Immunol 23:242-247

Dawes PJD, Petersen VB, Rees Smith B, Hall R 1978 Solubilization and partial characterization of human and porcine thyrotrophin receptors. J Endocrinol 78:89-102

Dorrington KJ, Munro DS 1966 The long-acting thyroid stimulation. Clin Pharmacol Ther 7:788-806

Endo K, Kasagi K, Konishi J, Ikekubo K, Okuno T, Takeda Y, Mori T, Torizuka K 1978 Detection and properties of TSH-binding inhibitor immunoglobulins in patients with Graves' disease and Hashimoto's thyroiditis. J Clin Endocrinol Metab 46:734-739

Hales IB, Luttrell BM, Saunders D M 1980 In: Stockight JR, Nagataki S (eds) Proceedings of the VIIIth International Thyroid Congress, Sydney, Australia. Australian Academy of Sciences, Canberra, p 591-593

Hall R, Rees Smith B, Mukhtar ED 1975 Thyroid stimulators in health and disease. Clin Endocrinol 4:213-230

Karem S 1979 The binding of human chorionic gonadotrophin to the rat testis. MSc Thesis, University of Newcastle upon Tyne

Kendall-Taylor P 1972 Adenyl cyclase activity in the mouse thyroid. J Endocrinol 52:533-540

Kendall-Taylor P 1973 Effects of long-acting thyroid-stimulator (LATS) and LATS protector on human thyroid adenyl cyclase activity. Br Med J 3:72-75

Konishi J, Kasagi K, Endo K et al 1980 In: Stockight JR, Nagataki S (eds) Proceedings of the VIIIth International Thyroid Congress, Sydney, Australia. Australian Academy of Sciences, Canberra, p 555-558

Manley SW, Bourke JR, Hawker RW 1974 The thyrotrophin receptor in guinea pig thyroid homogenate: general properties. J Endocrinol 61:419-436

McLachlan SM, McGregor AM, Rees Smith B, Hall R 1979 Thyroid-autoantibody synthesis by Hashimoto thyroid lymphocytes. Lancet 1:162-163

Mukhtar ED, Rees Smith B, Pyle GA, Hall R, Vice P 1975 Relation of thyroid-stimulating immunoglobulin to thyroid function and effects of surgery, radioiodine and antithyroid drugs. Lancet 1:713-715

Ochi Y, Yoshimura M, Hachiya T, Miyazaki T 1977 Distribution of LATS activity in immunoglobulin G subclass. Acta Endocrinol 85:791-798

Povey PM, Rees Smith B, Davies TF, Hall R 1976 Thyrotrophin receptor binding, intracellular cyclic AMP levels and iodine release in isolated thyroid cells. FEBS (Fed Eur Biochem Soc) Lett 72:251-255

Petersen VB, Dawes PJD, Rees Smith B, Hall R 1977 The interaction of thyroid-stimulating antibodies with solubilised human thyrotrophin receptors. FEBS (Fed Eur Biochem Soc) Lett 83:63-67

Rees Smith B 1981 Thyrotropin receptor antibodies. In: Lefkowitz RJ (ed) Receptor regulation. Chapman & Hall, London (Receptors and recognition, Series B vol 13) p 213-244

Rees Smith B, Pyle GA, Petersen VB, Hall R 1977 Interaction of thyroid-stimulating antibodies with the human thyrotrophin receptor. J Endocrinol 75:401-407

Rees Smith B, Pyle GA, Petersen VB, Hall R 1977 Interaction of thyrotrophin with the human thyrotrophin receptor. J Endocrinol 75:391-400

Rickards C, Buckland P, Rees Smith B, Hall R 1981 The interaction of Graves' IgG with the thyrotrophin receptor. FEBS (Fed Eur Biochem Soc) Lett 127:17-21

Shuman SJ, Zor U, Chayoth R, Field JB 1976 Exposure of thyroid slices to thyroid-stimulating hormone induces refractoriness of the cyclic AMP system to subsequent hormone stimulation. J Clin Invest 57:1132-1141

Smith BR 1971 Characterisation of long-acting thyroid stimulator γG binding protein. Biochim Biophys Acta 229:649-662

Smith BR, Dorrington KJ, Munro DS 1969 The thyroid-stimulating properties of long-acting thyroid stimulator γG-globulin subunits. Biochim Biophys Acta 192:277-285

Smith BR, Hall R 1974 Thyroid-stimulating immunoglobulins in Graves' disease. Lancet 2:427-431

Teng CS, Rees Smith B, Anderson J, Hall R 1975 Comparison of thyrotrophin receptors in membranes prepared from fat and thyroid tissue. Biochem Biophys Res Commun 66:836-841

Teng CS, Rees Smith B, Clayton B, Evered DC, Clark F, Hall R 1977 Thyroid-stimulating immunoglobulins in ophthalmic Graves' disease. Clin Endocrinol 6:207-211

Verrier B, Fayet G, Lissitzky S 1974 Thyrotropin binding properties of isolated thyroid cells and their purified plasma membranes. Eur J Biochem 42:355-365

Zakarija M, McKenzie JM 1978 Isoelectric focusing of thyroid-stimulating antibody of Graves' disease. Endocrinology 103:1469-1475

DISCUSSION

Kahn: I have a technical question about the experiment in which you tried to form a complex of TSH with anti-receptor antibody and receptor. As a control for that, do you test to see that the anti-receptor antibody will immunoprecipitate the *unlabelled* receptor? In this case it shouldn't make any difference if the receptor is not labelled with TSH; that is, if the antibodies in Graves' disease are precipitating antibodies you should be able to deplete TSH-binding activity in the supernatant with the anti-receptor antibodies, using labelled, soluble TSH receptor preparations, and a second antibody.

Rees Smith: The experiment is difficult to do exactly as you suggest, but detergent-solubilized TSH receptors can be absorbed onto columns of receptor antibody coupled to Sepharose. We have not yet been able to dissociate active receptors from the antibody columns.

Kahn: The question is whether the anti-receptor antibody is directed to the receptor subunit that contains the TSH-binding site. If so, you should be able to deplete the TSH-binding sites. If the binding activity persists in the supernatant, maybe the antibodies are not directed at the TSH-binding subunit of the receptor.

Mitchison: The problem is that the anti-receptor antibody blocks binding anyway.

Venter: This would be the same assay we use for detecting monoclonal antibodies to the β-adrenergic receptor (Fraser & Venter 1980). If you add sufficient second antibody (anti-mouse IgG) to precipitate all the IgG–receptor complexes as well as uncoupled IgG, you should be able to demonstrate the receptor–IgG complexes in the pellet, or even more simply by assaying for loss of receptor from the supernatant by doing a binding assay on what remains. These assays are very simple and we use them to detect monoclonal antibody FV-104, which competes directly with ligands for receptor binding, as is the case with autoantibodies to the TSH receptor.

Rees Smith: As I said, we have been able to absorb TSH receptors with columns containing receptor antibody conjugated to Sepharose. We have been unsuccessful in dissociating the antibody–receptor complex in such a way as to retain the hormone-binding properties of the receptor.

Roitt: The fascinating point here is the effect of Fab (as distinct from F(ab′)$_2$), where Fab fragments of the receptor antibodies are as effective in inhibiting TSH binding as the intact IgG. Presumably, anti-TSH receptor antibody acts at the precise site where the hormone binds, whereas with the insulin receptor this is suggested not to be the case. The fact that with some receptors, such as insulin, (Fab′)$_2$ can trigger the receptors, when it (presumably) cross-links them, whereas in other instances, like TSH, the Fab fragment alone may trigger by direct reaction with the site where the hormone binds, raises the question of whether a first signal causes aggregation of receptors and this aggregation initiates a second signal. Perhaps cross-linking, bivalent antibodies are able to by-pass what a hormone such as insulin may do in a univalent way. Unfortunately, it's unlikely that you could do studies with electron microscopically visible labelled tags on the Fab fragment, to see if the receptors do aggregate. There are so few TSH receptors on the cell that it would be difficult to detect them against the background noise.

Mitchison: Do we know much about the distribution of receptors for TSH, in fact?

Rees Smith: No. All we can say is that there are very small numbers of receptors on the surfaces of isolated thyroid cells.

Bitensky: Kotulla et al (1976) found that when they attempted to purify human thyroid plasma membrane fractions from homogenates of the gland, the fraction which had the highest content of the plasma membrane marker, namely 5′-nucleotidase, was different from the fraction to which TSH was bound. One can assume that the fraction that binds TSH is the one that contains the receptors. So it seems that the receptors are not distributed uniformly in the plasma membrane and this result might imply that they may be concentrated on one side, which might be the basal, or vascular, pole.

On cross-linking and the bivalency of the interaction between the receptor and the antibody, or hormone and receptor, could the difference between the TSH receptor and the insulin receptor be related to the fact that the TSH molecule itself has two subunits? Is it possible that the antibodies are binding across a two-subunit binding site, and that the hormone receptor in itself already has the bivalency built into it, because of the subunit character of the hormone?

Rees Smith: To me it's significant that the TSH receptor does seem to be monovalent for the hormone (i.e., one molecule of TSH receptor appears to have only one binding site for TSH), whereas the insulin receptor is established to be divalent for insulin. This may explain why cross-linking is involved in insulin receptor stimulation by insulin receptor antibodies but not in the binding of TSH receptor antibodies to the TSH receptor.

Bitensky: To amplify, TSH has two subunits, α and β, both of which need to be present in order for TSH to be active, but we don't know exactly where these two subunits bind to the receptor.

Kahn: The α subunit of TSH is the same as the α subunit of human chorionic gonadotropin (hCG), luteinizing hormone (LH) and follicle-stimulating hormone (FSH). If the α subunit has a binding site and the β subunit has a second binding site, you would expect that in binding studies the other glycoprotein hormones that contain the same α subunit would compete at least partially with TSH. I don't believe they do, in your system?

Rees Smith: Very high doses of LH and hCG do appear to bind to the TSH receptor and induce a stimulating signal. However, the amounts required are in the region of 10^4 times the amounts of TSH required to cause the same effect.

Mitchison: Does this make Dr Bitensky's hypothesis about a divalent hormone less likely?

Jacobs: It depends what you mean by 'divalent hormone'. The TSH molecule is so big ($M_r = 28\,000$) that there may be more than one region of the hormone which is in contact with the receptor. I wouldn't be surprised if there were two contact regions separated by some distance. Would that make it bivalent?

Rodbell: As I said earlier (p 19), the term 'bivalency' appears to be rather ambiguous in its meaning. Any structure, even the simplest catecholamine, can be looked upon as having distinct functional regions for binding and action. This is precisely what we (Wright & Rodbell 1979) have shown for glucagon. With a large two-subunit molecule such as TSH, one could understand how one segment could bind to one receptor subunit while the other sits on the other. The combined interactions of the TSH subunits and the hypothetical receptor subunits would then yield a structure that we would call 'active'.

Mitchison: Wasn't Dr Bitensky talking about the possibility of cross-linking two receptors, not two subunits of one receptor?

Bitensky: You are making too clear what was a fuzzy idea in my mind! I was simply wondering whether the difference between the experiments with the insulin receptor antibody and the TSH receptor antibody was the fact that the hormones are of such different chemical structure.

Davies: We should not underestimate the concept of specificity cross-over at the TSH receptor. By this I mean that hormones whose primary binding site may be in the testis or ovary—such as hCG—can, when present in sufficient concentrations, interact at the TSH receptor. There is much evidence for such cross-over between hCG and TSH both at the binding sites and in bioassays. If you consider the LH molecule alone, then the potency at the TSH receptor is considerably more than that of hCG (Williams et al 1980). It remains orders of magnitude less than the sensitivity of the site to TSH, but there is clear specificity cross-over. Hence, the idea that there is no interaction of the α subunit with the TSH receptor remains uncertain.

Roitt: If the Fab fragment can do what TSH can do, do we need also to postulate that the Fab fragment has some type of bivalency?

Davies: The Fab fragment does produce TSH-like activity.

Jacobs: Does the light chain of Fab produce TSH-like activity?

Rees Smith: No, only the heavy chain.

Kahn: I was interested in your suggestion that the TSH receptor may have only one antigenic determinant, and that that is the TSH-binding site. I believe that the bulk of experience is against that. If one looks at the history of the bioassays designed to detect long-acting thyroid stimulator (LATS) and LATS protector, and then going from animal to human thyroid tissue, we know that sera can be positive in one assay and negative in another. This suggests that each antiserum is seeing antigenic determinants that are slightly different from those seen by the other. With human thyroid tissue there are many more positives than with rodent thyroid. Also, among the purified IgG fractions, you said yourself that some are agonists, and some are partial agonists or antagonists; some are positive in the adenylate cyclase assay and some are not. This suggests that there is heterogeneity in the antibody-binding sites.

Rees Smith: If we look at TSH receptors from a wide variety of species (mouse, man, pig, guinea-pig, dog, cattle) and study the binding of labelled

TSH, we find that antibodies from different patients show similar inhibitory effects. So the actual binding site for the antibody, and for the hormone, seems to be highly conserved.

If we now consider the next stage after binding, namely stimulation, we see a difference between species. For example, with the mouse TSH receptor, a TSH receptor antibody from one patient will bind to the receptor but will not induce a stimulating signal. The same antibody will however bind to the human TSH receptor and induce a stimulating signal. I am suggesting that in this case antibodies are essentially interacting with the same sites on the receptors in different species, but the nature of the interaction is slightly different leading to (in this example) an antagonistic action in the mouse and an agonistic one in man.

Mitchison: How can you have a receptor that is made up of two identical subunits and where the antibody can react only with a single determinant?

Rees Smith: I don't know that the receptor has *two* subunits; but I am suggesting that it has more than one, simply by analogy with other receptors, like the ACh receptor. The TSH receptor does appear to be a large membrane protein with a relative molecular mass (M_r) of 200 000, at least as judged by gel filtration. The chances that it has a subunit structure are high. Perhaps the hormone binds to a site contributed to, or situated between, the two subunits?

Harrison: When you compare stimulation of say mouse and human TSH receptors, are you certain it is the *same* antibody in each case?

Rees Smith: No, I'm not sure.

Jacobs: I believe antibodies from patients with Graves' disease have been described that don't inhibit binding of TSH but do stimulate the receptor (Sugenoya et al 1979)?

Rees Smith: There is good evidence for the existence of antibodies that bind but do not stimulate, but there is as yet no convincing evidence that patients' sera contain antibodies which stimulate the thyroid without interacting with the TSH receptor.

Jacobs: But there is heterogeneity among patients, in that antibody from some patients stimulates TSH receptors but antibody from some other patients does not. Those antibodies cannot be directed against exactly the same site.

Rees Smith: In a situation where we have antibodies acting as agonists and antagonists, the antibodies with different properties are going to be slightly different. I think the analogy with conventional agonists and antagonists of, for example the β-receptor, is a good basis for proposing that ligands binding to the same site can induce different effects.

Mitchison: To return to the hypothetical single binding site made by the interaction of two identical protein chains in the receptor: is there any precedent for that?

Rees Smith: Unfortunately, we don't know enough about the structure of the TSH receptor. This suggestion was basically a guess!

Fuchs: Perhaps it is a question of steric hindrance? With an M_r of TSH as high as 28 000, there might be two subunits and two binding sites on the receptor. It is possible that when one molecule of TSH binds to one subunit, another TSH molecule cannot get close enough to bind to the other subunit. The TSH hormone is a very large molecule, in comparison with acetylcholine or even insulin.

Bottazzo: What is the reason why the TSH receptor has not yet been analysed into subunits by the methods used for the extraction of insulin and acetylcholine receptors? In all these cases the purified hormone and receptor antibodies are available.

Crumpton: Several things could be done towards elucidating the structure of the TSH receptor. For instance, you could try to label the receptor either with a photoaffinity probe or biosynthetically with [^{35}S]methionine, using thyroid slices or cells grown in culture. Labelled cells can then be lysed in non-ionic detergent prior to immunoprecipitation and subsequent analysis of the labelled immunoprecipitate by polyacrylamide gel electrophoresis in sodium dodecyl sulphate. Such studies should provide some fairly definitive information on the number of subunits and whether they are identical, their molecular weights, whether they are linked by disulphide bridges, and so on.

Harrison: This all seems to revolve around the apparent inability to immunoprecipitate the receptor. Differences in the size of structures if you label them pre- and post-extraction may also be involved. Have you pre-labelled the receptor with TSH and *then* solubilized the complex, as well as solubilizing the cell membrane and trying to postlabel it with TSH?

Rees Smith: Yes.

Harrison: And you still can't immunoprecipitate the receptor?

Rees Smith: No; one can't precipitate the receptor either way. Dr Paul Buckland in our laboratory has successfully linked labelled TSH to the receptor using the cross-linking reagents, hydroxysuccinimidyl-4-azidobenzoate and disuccinimidyl suberate. His studies suggest that the receptor contains two subunits both with M_r values of 45 000.

Drachman: You suggested that most if not all the lymphocytes producing anti-thyroid antibody are located within the thyroid. What is the evidence that they are there, and *not* elsewhere?

Rees Smith: There is good evidence that the thyroid in Graves' disease is a major site of TSH receptor antibody synthesis. This is principally derived from studies of the effects of anti-thyroid treatment on synthesis of this antibody, as I discussed in my paper.

McLachlan: Our studies suggested that the thyroid was a major site of autoantibody synthesis; the lymphocytes were able to produce thyroid autoantibodies in culture in the absence of mitogen and we were able to stimulate thyroglobulin antibody production using thyroglobulin (McLachlan et al 1979).

Hall: After thyroidectomy for Graves' disease, levels of receptor antibody fall during the next few months.

Roitt: That could be due to two things, since you take away both the antigen and the lymphocytes.

Davies: We have been looking at arterio-venous differences in antibody levels after thyroidectomy for Graves' disease. This may not be the right approach, because of the anti-thyroid drug treatment, but we found no differences between thyroid arterial and thyroid venous titres, in six patients.

Rees Smith: The effects of conventional forms of treatment on TSH receptor antibody levels, and levels of other thyroid antibodies, in Graves' disease, are striking, as I described (p 122). It is difficult to explain the changes unless you postulate that the antibodies are, to a considerable extent, made in the thyroid.

Newsom-Davis: Have you determined whether there are sites of anti-receptor antibody production additional to the thyroid, by looking for antibody synthesis in cells cultured from the draining lymph nodes?

Roitt: Bob White a long time ago showed plasma cells in the lymph nodes draining the thyroid in Hashimoto patients who were making anti-thyroglobulin antibody (White 1957).

McLachlan: We have tried to obtain lymph nodes from Graves' patients undergoing subtotal thyroidectomy, but without success.

Drachman: In a recent paper on pulmonary sarcoidosis, an excess of helper T cells were found in the lung in active cases, but not in relatively inactive cases (Hunninghake & Crystal 1981). Has anyone determined the proportion of helper T cells in the thyroid in Hashimoto's thyroiditis?

McLachlan: We are currently investigating cell markers on lymphocytes extracted from thyroid tissue of patients with autoimmune thyroid disease. In the lymphocyte suspensions extracted from thyroid tissue of two Graves' patients there were fewer total T cells, in agreement with published data (Totterman 1978), but no significant changes in OKT4-positive or OKT8-positive (that is, T helper and T cytotoxic/suppressor) cells compared with peripheral blood lymphocytes.

Drachman: It would be interesting to know if there is a difference in the proportion of helper T cells found in patients with active thyroiditis as compared with those with relatively inactive disease, as was reported in the sarcoidosis study.

McLachlan: We cannot draw such conclusions yet, as we have results from only two patients.

REFERENCES

Fraser CM, Venter JC 1980 Monoclonal antibodies to β-adrenergic receptors: use in purification and molecular characterization of β-receptors. Proc Natl Acad Sci USA 77:7034-7038

Hunninghake GW, Crystal RG 1981 Pulmonary sarcoidosis: a disorder mediated by excess helper T-lymphocyte activity at sites of disease activity. N Engl J Med 305:429-434

Kotulla P, Aulbert E, Meinhold H, Adlkofer F, Wenzel KW, Schleusener H, Kruck I, Kruck G 1976 Methodological approaches to measuring thyroid stimulating factors with a radioligand receptor assay. In: Muhlen A von zur, Schleusener H (eds) Biochemical basis of thyroid stimulation and thyroid hormone action. Thieme, Stuttgart

McLachlan SM, McGregor A, Rees Smith B, Hall R 1979 Thyroid-autoantibody synthesis by Hashimoto thyroid lymphocytes. Lancet 1:162-163

Sugenoya A, Kidd A, Row VV, Volpé R 1979 Correlation between thyrotropin-displacing activity and human thyroid-stimulating activity by immunoglobulins from patients with Graves' disease and other thyroid disorders. J Clin Endocrinol Metab 48:398-402

Totterman TH 1978 Distribution of T-, B- and thyroglobulin-binding lymphocytes infiltrating the gland in Graves' disease, Hashimoto's thyroiditis and de Quervain's thyroiditis. Clin Immunol Immunopathol 10:270-277

White RG 1957 An immunological investigation of Hashimoto's disease. Proc R Soc Med 50:953-954

Williams JF, Davies TF, Catt KJ, Pierce JG 1980 Receptor-binding activity of highly purified bovine luteinizing hormone and thyrotropin, and their subunits. Endocrinology 106:1353-1359

Wright DE, Rodbell M 1979 Glucagon$_{1-6}$ activates adenylate cyclase and binds to the glucagon receptor. J Biol Chem 254:268-269

Thyrotropin receptor antibodies: clinico-pathological correlations

R. HALL, S. McLACHLAN,* A. M. McGREGOR, A. P. WEETMAN and B. REES SMITH

*Department of Medicine, Welsh National School of Medicine, Heath Park, Cardiff, CF4 4XN and *Department of Medicine, University of Newcastle upon Tyne, Royal Victoria Infirmary, Newcastle upon Tyne, NE1 4LP, UK*

Abstract Immunoglobulins which interact with thyroid membrane receptors can be detected in all of the autoimmune thyroid diseases, namely Graves' disease and its variants, Hashimoto's disease and myxoedema. In Graves' disease it is generally accepted that specific immunoglobulins interacting with the thyrotropin (TSH) receptor, or a closely related site, are responsible for the hyperthyroidism. Receptor antibodies, which inhibit labelled TSH binding but lack biological activity, can also be detected in Graves' disease, ophthalmic Graves' disease and in Hashimoto's disease. Such antibodies can inhibit TSH action and may contribute to the hypothyroidism seen in some cases of Hashimoto's disease and of neonatal hypothyroidism.

Detection of these receptor antibodies is of value in the diagnosis of Graves' disease and its variants, in predicting the risk of neonatal hyperthyroidism or hypothyroidism and in predicting relapse after anti-thyroid therapy.

Treatment with carbimazole or methimazole leads to a fall in the level of receptor and other thyroid antibodies and reduced lymphocytic infiltration of the thyroid, and similar effects can also be demonstrated in an animal model of autoimmune thyroid disease. The mechanism by which this effect is brought about is unknown. It could result from a general immunosuppressive action of the drug or from a direct action on thyroid lymphocytes, though current evidence suggests that methimazole might interfere with the processing of thyroid antigens by monocytes.

It is now widely accepted that the hyperthyroidism and goitre of Graves' disease result from the action of specific immunoglobulins which bind to the thyroid cell membrane and cause activation of adenylate cyclase. There is still some disagreement about the site of action of Graves' immunoglobulins but the evidence is now compelling (Rees Smith & Buckland 1982) that they react with the thyrotropin (TSH) receptor. Hence it seems appropriate to refer to

1982 Receptors, antibodies and disease. Pitman, London (Ciba Foundation symposium 90) p 133-152

these Graves' Igs as receptor antibodies, though this term should not be taken to imply that all of the antibodies which bind to the TSH receptor cause activation of adenylate cyclase. Indeed, it is well known that in some patients with Graves' disease, and particularly in its ophthalmic variant, receptor antibodies are present which inhibit TSH binding but do not activate the cyclase. Such blocking antibodies may inhibit the action of endogenous TSH and contribute to the development of hypothyroidism in some cases of Hashimoto's disease. Transplacental passage of such blocking antibodies has been shown to be a rare cause of transient neonatal hypothyroidism (Matsuura et al 1980).

Our current view is that the serum of patients with Graves' disease contains a variable mixture of stimulating and blocking antibodies capable of interacting with the TSH receptor. In the untreated patient with hyperthyroid Graves' disease the action of stimulating antibodies is obviously dominant, whereas in ophthalmic Graves' disease blocking antibodies are more common. It seems likely that the balance of these two types of antibody may change either spontaneously with time or as a result of various treatment regimens.

Phylogenetic specificity of receptor antibodies

Although the original bioassay for receptor antibodies (long-acting thyroid stimulator, LATS) depended on their interaction with animal thyroid glands, only a proportion of sera from Graves' disease patients (< 50%) gave positive results. More frequent positive results can now be obtained using assays depending on human thyroid tissue (70–95%). It has been assumed that only some of the receptor antibodies cross-react with the antigen (the TSH receptor) in other species, and then usually with lower avidity. However, there are recent reports of high frequencies of positive results in more sensitive bioassays using animal tissue, such as the cytochemical bioassay using guinea-pig thyroid and an assay based on the release of triiodothyronine (T3) from porcine thyroids. These reports raise the possibility that most receptor antibodies will cross-react with animal thyroid tissue if a sufficiently sensitive assay is used, suggesting close similarities in the structure of the TSH receptor from species to species.

Assays for receptor antibodies

The wide variety of assays used testifies to their many deficiencies. Assays for receptor antibodies are shown in Table 1. They can be divided into bioassays

TABLE 1 Assays for anti-thyrotropin receptor antibodies

Method	Species used for detection	Parameter measured	Term applied to stimulator	Advantages	Disadvantages
Bioassays					
McKenzie	Mouse	Iodine release from thyroid	LATS[a]	Bioassay	Laborious, mouse assay
Cytochemical bioassay	Guinea-pig	Alteration in lysosomal permeability	TSAb[b]	Bioassay, very sensitive	Technically difficult, low throughput, guinea-pig assay
T3 release[c]	Pig	Release of T3 by porcine thyroid slices	TSAb	Bioassay, quite sensitive	Porcine assay, rather low throughput
Cyclic AMP	Man	Either activation of adenylate cyclase in membranes, or increase in cyclic AMP in slices or in human thyroid cells in tissue culture	TSAb	Bioassay, human	Laborious, needs normal human thyroid tissue
Receptor assays					
LATS-P[d]	Man	Inhibition of binding of LATS	LATS-P	Human	Laborious, not a bioassay
Receptor	Man	Inhibition of labelled TSH binding	Receptor antibodies or TBII[e]	Simple, human	Not a bioassay

[a] LATS, long-acting thyroid stimulator.
[b] TSAb, thyroid-stimulating antibody.
[c] T3, triiodothyronine.
[d] LATS-P, LATS-protector.
[e] TBII, TSH-binding-inhibiting immunoglobulin.

and receptor assays. Comparisons of results in these various assays have preoccupied workers in many laboratories. Correlations and lack of correlation have been reported, which is not surprising, given the differences in the assay methodology and their precision. Assays based on sensitive estimation of cyclic AMP concentrations in cultured human thyroid cells now appear to be the most precise and possibly the most sensitive of the feasible bioassays (Stöckle et al 1981). Receptor assays using solubilized or purified receptors are also more precise and less affected by normal IgG than the earlier membrane assays.

A new generation of assays is now being developed to screen for monoclonal antibodies produced by hybridomas. ELISA (enzyme-linked immunosorbent) assays based on solubilized receptors and inhibition of TSH binding should prove valuable. The observation that TSH binds to fat cells which are not involved in other thyroid antigen–antibody-related events has been used to develop rapid, specific assays for receptor antibodies (Tao et al 1981). It seems likely that further progress in assay methodology will result from current attempts to purify the receptor and to produce monoclonal antibodies reacting with it.

Conditions in which receptor antibodies are detected

Depending on the series, some 70 to 90% of patients with untreated Graves' hyperthyroidism have antibodies to the TSH receptor, measured by the receptor assay of Smith & Hall (1974) (Fig. 1). If the assay is repeated on several occasions before and during the early phases of therapy, up to 95% positive results are obtained. The reason for this variability is uncertain but it may merely represent random fluctuations or the variable formation of immune complexes. In neonatal Graves' disease it is generally accepted that the hyperthyroidism that occurs *in utero* or neonatally is the result of the transplacental passage of the stimulating antibodies. In ophthalmic Graves' disease, receptor antibodies can be detected in just less than half the patients. It is not uncommon for the antibodies in this group of patients to be biologically inactive, which probably explains why the patients do not usually become hyperthyroid. Biologically active antibodies can also be detected in ophthalmic Graves' disease but they are unable to produce hyperthyroidism because of the presence of extensive autoimmune thyroiditis.

In Hashimoto's disease, receptor antibodies can be detected in 10 to 15% of cases. As in ophthalmic Graves' disease they are often biologically inactive and these blocking antibodies may contribute to the development of hypothyroidism (Endo et al 1978). The recent report of neonatal hypothyroidism in the offspring of a woman with Hashimoto's thyroiditis who had

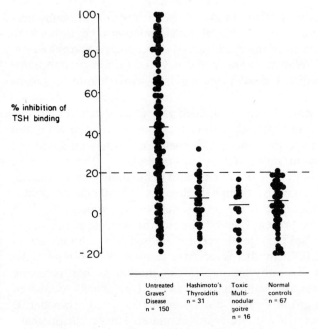

FIG. 1. TSH receptor antibody activity in different groups of patients.

circulating receptor antibodies illustrates the effect of the transplacental passage of blocking receptor antibodies (Matsuura et al 1980).

We have found receptor antibodies in a few patients with thyroid cancer. Whether this results from destructive therapy to the thyroid, or from an association with autoimmune thyroid disease, awaits further study.

In subacute thyroiditis, receptor antibodies may appear transiently in the circulation. The reason for this is uncertain. It could reflect the release of thyroid antigens in genetically predisposed individuals. It is of interest that an association has been described between this disease and the HLA type BW 35, which is itself associated with Graves' disease in the Japanese.

The finding of receptor antibodies in some series of patients with toxic multinodular goitre (Brown et al 1978) probably reflects differences in selection criteria as well as geographical factors relating to iodine intake and ethnic origin.

Clinical applications

In patients with hyperthyroidism without the eye signs of Graves' disease, it is sometimes helpful to have confirmation that the hyperthyroidism is in fact caused by Graves' disease. Diffuse uptake of radioisotope on scanning may help to confirm Graves' disease, but it may sometimes be difficult to distinguish this condition from the syndrome of disseminated thyroid autonomy seen in areas of relative iodine deficiency. The finding of receptor antibodies is strong confirmation that the patient's hyperthyroidism results from Graves' disease.

Ophthalmic Graves' disease may be defined as the occurrence of the eye signs of Graves' disease in a patient who is not clinically hyperthyroid and gives no past history of hyperthyroidism. The condition is often unilateral and there may be difficulty in ruling out an orbital tumour. The finding of receptor antibodies in about 45% of patients with ophthalmic Graves' disease helps to support this diagnosis, though if there is still significant doubt, computerized axial tomography of the orbit should be performed.

All women with past or present Graves' disease who become pregnant are at risk of the transplacental passage of receptor antibodies which may act on the thyroid of the fetus. If the mother is receiving carbimazole this crosses the placenta and prevents hyperthyroidism. If the mother is not receiving carbimazole, hyperthyroidism can occur *in utero*. This usually occurs in women who have eye signs of Graves' disease and/or localized myxoedema, when high levels of receptor antibodies are common. Hence, all pregnant women with Graves' disease should be tested for receptor antibodies. Positive findings indicate that the child is at risk for the development of hyperthyroidism *in utero* (if the mother is not receiving carbimazole) or of neonatal hyperthyroidism if the mother is being treated.

Recent studies suggest that women with Hashimoto's disease, myxoedema or any of the autoimmune thyroid diseases who become pregnant should also be tested for receptor antibodies. High levels of blocking receptor antibodies are one cause, albeit rare, of neonatal hypothyroidism (Matsuura et al 1980).

The use of receptor antibody measurements in the prediction of relapse will be considered later.

Effects of therapy

The hyperthyroidism of Graves' disease can be treated by anti-thyroid drugs, by partial thyroidectomy or by radioactive iodine. Until recently all these modes of therapy were believed to act solely on the thyroid follicular cell. Anti-thyroid drugs, such as the thionamides—carbimazole, methimazole or propylthiouracil—and iodides, block the organification of iodine; iodine and lithium, in addition, impair the release of thyroid hormone. Partial thyroidectomy removes a large proportion of the functioning thyroid tissue and radioiodine causes damage to the follicular cells and prevents their replication. However, it is now known that all these forms of treatment have effects on the interaction between the immune system and the thyroid which could contribute to their action.

Anti-thyroid drugs

During treatment of hyperthyroidism with carbimazole there is a parallel fall in the concentrations of receptor and thyroid microsomal antibodies (McGregor et al 1980a). Methimazole, the active metabolite of carbimazole, inhibits thyroid antibody production by lymphocytes *in vitro*. It seems likely therefore that carbimazole, which is known to be concentrated in the thyroid, inhibits thyroid antibody production by an action on lymphocytes within the thyroid, the major source of thyroid antibodies in man. Swanson Beck et al (1975) have shown a reduction of lymphocytic infiltration in the thyroid of patients with Graves' disease treated with carbimazole. Propylthiouracil probably has a similar type of action to carbimazole.

We have been unable to demonstrate any concentration of methimazole by lymphocytes. We are now using an antigen-driven autoantibody system, in which small amounts of thyroglobulin stimulate thyroglobulin antibody and IgG synthesis by lymphocytes from patients with Hashimoto's disease. We have shown that incubation of monocytes with 10^{-4} M-methimazole can prevent the stimulatory effects of thyroglobulin (Weetman et al 1982). This finding suggests that an interaction between methimazole and monocytes could be a key factor in the local immunosuppressive effect of the drug.

We have also some evidence that iodides and lithium enhance thyroid autoantibody production both *in vivo* and *in vitro*, which is an interesting discrepancy in the immunological effects of different classes of anti-thyroid drugs.

Using an animal model of autoimmune thyroiditis we have been able to show that treatment with methimazole either before or after induction of thyroiditis reduces the severity of the thyroiditis, as shown by thyroid histology and by measurements of thyroglobulin antibody levels (Rennie et al 1982).

The evidence for an immunological action of the thionamides can be summarized as follows. Administration of carbimazole causes a parallel fall in levels of receptor and microsomal antibodies. The fall continues when thyroxine replacement is added to a blocking dose of carbimazole, which suggests that lowering of thyroid hormone levels is not responsible. In patients whose hyperthyroidism recurs after drug withdrawal there is a prompt rise in receptor antibody levels. Administration of carbimazole in man leads to a fall in the number of thyroid and thymic lymphocytes. In an animal model of autoimmune thyroid disease, methimazole treatment diminishes the extent of the thyroiditis.

Thionamides decrease [³H]thymidine incorporation into lymphocyte DNA *in vitro*. Likewise, methimazole decreases thyroglobulin and microsomal antibody production by lymphocytes. Treatment of macrophages with methimazole reduces the production of thyroglobulin-stimulated thyroglobulin antibody and IgG.

Partial thyroidectomy

Partial thyroidectomy renders the majority of patients euthyroid, only some 20% developing hypothyroidism and less than 5% having a relapse of their hyperthyroidism. Receptor antibody levels show a transient rise and then a gradual fall after operation (Fig. 2), and six months later very few patients

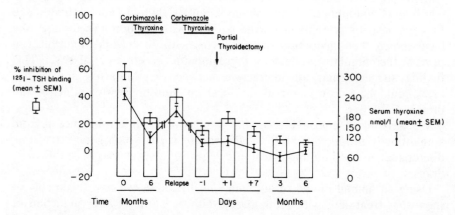

FIG. 2. Mean levels of TSH receptor antibody and serum thyroxine in 30 patients with Graves' disease treated by partial thyroidectomy.

show persistence of antibody. The mechanism responsible for the fall in receptor antibody levels is uncertain, though removal of antibody-producing thyroid lymphocytes is likely to be at least partly involved. Relapse of hyperthyroidism after operation is known to be associated with the presence of high levels of receptor antibody.

Radioactive iodine

Receptor and microsomal antibody levels rise after radioiodine therapy (McGregor et al 1979a), though the frequency and extent of this rise is to some extent dose-related, occurring more consistently with higher doses of ^{131}I (e.g. 15 mCi). Levels peak at about three months and then show a progressive fall, so that in most patients antibodies are undetectable two years later. The mechanism responsible for the rise in antibodies after ^{131}I treatment is still uncertain. It could reflect release of thyroid antigens by the damaged follicular cells, but other more complex possibilities might be involved. McGregor et al (1979b) have shown that though immunoglobulin and autoantibody synthesis can be inhibited by irradiation *in vitro*, the irradiated lymphocytes in co-culture can strongly enhance antibody production by non-irradiated lymphocytes. By analogy with this situation, radioiodine given *in vivo* could selectively kill suppressor T cells in the thyroid. Radioresistant helper T cells which survive in the thyroid could then stimulate antibody production as the thyroid is repopulated with B cells.

Prediction of relapse in hyperthyroidism

Treatment of patients with hyperthyroidism attributable to Graves' disease for six months to two years is followed by a recurrence of the hyperthyroidism in at least 50% of patients. Various clinical signs and laboratory tests have been used in an effort to predict which patients are likely to relapse, but the results have until now been disappointing. Patients with large goitres which do not decrease in size during therapy and those with severe disease are more likely to relapse.

Although patients who fail to show normal thyroid suppressibility of thyroidal radioisotope uptake by T3 during and at the end of a course of anti-thyroid drugs are more prone to relapse, this is not always the case. Conversely, those who show suppressibility may also relapse. Significant differences in course can be demonstrated between the non-suppressible (relapse-prone) and the suppressible (remission-prone) groups, but because of the overlap this method has not been widely adopted.

Measurements of serum thyroglobulin have been used in an effort to predict patients more likely to relapse, using thyroglobulin levels as an index of thyroid stimulation. Special methods are required to measure thyroglobulin in the presence of thyroglobulin antibodies. In general, patients with high pretreatment levels of thyroglobulin which persist during therapy are more prone to relapse, but again many exceptions occur.

Measurements of receptor antibodies at the end of a course of anti-thyroid therapy give some help in prediction. Virtually all patients with high antibody levels relapse, but patients with low or undetectable levels may also relapse (Fig. 3).

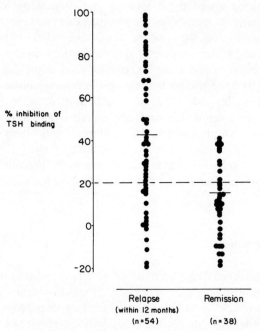

FIG. 3. TSH receptor antibody activity as a predictor of early relapse after six months of carbimazole treatment.

Following up the observation that Graves' disease is associated with the HLA type DRw3, McGregor et al (1980b) showed that patients who are HLA-DRw3 positive are very likely to relapse. By combining HLA typing with receptor antibody measurement they were able to predict the occurrence of remission or relapse in some 95% of cases (Fig. 4). Further studies are obviously required to confirm the generality of these observations.

Recent studies by Schleusener et al (1981) confirm the higher relapse rate of B8/DR3-positive patients. They have also found that in hyperthyroid patients without ophthalmopathy or receptor antibodies, HLA-DR5 patients had a greater frequency of relapse. It is possible that these patients represent another subgroup of autoimmune hyperthyroidism or even a separate disease entity.

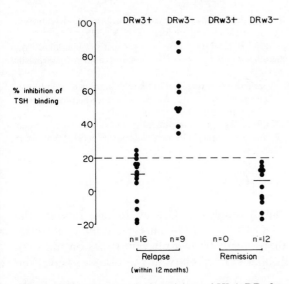

FIG. 4. TSH receptor antibody activity and HLA-DRw3 status as predictors of relapse after six months of carbimazole treatment.

REFERENCES

Brown RS, Jackson IMD, Pohl SL, Reichlin S 1978 Do thyroid-stimulating immunoglobulins cause non-toxic and toxic multinodular goitre? Lancet 1:904-906

Endo K, Kasagi K, Konishi J et al 1978 Detection and properties of TSH-binding inhibitor immunoglobulins in patients with Graves' disease and Hashimoto's thyroiditis. J Clin Endocrinol Metab 46:734-739

McGregor AM, Petersen, MM, Capiferri R, Evered DC, Rees Smith B, Hall R 1979a Effects of radioiodine on thyrotrophin binding inhibiting immunoglobulins. Clin Endocrinol 11:437-444

McGregor AM, McLachlan SM, Rees Smith B, Hall R 1979b Effect of irradiation on thyroid-autoantibody production. Lancet 3:442-443

McGregor AM, Petersen MM, McLachlan SM, Rooke P, Rees Smith B, Hall R 1980a Carbimazole and the autoimmune response in Graves' disease. N Engl J Med 303:302-307

McGregor AM, Rees Smith B, Hall R, Petersen MM, Miller M, Dewar PJ 1980b Prediction of relapse in hyperthyroid Graves' disease. Lancet 2:1101-1103

Matsuura N, Yamada Y, Nohara Y et al 1980 Familial neonatal transient hypothyroidism due to maternal TSH-binding inhibitor immunoglobulins. N Engl J Med 303:738-741

Rees Smith B, Buckland PR 1982 Structure–function relationships of the thyrotropin receptor. This volume, p 114-125

Rennie DP, McGregor AM, Keast D, Weetman AP, Foord S, Dieguez C, Williams ED, Hall R 1982 The influence of methimazole on thyroglobulin-induced autoimmune thyroiditis in the rat. Endocrinology, in press

Schleusener H, Schernthaner G, Mayr W et al 1981 HLA-DR3 and HLA-DR5 associated thyrotoxicosis—two different types of toxic diffuse goitre. Annales d' Endocrinologie 42:14A (abstr 8)

Smith BR, Hall R 1974 Thyroid-stimulating immunoglobulins in Graves' disease. Lancet 2:427-431

Stöckle G, Wahl R, Seif FJ 1981 Micromethod of human thyrocyte cultures for detection of thyroid-stimulating antibodies and thyrotrophin. Acta Endocrinol 97:369-375

Swanson Beck J, Elmslie WH, Harbitz TLB et al 1975 The influence of pre-operative drug treatment on the histological appearances and in vitro ^{131}I uptake of human hyperplastic thyroid gland. Clin Endocrinol 4:469-475

Tao TW, Peterson KM, Kriss JP 1981 A sensitive new assay for antibodies binding to membranes containing TSH receptors in patients with Graves' disease. Abstracts of the American Thyroid Association, Minneapolis, Minnesota, September 1981, T-8

Weetman AP, McGregor AM, Hall R 1982 Thyroglobulin-primed monocytes enhance human thyroglobulin autoantibody synthesis and are inhibited by methimazole. Proc 64th American Endocrine Society Meeting, June 1982 (abstr 553)

DISCUSSION

Newsom-Davis: Japanese family studies of Graves' disease indicate the importance not only of HLA-DR5 but also of Gm allotypes (Uno et al 1981). The analysis suggested that there might be *two* relevant genes on the sixth chromosome that were controlling susceptibility to the disease. Have you looked at any Gm allotypes?

Hall: We haven't done this yet, but we are adding this into our screening in our further treatment trial.

Davies: It should be stressed that these were family studies of Gm typing, and there was no clear link for the whole population.

Harrison: Is the Gm locus known to be on chromosome 6?

Newsom-Davis: Studies on man–mouse hybrid clones indicate this (Smith & Hirschhorn 1978).

Knight: Croce et al (1979) conclude that the genes for human Ig heavy chains are located on chromosome 14.

Engel: Does Graves' disease IgG also have a pathogenetic role in ophthalmic Graves' disease?

Hall: There is a big debate about this. As I stated, about 45% of patients with the ophthalmic form have receptor antibodies, but there is no correlation between the eye signs and levels of receptor antibody.

Knight: Then presumably you are measuring the wrong antibody?

Davies: The ophthalmic and the thyroidal form of Graves' disease seem to follow different natural histories. One could even argue that they are two different diseases that are closely linked and, therefore, seen often together.

Hall: I don't think there is good evidence that the receptor antibodies *are* involved in the pathogenesis of the eye signs.

Knight: This revolves round the definition of whether 'the' receptor antibody is the *same* antibody that causes the eye signs. You could have a slightly variant autoantibody that doesn't cross-react with thyroid tissue.

Rees Smith: Patients can have severe eye signs without any evidence of thyroid autoimmunity.

Hall: We have no good assays for the factors responsible for the eye signs. Dr J. P. Kriss has investigated the role of thyroglobulin/anti-thyroglobulin complexes in the pathogenesis of the eye signs. He has evidence that these complexes bind to orbital tissue, but it is difficult to see the mechanisms responsible for all the varieties of eye signs in Graves' disease.

Mitchison: Is Knight suggesting that there may be a different receptor molecule in eye tissue from the receptor in the thyroid?

Knight: Yes; and then variants of thyroid-stimulating antibody clones could produce antibodies (or perhaps it could be T cell-mediated) against the slightly different receptor in the eyes (Knight & Adams 1980). This doesn't preclude the idea that you do get the eye signs alone, without thyrotoxicosis.

Mitchison: Is there any example, for any hormone, of different receptor molecules in different tissues?

Kahn: Yes. The pituitary hormones vasopressin and oxytocin have overlapping structure and activity. If one looks at vasopressin and oxytocin receptors in different tissues, where the expression of their actions is different, these receptors have different binding characteristics (Roy et al 1975). The lactogenic hormones and growth hormone are also structurally related hormones. Again there are similar but separate receptors, with overlapping binding specificities (Roth et al 1975). Insulin and the insulin-like growth factors also show this behaviour.

Rees Smith: If you look at, say, insulin receptors in a range of different tissues, are the binding characteristics different?

Kahn: They are very similar, if not identical.

Friesen: In the case of prolactin, the receptor in the kidney seems immunochemically different from the receptor for this hormone in the mammary gland (M. J. Waters & H. G. Friesen, unpublished observations).

Knight: So it could be antigenically different?

Friesen: Yes, it appears to be different both immunologically and also electrophoretically.

Mitchison: We have heard already of several instances where the environment of an antigen may affect the exposure of antigenic determinants. We heard about the impact of viral infection on the insulin receptor. We also discussed the impact of viral infection on HLA molecules and there was a suggestion that the environment in which a receptor molecule finds itself may affect the accessibility to antibody of that molecule. So this is a general point, outside the particular context of the thyroid-stimulating antibody.

Friesen: Is the proposition that there may be isoreceptors in the same way that there are isoenzymes? Perhaps such isoreceptors evolved structurally over a period of time? We have speculated that one of the primitive functions of prolactin is in salt and water regulation, hence the first receptor for prolactin may have developed in the kidney. With mammalian evolution the mammary gland receptor may have been a later development, which is perhaps why it appears to be different structurally.

Mitchison: That is one possibility. The other possibility is some difference in exposure, so that one molecule may be presented in a different way on different membranes.

Crumpton: There is a specific example of that. A number of monoclonal antibodies against human class II histocompatibility (HLA-DR) antigens are bound by B lymphoblastoid cells but do not react with peripheral blood B lymphocytes (personal communications from Dr Julia G. Bodmer & Dr Veronica van Heyningen).

Rodbell: An excellent example of how a receptor may behave differently, depending on the environment in which its function is measured, is that of the receptor for cholecystokinin (reference quoted in Rodbell 1980). This hormone stimulates the secretion of enzymes from the acinar pancreas by a process that does not involve cyclic AMP production. In the same cells, secretin stimulates ion fluxes. Yet when acinar cells are broken and membranes are isolated, cholecystokinin is a powerful activator of adenylate cyclase, even more so than secretin. Clearly, something has happened subsequent to cell breakage in which the receptor for cholecystokinin operates through the cyclase system, whereas before cell breakage the receptor was linked to another, as yet unidentified process. An explanation for this paradox might also explain some of the equally interesting phenomena described here.

Michison: Dr Friesen, granted that there are situations where there are differences in exposure of antigens, do you think that there are *also* isoreceptors?

Friesen: I think that the present evidence for this concept is suggestive.

Roitt: David El Kabir did studies of long-acting thyroid stimulator (LATS), and obtained evidence for stimulation of the adrenal (El Kabir & Hockaday 1969). This was interpreted as some degree of cross-reaction, with, I presume, the ACTH receptor.

Hall: Professor G. M. Besser looked at the effect of LATS-positive sera on his ACTH bioassay in rats and was unable to demonstrate any effect (personal communication).

Bitensky: We tried this in the cytochemical assay for ACTH. In fact, LATS-positive sera do cause ascorbate depletion in guinea-pig adrenal (Loveridge 1981). Interestingly, the time course is not identical with that of ACTH, and if ACTH is present (which may be why those experiments that Professor Hall quotes did not succeed) it entirely abolishes the response to LATS. So there is a selective response in the adrenal.

Davies: You discussed the mode of action of the anti-thyroid drugs, Dr Hall, but there is another piece of evidence for immunosuppression by these compounds. Peter Wise followed early ^{99m}Tc uptake (40 min) throughout an 18-month course of carbimazole (40 mg daily) supplemented with T3. The uptakes did not fall suddenly at the beginning but fell slowly over 12 months, suggesting a loss of stimulator at the pre-biosynthetic level (Wise et al 1979).

Mitchison: I didn't really understand Professor Hall's idea here. He appeared to be suggesting that these drugs were acting selectively on cells of the immune system that had accumulated inside the thyroid, but then he referred to studies with peripheral blood leucocytes, so that evidently wasn't the idea. Do you view these drugs as *general* immunosuppressive agents? You surely can't be thinking that there is something unique in the physiology of a plasma cell that is making one particular kind of antibody?

Hall: There is the observation that methimazole treatment is associated with a reduction in the anti-thyroid antibody level. We know that this drug is concentrated within the thyroid, and that at least in many patients with Graves' disease the thyroid is a major site of thyroid antibody production. We are therefore suggesting that methimazole is acting on thyroid lymphocytes, perhaps because it reaches a sufficiently high level in the thyroid, to cause a fall in their production of thyroid antibodies. That is not to say that it is not also acting on lymphocytes elsewhere in the body.

Mitchison: You mentioned studies on peripheral lymphocytes, where there seemed to be a selective action against lymphocytes synthesizing anti-thyroid antibodies.

McLachlan: Unfortunately we do not have regular access to lymphocytes from thyroid tissue. Our *in vitro* system for studying autoantibody synthesis is therefore based on peripheral blood lymphocytes (McLachlan et al 1977, McGregor et al 1979). We have evidence to suggest that the antibody synthesized by peripheral blood lymphocytes *in vitro* is similar to the antibody in serum, so we are assuming that the *in vitro* experiments provide information on the response of thyroid-specific lymphocytes when they reach the thyroid. We generally culture Hashimoto lymphocytes, which synthesize microsomal and thyroglobulin antibodies.

The *in vivo* study with carbimazole was done initially in Graves' disease patients with microsomal and TSH receptor antibodies (McGregor et al 1980a), and essentially similar results were later demonstrated for microsomal antibodies in patients with Hashimoto's disease (McGregor et al 1980b).

Newsom-Davis: Do these peripheral blood lymphocytes ever make anti-thyroid antibodies spontaneously, or do they always require stimulation either with antigen (thyroid) or with pokeweed mitogen?

McLachlan: The studies referred to were done with pokeweed mitogen in the culture medium and the levels of thyroid autoantibody were measured by haemagglutination tests. We have recently developed more sensitive assays for thyroglobulin and microsomal antibodies; using the enzyme-linked immunosorbent assay (ELISA), readily detectable amounts of thyroid autoanti-body are produced in culture by peripheral blood lymphocytes from some Hashimoto patients in the absence of mitogen (McLachlan et al 1982).

Mitchison: So, to make the rationale of your experiment clear, there was no reason, in this experiment on *peripheral blood* lymphocytes, to use an antibody against thyroid antigens; you could have chosen an antibody against herpes zoster, for instance? That just happened to be the assay that you use. There is no suggestion of selectivity among antibody-forming cells?

McLachlan: Yes; to determine the effect of carbimazole on antibody production we could have selected any antibody or we could have simply measured total immunoglobulin production (we routinely monitor total IgG synthesis). However, the relevant antibodies to measure in this situation were antibodies to thyroglobulin and thyroid microsomes.

Davies: We have recently confirmed some of these findings using a quite different system, that of haemolytic plaque-forming cell assays, with protein-A as a non-specific end-point for all secreted immunoglobulin and thyroglo-bulin-linked sheep red blood cells as a specific thyroid antibody assay. We investigated the influence of both methimazole and propylthiouracil on specific and non-specific immunoglobulin secretion *in vitro*. Both these drugs inhibited such secretion at doses compatible with intrathyroidal levels (Weiss & Davies 1981). This does not, however, tell us what these drugs do to antibody levels *in vivo*. In fact, our own results on antibody levels during anti-thyroid drug therapy are somewhat contradictory, with some patients showing a fall in antibody titres and others showing no change at all.

Hall: In other words, we don't know yet whether there is selectivity of action against lymphocytes making anti-thyroid antibodies. The obvious control experiment is to look at gastric parietal cell antibodies to see if methi-mazole affects titres of these. Dr Bottazzo is doing that for us (see p 150).

Mitchison: It is highly unlikely that a drug would have a selective action on the production of one particular antibody.

Hall: We haven't observed any general immunosuppressive effect in patients being treated with carbimazole, but we need to look at other autoantibodies, as we are now doing.

Mitchison: So the idea is that these drugs 'target'—that is to say, they go specifically to a particular cell or organ. But this is an unusual instance of targeting, because the drug is 'targeted' by one cell type, the acinar cell, and then it acts on *another* cell, the lymphocyte.

Harrison: Ehrlich must be turning in his grave! At a meeting where we are looking at molecular mimicry—antibodies mimicking natural ligands—and we know that for many natural ligands there are drug analogues, and vice versa, you are claiming that specificity is out of the question.

Davies: We have some evidence for antigen specificity of drug action in an animal model. When we immunize A/J mice with human thyroglobulin and treat one group with methimazole we see no change in total plaque-forming cells in the spleen but we see a gross reduction in specific anti-thyroglobulin antibody-producing plaques in the spleen (unpublished results).

Mitchison: So you are suggesting that these drugs interact directly with the combining sites of the antibody?

Harrison: Why not? Molecular mimicry between drugs and receptors and antibody combining sites is a possibility, but antibody expression could also be altered indirectly. By analogy, there are many agents that specifically affect the number and affinity of hormone receptors without necessarily interacting directly with the receptors. Some drugs do block receptors—for example, propranolol on β-adrenergic receptors, spironolactone on mineralocorticoid receptors, and cimetidine on histamine receptors. Other drugs, such as the sulphonylureas and glucocorticoids, increase the numbers of insulin and β-adrenergic receptors, respectively, but indirectly, presumably via an action on the pathways of receptor synthesis or degradation.

Rees Smith: We have results that have to be explained. The effects of treatment of Graves' disease are very marked. With radioiodine, circulating levels of antigen go up, with a massive release of thyroglobulin. Levels of autoantibody go up. If you treat the patient by partial thyroidectomy, so there is plenty of thyroid antigen left in the body, levels of thyroglobulin go up as they do after radioiodine, but levels of the autoantibodies fall.

Vincent: Do the levels of all three antibodies (anti-thyroglobulin, anti-TSH receptor and anti-microsomal antigen antibody) fall together?

Rees Smith: The microsomal and the TSH receptor antibody showed a remarkable parallelism and show similar changes in almost all patients. It is more difficult to measure anti-thyroglobulin antibody, as high levels of thyroglobulin are released into the circulation after thyroidectomy or ^{131}I treatment. After treatment with drugs such as carbimazole, antigen levels (monitored by serum thyroglobulin), show only small changes but thyroid autoantibody levels fall. This can be explained most simply by postulating that lymphocytes in the thyroid are making the antibody. But I want to stress that the effects of treatment on serum autoantibody levels are not seen in every patient. I explain this discrepancy by postulating that in some patients the thyroid is not a major site of autoantibody synthesis.

Mitchison: Is there an additional idea here that these drugs cause a local release of antigen, and that a drug that is otherwise relatively ineffective on resting lymphocytes may be more effective on a lymphocyte that has been brought into mitotic cycle by antigenic stimulation?

Rees Smith: The lymphoid cells making IgG antibodies in the thyroid are already in close proximity to the thyroid follicle cells. Perhaps we can envisage that after the drug is concentrated in the thyroid follicular cells, a toxic metabolite of methimazole is released from these cells and locally influences lymphocyte function.

Bottazzo: Carbimazole suppresses thyroid antibody synthesis by its local concentration in the thyroid gland, since it does not reduce the gastric parietal cell antibodies in the same thyrotoxic sera (A. M. McGregor et al, in preparation). Therefore the drug will not be useful for preventive immuno-suppression in conditions such as prediabetes or for the prevention of exophthalmos.

Kahn: Patients with Graves' disease frequently show changes in their white cell populations. Do we know which white cell populations are being changed? We also need to know about IgG turnover in hyperthyroid and hypothyroid states, since they might affect measurements of antibodies. Is there any information on either the cell populations or IgG turnover?

Hall: We have no information on lymphocyte populations.

McLachlan: Dr Thielemans and his group (Thielemans et al 1981) have evidence for a reduction in the proportion of the T cytotoxic/suppressor (OKT8-positive) subset in patients with autoimmune thyroid disease. Our own preliminary studies indicate that there is considerable overlap with the values from normal individuals.

Rees Smith: Thyroid hormone levels are not important here. We have treated patients with Hashimoto's disease by anti-thyroid drugs in addition to replacement doses of thyroxine. Thyroid microsomal antibody levels fell, even though serum thyroid hormone levels were unchanged.

Bottazzo: In autoimmune thyroiditis, thyroxine replacement does not have a direct effect on thyroid antibody levels.

Engel: The question of whether methimazole is a non-specific or specific immunosuppressant might be investigated by trying to immunosuppress a different disease, such as experimental autoimmune myasthenia gravis, with this drug.

Hall: I'm sure that should be done. The other experiment is to immunize animals with bovine serum albumin and examine the antibody level during administration of the drug.

McLachlan: We are currently investigating this point by studying tetanus toxoid antibody levels after immunization with toxoid in Hashimoto patients treated with carbimazole. It is clear that some patients can produce an anti-tetanus toxoid antibody response, but it is not yet known whether their response is less than that in untreated patients.

Roitt: It will be important to do the right control experiment here. The effects of the drugs on autoantibody production were not marked; I don't call a reduction of a half in an antibody level very significant. What was significant was the pathology in the thyroid. Assuming that you are right about local targeting, you may be seeing an effect not on antibody production but on effector T cells. This is why it might be important to study a different sort of autoimmune condition, something like allergic encephalomyelitis which depends on T cell effectors.

Vincent: In myasthenia gravis, the failure of thymectomy to produce a long-lasting remission is usually thought to be associated with thymic remnants, yet in Graves' disease you get remissions in a large proportion of patients after partial thyroidectomy. Your data might also be interpreted as showing that *any* treatment which causes a temporary fall in antibody may be able to produce a long-lasting remission. Do you think this is a self-perpetuating system and that if you can lower antibody levels, by whatever means, you might induce a remission?

Hall: I don't think so. You can treat patients with carbimazole and most of them show a fall in receptor antibody level, but if you stop the drug there is a rise in receptor antibody levels in the majority of patients who relapse.

The effects of partial thyroidectomy are fascinating and baffling. Why does one see a long-lasting remission in 95% of patients after removing three-quarters or two-thirds of the thyroid? Some sort of immunological mechanism appears to be involved, because after partial adrenalectomy in Cushing's disease, the disease *always* recurs. I think we have to look for immunological answers here.

REFERENCES

Croce CM, Shander M, Martinis J, Cicurel L, D'Ancona GG, Dolby TW, Koprowski H 1979 Chromosomal location of the genes for human immunoglobulin heavy chains. Proc Natl Acad Sci USA 76:3416-3419

El Kabir DJ, Hockaday TDR 1969 Morphological changes in the adrenal cortex of experimental animals after injection of sera containing the long acting thyroid stimulator. Nature (Lond) 224:608-609

Knight A, Adams DD 1980 Autoantibodies with intrinsic biological activity. Horm Res 13:69-80

Loveridge N 1981 Studies on the mode of action of polypeptide hormones. Ph.D. thesis, Brunel University

McGregor A, McLachlan S, Clark F, Rees Smith B, Hall R 1979 Thyroglobulin and microsomal autoantibody production by cultures of Hashimoto peripheral blood lymphocytes. Immunology 36:81-85

McGregor AM, Petersen MM, McLachlan SM, Rooke P, Rees Smith B, Hall R 1980a Carbimazole and the autoimmune response. N Engl J Med 303:302-307

McGregor AM, Ibbertson HK, Rees Smith B, Hall R 1980b Carbimazole and autoantibody synthesis in Hashimoto's disease. Br Med J. 281:968-969

McLachlan SM, Rees Smith B, Petersen VBP, Davies TF, Hall R 1977 Thyroid-stimulating antibody production *in vitro*. Nature (Lond) 270:447-449

McLachlan SM, Clark S, Stimson WH, Clark F, Rees Smith B 1982 Studies of thyroglobulin autoantibody synthesis using a micro-ELISA assay. Immunol Lett, in press

Rodbell M 1980 The role of hormone receptors and GTP-regulatory proteins in membrane transduction. Nature (Lond) 284:16-22

Roth J, Kahn CR, Lesniak MA, Gorden P, DeMeyts P, Megyesi K, Neville DM, Jr, Gavin JR, III, Soll AH, Freychet P, Goldfine ID, Bar RS, Archer JA 1975 Receptors for insulin; NSILA-s, and growth hormone. Recent Prog Horm Res 31:95-139

Roy C, Barth T, Jard S 1975 Vasopressin-sensitive kidney adenylate cyclase: studies with oxytocin analogues. J Biol Chem 250:3157-3168

Smith M, Hirschhorn K 1978 Localization of the genes of human heavy chain immunoglobulin to chromosome 6. Proc Natl Acad Sci USA 75:3367-3371

Thielemans C, Vanhaelst, L, De Waele M, Jonckheer M, Van Camp B 1981 Autoimmune thyroiditis: a condition related to a decrease in T-suppressor cells. Clin Endocrinol 15:259-263

Uno H, Sasazuki T, Tamai H, Matsumoto H 1981 Two major genes, linked to HLA and Gm, control susceptibility to Graves' disease. Nature (Lond) 292:768-770

Weiss I, Davies TF 1981 Inhibition of immunoglobulin-secreting cells by antithyroid drugs. J Clin Endocrinol Metab 53:1223-1228

Wise PH, Marion M, Pain R 1979 Mode of action of carbimazole in Graves' disease. Clin Endocrinol 10:655-664

Thyroid antibodies in thyroid diseases

G. F. BOTTAZZO*, H. A. DREXHAGE** and E. L. KHOURY†

*Department of Immunology, Middlesex Hospital Medical School, London W1P 9PJ, UK, **Department of Pathology, The Free University, Amsterdam, Holland and †C.E.M.I.C., Sanchez de Bustamante, Buenos Aires, Argentina

Abstract The cell surface expression of the thyroid microsomal antigen is confined to the apical microvilli of the polarized cells in intact or semi-intact thyroid acini. This makes it possible to envisage a pathogenetic role for the commonest antibodies found in thyroid autoimmunity by mechanisms involving complement- and antibody-dependent cytotoxicity. TSH receptor antibodies can now be differentiated into those that stimulate hormone synthesis and release (TSI), and those which mimic TSH in its growth-promoting function (TGI). TGI were demonstrated in goitrous Graves' disease and in some patients with euthyroid non-toxic goitres, diffuse or nodular, defining a new variety of thyroid autoimmunity. In patients with non-toxic goitre there is hardly any lymphoid thyroiditis and a low incidence of thyroglobulin or microsomal antibodies, the main expression of autoimmunity being the impetus to thyroid hyperplasia and hypertrophy. TSH receptor antibodies of both types, TSI and TGI, can either be stimulating or have blocking effects (TSI block and TGI block). Atrophy of the thyroid gland in myxoedema is due to blocking of the normal pituitary-controlled repair mechanism. In goitrous thyroiditis cell re-growth as a result of increased TSH can occur, as there are no blocking antibodies. In some patients with 'simple' euthyroid goitres, TSI blockers prevent the onset of hyperthyroidism while growth-promoting antibodies give rise to the goitre.

The autoantibodies to thyroglobulin and to the 'microsomal' cytoplasmic antigen in autoimmune thyroid diseases are characterized by an unrestricted polyclonality, and after 25 years of studies it is still thought that tolerance is lost to only two pairs of epitopes on each half of the thyroglobulin molecule. The number of antigenic specificities among microsomal antibodies is probably equally limited but direct demonstration is still uncertain. By contrast, antibodies to the thyrotropin (TSH) receptor appear to be more restricted in their clonality, as shown on electrofocus analysis of thyroid-stimulating antibodies; yet their varied biological activities suggest that a larger number of epitopes is involved.

1982 Receptors, antibodies and disease. Pitman, London (Ciba Foundation symposium 90) p 153-177

This review will concentrate on two main aspects: first, the demonstration that the 'microsomal' antigen is only partly intracytoplasmic and, being expressed on the thyroid cell surface, is accessible to sensitized immunocytes. The second topic is the division of thyroid-stimulating immunoglobulins into those that increase triiodothyronine/thyroxine (T3/T4) synthesis and release (TSI), and some that transmit mainly trophic signals and contribute to goitre formation (TGI). We shall also give evidence that each of these pathways may be either 'turned on' or biologically inactivated (TSI block or TGI block), possibly depending on the exact location of the reacting epitope on the hormone-receptor molecules.

Cell surface expression of the thyroid microsomal antigen

Endocrine autoimmunity is characterized by the appearance of strictly organ-specific, or even cell-specific antibodies in the patient's serum, reacting with apparently 'normal' constituents of the affected gland. Some antibodies are directed against the secretory product (hormone or prohormone), but in human autoimmune diseases the chief serological markers are against antigens which by traditional cell fractionation procedures segregate in the 'microsomal' fraction. These 'microsomal' antigens form a closely knit family with many biochemical properties in common yet differing in that each has its specific organ attachment site. It is likely that they represent integral membrane proteins or glycolipids with hydrophobic domains which lose their antigenic properties when removed from their normal position in the lipid bilayer. The small vesicles which carry the hormone precursor to the plasma membrane become fused with it during exocytosis and recent tissue culture work has shown that 'microsomal' antibodies attach themselves to the surface of living cells. This has been demonstrated for human thyroid, pancreatic islets, adrenal cortex and gastric parietal cells. The fact that 'microsomal' antigens are also represented on the cell surface implies that either activated T or K (killer) lymphocytes can exert a cytopathic effect directly, *in vivo*, whereas if the antigens were purely intracellular, as was previously thought, the only pathogenetic role envisaged for microsomal antibodies would be through complement-mediated mechanisms in dying cells permeable to antibodies.

In the case of thyroid epithelial cells, tissue cultures have revealed interesting new phenomena. It was found that blood group ABH antigens become re-expressed on thyroid cell monolayers and, if the test serum contains natural isoagglutinins, these produce a typical immunofluorescence surface-staining pattern, making it preferable to use group O glands for such studies, though the organ-specific 'microsomal' surface antibodies give a different staining pattern. This thyroid cell surface reactivity correlates closely with the microsomal haemagglutination titres and with the cytotoxic properties of the patients' sera, whereas thyroglobulin antibodies are totally unreactive in these test systems (Khoury et al 1981).

The most interesting finding was that in partially disrupted thyroid follicles, where the cells are still organized in their natural setting, the 'microsomal' antigen is strictly polarized to the apical, microvillar border of the cells. We suggest that the surface antigen should now be called 'microvillar', to distinguish it from the intracellular 'microsomal' portion (E. L. Khoury et al, unpublished). The polarization of the thyroid cells is partly maintained in monolayers. When the cells are fully dispersed and rounded up, the antigen becomes redistributed over the entire plasma membrane. Many thyrotoxic glands contain areas with 'microvillar' antibodies deposited in vivo on the apical cell borders in thyroid sections. This finding is complementary to the previous demonstration of antigen–antibody complexes around the acinar basement membrane in diseased glands. However, whereas the microvillar antibodies are attached directly to the antigen and produced a thin linear immunofluorescence on the inner border of acinar cells, the complexes seen on the basement membrane are coarse granular, resembling those of 'immune complex nephritis', and their antigen is not yet identified.

It is not known how the microvillar antibodies penetrate the acini in vivo, but this is likely to happen when a follicle is breached in one area of its surface by cell-mediated immune mechanisms, thus allowing antibodies to enter the colloid space, as shown previously for thyroglobulin and 'second colloid' antibodies. If microsomal antibodies are present in the circulation, they can reach the microvillar surface antigen directly in affected acini. This could have interesting implications in relation to both the secretion and the reabsorption of colloid and could also interfere locally with the effects of TSH or thyroid-stimulating immunoglobulins (TSI). However, the deposits on the microvilli are patchy and it might be difficult to demonstrate any possible metabolic consequences in the patient.

There is as yet no information as to how the organ-specific proteins are related to the cell-surface hormone receptors. Parietal cell antibodies are able to block the response of parietal cells to gastrin and also to inhibit their acid secretion (Loveridge et al 1980), which could imply that the gastric microsomal antigen is related to the gastrin receptor. If this were a general phenomenon it would form a satisfying conceptual link with the known receptor antibody diseases. Recent experimental findings emphasize the interrelation between the immune system and endocrine function. This supports the hypothesis of a network involving minute amounts of receptor antibodies in the physiological homeostasis of the organism, in line with the idiotype–anti-idiotype lymphocyte network. It is possible to conceive of endocrine autoimmunity as an exaggeration of normally occurring processes preserved in evolution, rather than as a purely pathological process (for references see Doniach et al 1982).

Many hormones transmit their signals to the cell machinery via the cyclic AMP pathway and some receptor antibodies are known to activate the membrane-bound adenylate cyclase. Cells from different organs can now be fused artificially, and it is of great interest for endocrine autoimmunity that the adenylate cyclase of one cell membrane can attach itself to hormone receptors from another tissue. This suggests that the receptors for various hormones are of similar chemical structure, apart from their individual binding sites. The signal does not pass directly from the individual receptor protein to the cyclase, but goes through a group of intramembranous regulatory proteins.

Evidence for new specificities of thyroid-stimulating and blocking antibodies

Autoantibodies to TSH receptors mimic pituitary thyrotropin (TSH) in various ways (Doniach & Marshall 1977) and may now be separated into those that stimulate thyroid hormone synthesis, the thyroid-stimulating immunoglobulins (TSI) (Zacharija et al 1980, Bech & Madsen 1980), and those that provoke thyroid growth—the thyroid growth immunoglobulins (TGI) (Editorial, *Lancet* 1981). In addition, 'blocking' antibodies for each of these separate receptor functions can now be distinguished—TSI block (Orgiazzi et al 1976) and TGI block (Drexhage et al 1981). These new results agree with recent ideas on hormone receptors including TSH receptors.

Cytochemical bioassay for TGI and TGI block

A cytochemical bioassay for thyroid-stimulating immunoglobulins was developed in the early 1970s and is the most sensitive method available (Bitensky et al 1974, Ealey et al 1981). It is thought to rely on the labilization of thyroid lysosomes by TSH or by TSI. This is one of the rapid effects of TSH and is connected with its thyroid hormone-stimulating properties. To assay cell growth, involving the slower actions of TSH and the effect of TGI, we studied a different cellular event, namely the synthesis of DNA.

Segments of guinea-pig thyroid glands were maintained for five hours in the presence of 125 μg/ml immunoglobulins (Ig) separated from the patients' sera by ammonium sulphate precipitation. DNA synthesis in sections from the thyroid segments was assessed by measuring the relative amount of DNA per nucleus as stained by the Feulgen reaction, a well-established histochemical technique used to assess cell growth (Sandritter 1979). 0.3 μU/ml of TSH standard was included as a positive control, and negative controls consisted of Igs from normal subjects and from goitre cases known to be unrelated to autoimmunity, such as dyshormonogenetic goitres and true hyperfunctioning tumours of the thyroid.

To further substantiate the growth-stimulating properties of TGI we used another quantitative cytochemical method for measuring activity of one of the dehydrogenases of the pentose shunt in the same guinea-pig thyroid segments (Drexhage et al 1982c). The pentose pathway yields ribose sugars required for DNA synthesis and provides cytosolic NADPH essential to many biosynthetic steps in cellular growth, as shown diagrammatically in Fig. 1. Glucose-6-

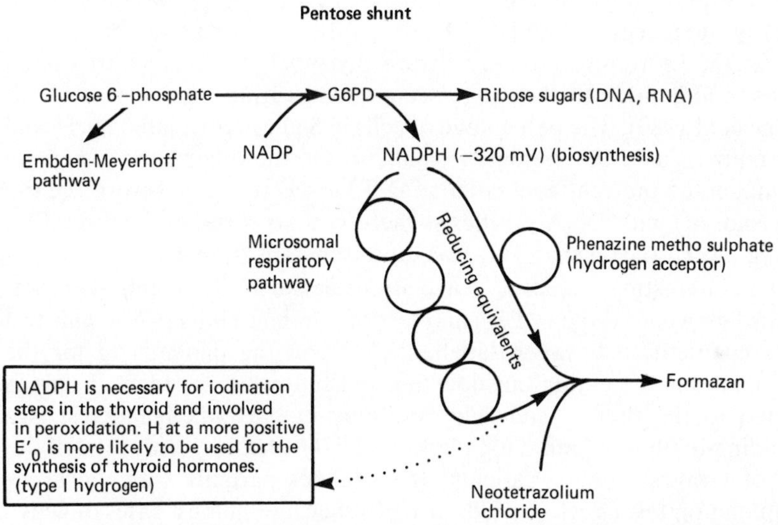

FIG. 1. Diagram showing the energy transfers measured in the glucose-6-phosphate dehydrogenase (G6PD) cytochemical test for thyroid-growth stimulating immunoglobulins and the NADPH-diaphorase test for type I hydrogen. When phenazine methosulphate is added to the reaction the total reducing equivalents are measured. In the absence of this hydrogen acceptor the energy is processed by microsomal enzymes to a lower (more positive) electrode potential, after which type I hydrogen is involved in the metabolic steps leading to thyroid hormone synthesis. In both instances neotetrazolium chloride is oxidized to the coloured reagent, formazan, which is measured cytophotometrically.

phosphate dehydrogenase (G6PD) is the rate-limiting step in this pathway. We also purified Igs on protein A–Sepharose columns and found all the TGI activity in the IgG1 fraction of active sera (Drexhage et al 1982a).

TGI and Graves' thyrotoxicosis

Most patients with Graves' disease have some enlargement of their thyroid gland but the size of the goitre bears little relation to the amounts of T3/T4 generated and about 2–10% of thyrotoxic patients have no goitre, yet the overproduction of thyroid hormones is such that they often present with heart failure (thyrocardiac disease). For these studies we selected the two extremes of this spectrum and compared cases having large or moderate goitres, as estimated by clinical palpation or at thyroidectomy, and patients with a just palpable or impalpable thyroid gland but proven raised T3/T4 concentrations and a negative response of their serum TSH levels to intravenous injections of 200 μg thyrotropin-releasing hormone (TRH). TSH itself produced an increase in the percentage of cells in S phase, and the Ig preparations from goitrous thyrotoxic cases stimulated DNA synthesis to a comparable extent. By contrast the Ig from seven non-goitrous thyrotoxic patients led to a small rise almost comparable to the range seen with Igs from normal individuals (Drexhage et al 1980). The percentage of cells in S phase correlated fairly well with the goitre size in the patients ($r = 0.76$). On the other hand, when we tried to match the pretreatment circulating T3 levels (i.e., the severity of the hyperthyroidism) with DNA synthesis, there was no correlation ($r = 0.01$), confirming our suspicion that TGI was quite separate from TSI.

Another interesting negative correlation between TGI and TSI was obtained when we used the radioligand test of Smith & Hall (1974). This test measures competition between labelled TSH and the patient's Ig for the thyroid membrane receptors but does not indicate what message, if any, is transmitted to the thyroid cell. The antibody in the radioligand test is a 'TSH-binding-inhibiting immunoglobulin' (TBII) and is positive in about 60–80% of Graves' disease patients. It correlates partially with the cyclic AMP stimulation test (Bech & Madsen 1980), because in most cases of active Graves' disease there are antibodies which activate thyroid hormone synthesis. Fig. 2 shows that when G6PD activity, expressed as total NADPH, is measured in guinea-pig thyroid segments exposed to Igs from goitrous and non-goitrous thyrotoxic patients there is also a good correlation with goitre size, whereas Igs from patients with goitres of non-autoimmune origin do not stimulate G6PD activity.

TGI in 'simple' non-toxic diffuse or non-toxic nodular goitre

The idea of looking for a growth-stimulating antibody originated from prolonged observation of patients with 'simple' goitres. The cases we see are familial or sporadic rather than endemic. We noted some 10 years ago that

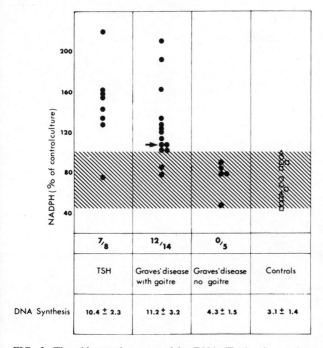

FIG. 2. Thyroid growth measured by DNA (Feulgen) cytophotometry correlates with total NADPH in thyroid segments assayed by cytochemical assay of G6PD. The two assays are positive with TSH itself and with Igs from goitrous Graves' disease patients. Both were negative with Igs from non-goitrous Graves' cases or from goitres of non-autoimmune origin, such as dyshormonogenesis (open squares), or 'single hot adenoma' (open triangles), or normal Igs (open circles). Arrow indicates the thyrotoxic Ig used for a dose–response curve. Shaded band indicates the normal range. (From Drexhage et al 1982a.)

euthyroid patients sometimes had flat TRH responses, and this has generally been observed in 10–20% of non-toxic nodular goitre (NTNG) patients (Emrich & Bähre 1978). In the UK very few of these patients ultimately progress to toxic nodular goitre, but this progression is well described (Miller 1978, Hamburger 1980). It is also known that non-toxic diffuse goitres (NTDG) progress to nodular goitres on prolonged follow-up. Although iodine deficiency plays an undoubted role in the aetiology of these goitres there is also an important genetic element involving an autoimmune pathogenesis. In our series specially selected for the TGI studies, half the cases had a close relative with thyrotoxicosis or with Hashimoto's disease.

Fig. 3 shows the effects of TGI from 10 of these cases on thyroid slices. The percentage of cells in S phase stimulated by Ig from these euthyroid patients was around 10%, similar to that obtained with the TSH standard, whereas the values from the non-autoimmune goitre controls were comparable to those of

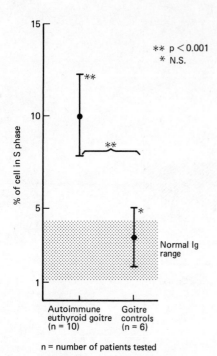

FIG. 3. Effect on guinea-pig thyroid segments of Ig from patients with sporadic non-toxic goitres and from patients with dyshormonogenetic (i.e. non-autoimmune) goitres, used as controls. DNA synthesis was measured by microdensitometry; nuclei containing 2.8–4C of DNA by Feulgen staining were considered to be in S phase (preparing for cell division). The shaded area represents the effects of normal Ig on DNA synthesis in the guinea-pig thyroid segments.

normal subjects ($P < 0.01$). The highest TGI values were seen in patients who had undergone subtotal thyroidectomies for non-toxic goitre in the past and whose goitres had regrown after 1–5 years. These patients were all given prolonged thyroxine treatment (0.2 mg daily) but their goitres did not shrink, since their serum TSH was already suppressed by the stimulating immunoglobulins present in the circulation. Positive TGI effects were obtained in some patients who had normal TRH responses and some with no response to TRH. This appeared to depend on the amount of T3 secreted; in some cases the serum concentration of this hormone was at the upper end of the normal range or even slightly above it. We have also seen patients with 'simple goitre' where the TRH response returned to normal after being flat, yet at no time were there any clinical signs of hyperthyroidism. We excluded patients showing eye signs. Such patients are classified as 'potential thyrotoxicosis' when they have a euthyroid goitre with trace or negative thyroglobulin or microsomal antibodies. When their antibody tests are strongly positive we call them Hashimoto's thyroiditis; if these patient's are thyrotoxic and have high titre thyroid antibodies they are classified as 'Hashitoxicosis'.

In classical Hashimoto's disease about 60–70% of the goitre volume consists of lymphoid cells and TSH itself is responsible for the regeneration of the thyroid acini. We found TGI only in patients in whom the goitre recurred after thyroidectomy or in those patients who failed to respond to full T4 replacement after some years. Microsomal antibodies do not affect the guinea-pig thyroid cultures and show no correlation with stimulation of DNA synthesis (Drexhage et al 1982b).

Tissue reoxidation of NADPH in thyroid hormone synthesis: a possible indication of TSI-like activity

As was shown in Fig. 1 (p 157), when no intermediate hydrogen acceptor (phenazine methosulphate) is added to the cytochemical test system, reducing equivalents from NADPH are processed in the cell through complex micro-somal enzyme systems to achieve a more positive electrode potential, at which point they may be used in the iodination steps necessary for hormone synthesis. The enzyme system mediating this is an NADPH-diaphorase and this proportion of the total NADPH generated has been termed type I hydrogen (Chayen et al 1974).

When type I hydrogen levels are compared in thyrotoxic and euthyroid patients (Fig. 4) it is seen that TSH itself and Ig from thyrotoxic Graves' disease patients and from 'Hashitoxics' increase the level, irrespective of the size of the goitres, whereas non-toxic goitre patients in whom TGI was demonstrated by DNA cytophotometry, and the euthyroid or hypothyroid Hashimoto patients and non-autoimmune goitre controls, were all in the normal range. A further indication that the type I hydrogen level reflects the hormonal synthesis pathway was the good correlation found between the severity of the hyperthyroidism, as measured by serum T3 levels, and type I hydrogen values obtained cytochemically ($r = 0.75$). These cytochemical studies need further elaboration before they can be considered as a potential test for TSI-related antibodies (Drexhage et al 1982d).

Blocking antibodies in primary myxoedema

Autoantibodies capable of blocking the cyclic AMP stimulation produced by TSH or TSI (TSI block) were described in sera from thyrotoxic patients (Orgiazzi et al 1976) and later in patients with primary myxoedema, one of whom gave birth to two babies with temporary neonatal hypothyroidism

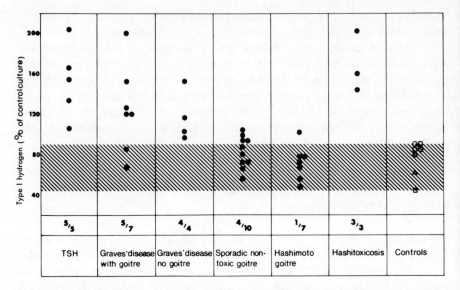

FIG. 4. Reoxidized NADPH represents 10–20% of the total reducing equivalents in the pentose shunt and is called type I hydrogen. This appears to be activated by TSH and by Igs from all thyrotoxic patients irrespective of whether their thyroid is enlarged or whether they have associated Hashimoto thyroiditis ('Hashitoxic' patients). This enzyme assay correlated better with hormone synthesis than with 'growth'. Shaded band represents the range obtained with normal Igs. (From Drexhage et al 1982b.)

(Endo et al 1978, Matsuura et al 1980). This is reminiscent of neonatal thyrotoxicosis caused by the transplacental passage of IgG with TSI activity. Blocking antibodies for the growth pathway (TGI block) can also be demonstrated in primary myxoedema (Drexhage et al 1981). That is, when Igs from such cases are tested in the cytochemical growth test, they do not stimulate DNA synthesis in guinea-pig thyroid segments. Furthermore, when Igs from primary myxoedema patients are incubated with the TSH standard, they depress the cell divison normally initiated by TSH (Fig. 5). The cultures containing only TSH (= 100%) were compared in each case with those where patients' Ig was added to the TSH. Up to 85% inhibition of the growth effect of TSH was seen. G6PD activity was similarly inhibited. Igs from patients with Graves' disease and Hashimoto goitre showed only one instance of slight inhibition of TSH growth stimulation. Ig from a patient with congenital myxoedema due to absence of the thyroid gland was negative in these tests, as were Igs from normal individuals.

It is likely that sera of myxoedematous patients contain one or both of the blocking antibodies and that this prevents activation of the TSH-mediated

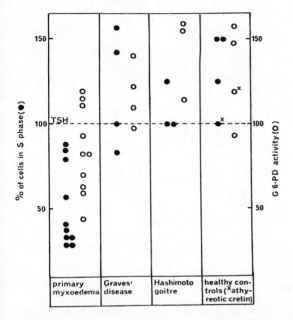

FIG. 5. When Igs from primary myxoedema patients were incubated with TSH they blocked the growth effect of TSH in the guinea-pig thyroid assay. Cells in S phase with TSH alone, 100%. These myxoedema Igs inhibited the trophic action of TSH by up to 85%. This was also seen with the G6PD assay for total NADPH. Similar preparations from patients with Graves' disease or Hashimoto goitre and from normal subjects did not have this inhibiting effect. TGI-blocking antibodies probably contribute to the atrophy of the thyroid gland, which is unable to regenerate in response to increased TSH secretion by the pituitary. (From Drexhage et al 1981.)

repair mechanisms necessary to counteract the constant cell destruction resulting from the lymphocytic thyroiditis in these glands. This is depicted in Fig. 6.

Some authors (Lamberg 1980) have suggested that cases of primary myxoedema showing no thyroglobulin or microsomal antibodies in their sera may perhaps have a 'pure' atrophy of the thyroid gland, unassociated with lymphocytic thyroiditis. This is still a possibility. However, receptor antibodies are not likely to overcome the TSH-independent autoregulatory mechanisms that are known to contribute to thyroid growth. Using sensitive radioimmunoassay tests for antibodies, practically 100% of myxoedema cases can be shown to have at least low titres of thyroglobulin or microsomal antibodies and on histological examination atrophic glands still show lymphocytic foci, even when the gland is difficult to locate, having atrophied to the stage of a fibrotic scar.

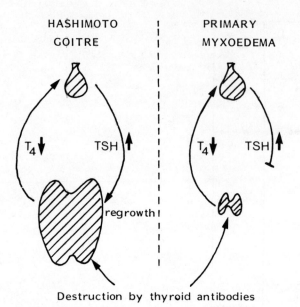

HASHIMOTO
GOITRE

PRIMARY
MYXOEDEMA

T_4↓   TSH↑ T_4↓   TSH↑

regrowth

Destruction by thyroid antibodies

FIG. 6. Diagram to show that both Hashimoto goitre and primary myxoedema are due to a destructive lymphoid invasion of the gland. This is counteracted by constant generation of new acini under the influence of TSH in Hashimoto's disease, whereas in primary myxoedema the repair mechanism is blocked. This ultimately leads to atrophy of the gland.

Conclusions

The work on thyroid growth-stimulating immunoglobulins and their blockers is still in its early and tentative stages, but it may involve a revision of accepted notions on the pathology of autoimmune thyroid diseases. It necessitates the inclusion of so-called 'simple' sporadic non-toxic goitre, with detectable thyroid growth-stimulating immunoglobulins, as a new variety of autoimmunity independent of destructive lymphocytic thyroiditis (Drexhage et al 1982b).

The detection of blocking antibodies may distinguish, well before any abnormalities of thyroid function become apparent, between non-progressive focal thyroiditis and the type of destructive lesion that leads to atrophy and myxoedema. Focal autoimmune thyroiditis is present in some 25% of glands examined at post mortem and thyroglobulin or thyroid microsomal antibodies can be detected in a similar proportion of the middle-aged female population, yet only 1–2% of women develop clinical hypothyroidism. Although three stages of 'asymptomatic autoimmune thyroiditis' (AAT) have been carefully evaluated, patients may have positive thyroglobulin and microsomal haemagglutinating titres for many years before showing an excessive secretion of

TSH in response to TRH. This represents Grade I AAT (the so-called 'low reserve thyroid'). It is at present impossible to predict its future progression and some cases even show remissions, with disappearance of antibodies and reversion to a normal TRH response. Our experience with autoimmune markers in other disorders, such as diabetes mellitus (Bottazzo et al 1982) or autoimmune adrenalitis, suggests that biologically active antibodies are present in the circulation for many years before the onset of clinical symptoms (Doniach et al 1982). Progressive and non-progressive asymptomatic thyroiditis cases show the same wide range of thyroglobulin and microsomal haemagglutinating titres, but if the positive sera could be tested for TSI block and TGI block, this might provide a better guide for selecting patients for follow-up, and will obviate unnecessary preventive treatment.

Another prospect arises from these new notions on the duality of hormone receptors in endocrine cells. This is the possibility that other organs, particularly the anterior pituitary, might be susceptible to receptor-stimulating and/or receptor-blocking autoantibodies. Some cases of Cushing's syndrome with bilateral adrenal hyperplasia may well turn out to be due to pituitary-stimulating antibodies, and microadenomas of the prolactin cells have many features in common with the 'autonomous' acini seen in the thyroid gland (Rentsch et al 1981). In the case of the thyroid, TGI may require the presence of another factor, for example iodine deficiency, to produce these effects. The unexpected finding of pituitary antibodies in 16% of recent-onset insulin-dependent diabetics and 36% of their unaffected relatives when these are selected for persistently positive islet cell antibodies (Bottazzo et al 1982) opens up a new field of endocrine autoimmune research with as yet unpredictable theoretical and practical consequences for the diagnosis or treatment of endocrine disorders.

Acknowledgements

We are extremely grateful to Mr R. C. G. Russell, FRCS, who provided many thyroidectomy specimens for this research. We also acknowledge the collaboration of Drs L. Bitensky and J. Chayen and of Professor D. Doniach. Mrs Linda Hammond gave expert assistance throughout this work. Miss Queenie Jayawardena typed the manuscript. This work was supported by The Wellcome Trust Foundation and The Royal Society.

REFERENCES

Bech, K, Madsen SN 1980 Influence of treatment with radioiodine and propylthiouracil on thyroid stimulating immunoglobulins in Graves' disease. Clin Endocrinol 13:417-424

Bitensky L, Alaghband-Zadeh J, Chayen J 1974 Studies on thyroid stimulating hormone and the long acting thyroid stimulating factor. Clin Endocrinol 3:363-371

Bottazzo GF, Mirakian R, Dean BM, McNally JM, Doniach D 1982 How immunology helps to define heterogeneity in diabetes mellitus. In: Tattersall RB, Koberling J (eds) The genetics of diabetes. Academic Press, in press

Chayen J, Bitensky L, Butcher RG, Altman FP 1974 Cellular biochemical assessment of steroid activity. Adv Steroid Biochem Pharmacol 4:1-60

Doniach D, Marshall NJ 1977 Autoantibodies to the thyrotropin receptors on thyroid epithelium and other tissues. In: Talal N (ed) Autoimmunity. Academic Press, New York, p 621-642

Doniach D, Cudworth AG, Khoury EL, Bottazzo GF 1982 Autoimmunity and the HLA-system in endocrine diseases. In: O'Riordan JLH (ed) Recent advances in endocrinology and metabolism. Churchill Livingstone, Edinburgh, p 99-132

Drexhage HA, Bottazzo GF, Doniach D, Bitensky L, Chayen J 1980 Evidence for thyroid-growth-stimulating immunoglobulins in some goitrous thyroid diseases. Lancet 2:287-292

Drexhage HA, Bottazzo GF, Bitensky L, Chayen J, Doniach D 1981 Thyroid growth-blocking antibodies in primary myxoedema. Nature (Lond) 289:594-596

Drexhage HA, Chayen J, Bitensky L, Bottazzo GF, Doniach D 1982a Application of cytochemical bioassay techniques to the study of thyrotropin-receptor antibodies. In: Chayen J, Bitensky L (eds) Cytochemical bioassay techniques and applications. Dekker, New York, in press

Drexhage HA, Doniach D, Bottazzo GF, Bitensky L 1982b Detection and clinical significance of antibodies stimulating or blocking thyroid growth in disorders of the thyroid gland. In: Williams ED (ed) Current endocrine concepts. Holt–Saunders, London, in press

Drexhage HA, Hammond LJ, Bitensky L, Chayen J, Bottazzo GF, Doniach D 1982c The involvement of the pentose shunt in thyroid metabolism after stimulation with TSH or with immunoglobulins from patients with thyroid disease. I. The generation of NADPH in relation to stimulation of thyroid growth. Clin Endocrinol 16:49–56

Drexhage HA, Hammond LJ, Bitensky L, Chayen J, Bottazzo GF, Doniach D 1982d The involvement of the pentose shunt in thyroid metabolism after stimulation with TSH or with immunoglobulins from patients with thyroid disease. II. The reoxidation of NADPH and stimulation of hormone synthesis. Clin Endocrinol 16:57-63

Ealey PA, Marshall NH, Ekins RP 1981 Time-related thyroid stimulation by thyrotropin and thyroid-stimulating antibodies as measured by the cytochemical section bioassay. J Clin Endocrinol Metab 52:483-487

Editorial 1981 Thyroid autoimmune disease: a broad spectrum. Lancet 1:874-875

Emrich D, Bähre M 1978 Autonomy in euthyroid goitre: maladaptation to iodine deficiency. Clin Endocrinol 8:257-265

Endo K, Kasagi K, Konishi J et al 1978 Detection and properties of TSH-binding inhibitor immunoglobulins in patients with Graves' disease and Hashimoto's thyroiditis. J Clin Endocrinol Metab 46:734-739

Hamburger JJ 1980 Evoluation of toxicity in solitary non-toxic autonomously functioning thyroid nodules. J Clin Endocrinol Metab 50:1088-1093

Khoury EL, Hammond L, Bottazzo GF, Doniach D 1981 Presence of the organ specific 'microsomal' autoantigen on the surface of human thyroid cells in culture. Its involvement in complement-mediated cytotoxicity. Clin Exp Immunol 45:316-328

Lamberg BA 1980 Hypothyroidism due to autoimmune thyroiditis. In: Bastenie PA et al (eds) Recent progress in diagnosis and treatment of hypothyroid conditions. Excerpta Medica, Amsterdam (International Congress Series 529) p 57-73

Loveridge NA, Bitensky L, Chayen J, Hausamen TU, Fischer JM, Taylor KB, Gardner JD, Bottazzo GF, Doniach D 1980 Inhibition of parietal cell function by human immunoglobulins containing gastric parietal cell antibodies. Clin Exp Immunol 41:264-272

Matsuura N, Yamada Y, Nohara Y, Konishi J, Kasagi K, Endo K, Kojima H, Wataya K 1980 Familial neonatal transient hypothyroidism due to maternal TSH-binding inhibitor immunoglobulins. N Engl J Med 303:738-741

Miller JM 1978 Hyperthyroidism from the thyroid follicle with autonomous function. Clinics Endocrinol Metab 7:177-197

Orgiazzi J, Williams DE, Chopra IJ, Solomon DH 1976 Human thyroid adenyl-cyclase stimulating activity in immunoglobulin G of patients with Graves' disease. J Clin Endocrinol Metab 42:341-348

Rentsch H, Studer H, Frauschiger B, Siebenhuner L 1981 Topographical heterogeneity of basal and thyrotropin-stimulated adenosine 3',5'-monophosphate in human nodular goiter. J Clin Endocrinol Metab 53:514-521

Sandritter WA 1979 A review of nucleic acid cytophotometry in general pathology. In: Pattison JR et al (eds) Quantitative cytochemistry, vol 1. Academic Press, London

Smith BR, Hall R 1974 Thyroid stimulating immunoglobulins in Graves' disease. Lancet 2:427-431

Zacharija M, McKenzie MJ, Banovac K 1980 Clinical significance of thyroid stimulating antibody in Graves' disease. Ann Intern Med 93:28-32

DISCUSSION

Kahn: The idea that there are anti-receptor antibodies that specifically stimulate growth is provocative, but there may be another interpretation of the results. You see an effect on the number of cells in S phase within five hours. With most cells in culture, when a mitogen is added the time until DNA synthesis begins is between 12 and 24 hours. Another explanation for your increased number of cells in S phase is that you are preventing the cells from moving from S phase into mitosis. If this is so, you are not stimulating growth, but accumulating cells in S phase by blocking the ultimate division of the cell. What is the rate of cell replication in the culture? Is there an increase in cell number in response to these antibodies?

Bottazzo: We have not assessed cell numbers but in parallel experiments we studied the incorporation of tritiated thymidine into guinea-pig thyroid segments. The autoradiographs showed more dividing cells after exposure to thyroid growth-stimulating immunoglobulin.

Bitensky: These aren't isolated *cells* in culture; they are cultured explants of thyroid segments. The speed of the response to Igs surprised us too. We didn't expect to see a response to TSH or to the immunoglobulins in five hours. The amount of DNA per nucleus in the cell population is increased; I don't think this is a block in mitogenesis, because the number of mitotic figures is low in the normal guinea-pig thyroid. There is evidence for a diurnal variation in mitotic activity in the rat thyroid, but this does not seem to have been looked at with the guinea-pig thyroid. All our animals, however, were killed in the morning, so that variable can be discounted. If we expose the gland or segments of it to TSH or to the Igs for longer than five hours we increase the percentage of cells in S phase, some of which reach the tetraploid level of DNA, but there is no further increase if we go up to 48 hours of exposure. Whatever is happening seems to be fairly rapidly switched on, and we don't see a pile-up of tetraploid cells; so it probably isn't a block of mitosis.

Knight: Have you tested whether the thyroid-stimulating antibodies compete with the thyroid growth-promoting antibodies for binding to receptor, in an assay system?

Bitensky: We have not yet done co-cultures with these two antibodies.

Bottazzo: Some of the growth-promoting sera also contained thyroid-stimulating antibodies, yet there was no correlation between the two specificities.

Roitt: What do the receptor biochemists think of the idea that the hormone, TSH, produces two quite different effects? TSH induces growth; it also stimulates the synthesis of thyroid hormones. Presumably, when a cell wants to divide it either puts on its surface a different TSH receptor which has the same binding site for TSH but communicates differently with the cell and triggers it in a different way; or it uses the same TSH receptor as usual but adds a new transducing protein. The fact that you find distinct antibodies, some of which promote growth and some of which promote thyroid hormone synthesis, suggests that they might react with different receptor molecules. The question is whether these receptors are reacting with an accessory or a subunit protein, or not. We need studies of exactly what is immunoprecipitated, or of how these two different types of antibody react with the purified receptor. We don't know yet even whether the antibodies block TSH binding.

Rees Smith: We really need good evidence that these antibodies do interact with the TSH receptor before we can begin to postulate how they can stimulate growth without stimulating function.

Davies: What happens to these IgG preparations in the more classical TSH cytochemical assay? Are they all negative?

Bottazzo: About 60 to 80% of the euthyroid cases are positive (P.A. Ealey et al, personal communication). The fact that some sera are negative in this sensitive test confirms that there is no correlation between the two activities.

Davies: What does cyclic AMP do to the growth-stimulating assay?

Bottazzo: We haven't investigated that.

Hall: The observations raise fundamental questions about hormone action. How often does one see a dissociation between a tropic hormone's stimulation of function and its stimulation of growth? There are parallel systems in the ovarian follicle, the testis, and the adrenal. Is there evidence for, say, ACTH stimulating growth separately from its stimulation of function, for example? If there were, I could accept your concept rather more easily.

Bitensky: When one starts to look at clinical syndromes, and basically these are the best experiments, there are suggestions, particularly in the adrenal—for example, the so-called 'non-functioning' nodule (Symington 1969). There is also suggestive evidence in the parathyroid, but here the possible action of Igs on growth is difficult to assess, because there is no known tropic hormone driving the parathyroid gland.

Mitchison: Have you thought about this concept in relation to R. T. Prehn's ideas about the immunostimulation of cancers? One could imagine that anti-receptor antibody might promote tumour growth and that this would explain why certain cancers grow more actively in the presence of an immune response.

Bottazzo: It is conceivable that growth-promoting immunoglobulins could contribute to tumour transformation.

Crumpton: The basic question that Ivan Roitt raised is whether there is more than one type of molecule (receptor) on the surface of a cell that can mediate growth of that cell. The answer to this question is surely yes. Two experimental systems are extensively used as models for studying cell growth. These are the stimulation of growth of quiescent fibroblasts by growth factors (Rozengurt 1980) and of normal lymphocytes by polyclonal mitogens (Owen & Crumpton 1981). In the fibroblast system, Henry Rozengurt (I.C.R.F.) has evidence that you can stimulate fibroblasts to multiply by a variety of factors, including insulin, vasopressin, epidermal growth factor, and phorbol esters. In some cases, combinations of different factors stimulate greater growth than either factor alone. These results provide strong evidence in support of the presence of more than one type of growth-mediating surface receptor.

In the lymphocyte system, human peripheral blood T lymphocytes are typically stimulated to grow by plant lectins, especially *Phaseolus vulgaris* phytohaemagglutinin (PHA). Recently two monoclonal antibodies have been described, namely OKT3 (Ortho Diagnostics Inc.) and UCH-T1 (P. C. L. Beverley), which are potent mitogens for human lymphocytes (Kanellopoulos et al 1982). In my laboratory we have evidence that PHA and the monoclonal antibody UCH-T1 react with different molecules on the lymphocyte surface. In view of these results you don't necessarily have to assume that it is an auto-antibody against the TSH receptor that is the growth-promoting antibody.

Reverting to our previous discussion on the role of receptor cross-linkage in cell activation, there is strong evidence (Maino et al 1975) that cross-linkage is essential in so far as growth-stimulating antibodies are concerned. In this respect, Dr Bottazzo, have you separated the Ig fraction from Graves' disease serum, digested it with papain and determined whether the Fab fragments stimulate growth of the thyroid segments? If the antibody interacts with the TSH receptor, it is conceivable that the Fab fragment will stimulate growth; either way, the result would be interesting.

Bottazzo: We have not studied Fab fragments, but we investigated the IgG subclasses in the growth response. We found that growth-promoting activity was mainly in the IgG1 fraction (Drexhage et al 1982). Similar subclass restrictions have been reported in Graves' thyrotoxicosis, where the thyroid-stimulating activity is said to be of IgG3 subclass, whereas in Type I (insulin-dependent) diabetes, IgG3 specificity is frequently lacking in islet cell antibodies and IgG2 is the predominant subclass (Dean et al 1980).

Davies: Can you absorb out the growth-promoting activity with thyroid tissue?

Bottazzo: Absorption experiments have not yet been done but we have demonstrated the organ-specificity of thyroid growth immunoglobulin. These antibodies did not increase the percentage of cells in S phase when applied to guinea-pig parathyroid or stomach segments.

Going back to the previous discussion, I also favour the hypothesis that a stimulating immunoglobulin should not necessarily recognize a specific hormone receptor expressed on the surface of the cell. As far as we can tell, any portion of the membrane can become an autoantigen and the interaction with its specific autoantibody might create a perturbation at the level of the cell membrane. It is this 'perturbation' which might give an intracellular signal capable of switching on either metabolic or growth activities. Sometimes we are too optimistic in thinking that an antibody molecule should have the same shape as the corresponding hormone and interact exactly with its receptor.

Engel: You mentioned that the antibody is localized on the microvillar, luminal border of the thyroid follicles in Graves' disease, where (presumably) the microsomal antigen is present in excess. Does this imply that the TSH receptor is present at that site? One could investigate this by studying the binding of Graves' disease IgG that had been absorbed with microvilli on normal thyroid slices.

Bottazzo: We have proof that the antibodies bound *in vivo* are localized at the apical pole of the thyroid cell. Presumably they are anti-microsomal (microvillar) antibodies. We have not dissected this reaction yet to see whether other antibodies with different specificities might be trapped at the level of the apical pole.

Engel: So you cannot conclude that the antibody binds to the TSH receptor on the thyroid cell?

Bottazzo: No, we cannot. We have applied to human thyroid cell mono-layers sera positive only for thyroid-stimulating immunoglobulins. The in-direct immunofluorescence technique did not reveal any surface reaction. The same negative results were obtained with sera positive only for thyroglo-bulin antibodies. It is also known that LATS does not give rise to surface fluorescence.

Mitchison: Dr Bottazzo, the ideas that you have proposed seem to belong to the category of things that are interesting to think about and make clinical observations on, but from a deeper point of view of understanding mechanisms, I suspect that they will be clarified only by means of monoclonal antibodies. The distinctions that you made are of a provisional character until you have demonstrated them with monoclonal antibodies. Is that a fair comment?

Bottazzo: Yes and no. Naturally occurring autoantibodies are incredibly specific. Thyroid antibodies, for example, do not cross-react with any other endocrine cell in the body. The same is true of other organ-specific antibodies.

Mitchison: You propose an antibody which reacts with a growth-control receptor as distinct from the hormone receptor. If you had two monoclonal antibodies, you could immediately ask whether they are reacting with the same target or not; you could do direct inhibition-of-binding studies and you could make predictions about which effect each antibody would have. Wouldn't you be in a much stronger position?

Bottazzo: Yes, certainly. Dr Leonard Kohn at NIH has produced two distinct monoclonal antibodies which have thyroid growth-stimulating and blocking activities. We hope to obtain these reagents to test them in our system.

Kahn: Monoclonal antibodies are wonderful probes from the molecular biochemists's point of view, but let me act as the devil's advocate and ask whether, in any situation, a monoclonal antibody has shed light on an autoimmune disease where there are naturally occurring autoantibodies and has clarified anything that wasn't already known about the mechanism of the disease. For example, the chemistry of the acetylcholine receptor is well known and monoclonal antibodies had been raised to individual subunits of the receptor, but what do we know about the immunopathology of myasthenia gravis that we didn't know from studies done using patients' serum?

Lindstrom: The monoclonal antibodies have been quite useful for defining antibody specificities that are present in the sera of myasthenia gravis patients (Tzartos et al 1982).

Kahn: But pathogenetically, I don't think we have learned anything more fundamental.

Mitchison: That's a fair point. You could say that about all the monoclonal antibodies.

Kahn: I would just like to make a comment about the insulin system. Insulin is a hormone with both metabolic and growth effects. We know that the cell contains a series of receptors for insulin-like growth factors as well as for insulin itself. These other receptors could be viewed as 'isoreceptors', because these are structurally related hormones and they appear to have structurally related but not identical receptors. In patients with an autoimmune syndrome with antibodies to the insulin receptor, there are varying degrees of cross-reactivity to the growth factor receptors. Because we lack purified antibody populations we cannot ask whether the same antibodies are cross-reacting to both receptors; but we also have the problem that the receptors are very similar too, so even if we had a single (monoclonal) antibody, the receptors might be like isoreceptors and would not be distinguishable.

Mitchison: May I raise another general issue, which seems to be a strong thread running through this meeting so far. Earlier Professor Hall spoke about the way in which the tissue slice assays are wanting, the animal experiments are difficult, and the human material is hard to come by. Dr Bitensky stresses that these aren't *cell* cultures but cultured tissue fragments, which are perhaps not satisfactory for answering all our questions. Now Dr Crumpton talks about Rozengurt's fibroblasts growing in cell cultures, and that is a different world, with a uniform cell population which is there every morning, ready for the next experiment! I am tremendously impressed, to take another example, by what Henry Metzger has been able to do by growing IgE receptors in tumour cell lines. What about cell lines from organs such as the pancreas or the thyroid? Are there cell lines—or, at least, are there tumours from which cell lines could be started?

Hall: A human thyroid adenoma cell line is being used by Basil Rappoport to assay receptor antibodies. Terry Davies and others are culturing human thyroid cells taken at thyroidectomy and getting reproducible results on them. This is the way the assay is going to evolve, because the thyroid slice system for thyroid stimulators is so poorly reproducible from thyroid to thyroid.

Mitchison: Are people trying transformations of responsive cells by SV40 virus?

Bottazzo: No. I agree with you that the present culture correlations are not ideal. Human thyroid cells in culture lose their surface and cytoplasmic autoantigens after seven days. We are now trying to reconstitute human thyroid follicles and obtain a system which is closer to the one *in vivo*.

McLachlan: What happens if you add serum from patients with growth-stimulating antibodies to the culture medium?

Bottazzo: We haven't done that yet.

Mitchison: Why can't one use the cell line from the thyroid adenoma?

Rees Smith: Unfortunately, thyroid cells don't divide very quickly; this is the basic problem. Professor E. D. Williams' group in Cardiff have produced guinea-pig thyroid tumours which are rich in TSH receptors, but these tumours have grown to only about 5 g in weight over two years.

Mitchison: Surely the lesson of the hybridomas is that if you know what you are looking for (in this case, a growth-control receptor), you should be able to rescue it from a non-dividing cell and immortalize it by fusion with a cell line. You don't need to have the property in a cell line; you can use a line to rescue anything you like out of normal cells by fusion, provided you know what you want.

Harrison: There is a limited supply of human cell lines available for cell fusions. It has been tried, but there hasn't been much success yet.

McLachlan: Preliminary studies done in collaboration with Stuart Clark and Bill Stimson at the University of Strathclyde have shown that human hybridomas produced by fusing peripheral blood lymphocytes from Hashimoto patients with the myeloma line 8226 are able to synthesize small amounts of thyroglobulin antibody (Report 1981).

Mitchison: The message of this meeting seems to be that everybody is trying, but nobody has yet done it!

Davies: There have been considerable advances in the use of human thyroid cells, based on Basil Rappoport's work. We have been extending this. Basically, you freeze the cells after seven days in culture. You can keep them in liquid nitrogen until you do the experiments. You also have improved precision for the thyroid-stimulating activity by keeping cell numbers down to 20 000–30 000 per well, and by having a very sensitive assay for the end-point, an acetylated cyclic AMP radioimmunoassay, which detects a few femtomoles of cyclic AMP in just a few thousand cells. This is the sort of direction in which work on thyroid bioassay will go now.

Knight: And is there any correlation, in that assay, between the severity of Graves' disease and the levels of circulating antibodies detected?

Davies: I don't know what you mean by severity, but such results correlate with circulating T3 levels.

Bitensky: May I voice one prejudice about isolated cells and cell lines, with respect to the thyroid, although this is a more generalized comment as well. If you take explanted cells from the thyroid that have been separated, and give them TSH, this has an extraordinary effect. TSH causes those cells to recombine back into follicles. I suspect that the behaviour of receptors, and the interaction between active molecules and cell membranes, might well be different when cells are combined within a tissue, in their normal matrix with their normal connective tissue surroundings, from when such cells are isolated. This presumably doesn't apply to lymphocytes or other cells which normally live as separate entities. When one is dealing with an organized tissue one should view with caution the fact that one can take that cell out of its normal milieu, grow it in a proliferative culture and say that it's the same cell.

Mitchison: I have heard recently of an epithelial cell line grown in culture which possesses polarity, in the sense that it establishes polarity between upper and lower surfaces when it reaches confluence in a culture dish.

Crumpton: Another instance of polarity is in respect of virus infection. Thus, infection of epithelial cells grown as monolayers with several different enveloped viruses results, for each virus type, in a characteristic asymmetrical budding of virions; that is, certain viruses bud from the upper cell surface whereas others bud from the surface in contact with the plastic culture dish (Rodriguez Boulan & Sabatini 1978).

Kahn: Franco Bottazzo showed that the cultured isolated human thyroid cell and the same cell in intact organ culture have very different polarity. We have looked in a culture system at the 3T3-L1 cell, which is a pre-adipocyte, at the distribution of insulin receptors, using our immunofluorescence technique. When the cells are grown attached to a dish, the receptors will 'patch' but not 'cap', but when the cells are detached from the dish they form distinct caps. So the state of growth of even a cultured cell may change the distribution of surface membrane proteins, or their ability to be redistributed in the plane of the membrane. One therefore has to be cautious about extrapolation to the *in vivo* condition.

Mitchison: That is a very good point, but in the present context of whether you can do things in culture, that flexibility actually gives an advantage. You are saying that if you pick the right culture system, it's remarkable what you can do with an apparently unpromising cell line.

Bottazzo: It is of interest that the ABH blood group system is re-expressed on thyroid monolayers. These isoantigens persist for up to 30 days and normal blood group O sera containing high titre isohaemagglutinins will stain group A or B thyroid cell monolayers. This can interfere with the microvillar specific surface staining (Khoury 1982).

Drachman: As a more general point, I am interested in how the autoimmune responses start in Hashimoto's and Graves' diseases. Robert Volpé has reported some interesting results relevant to this (Okita et al 1980, 1981), using an enriched preparation of human T lymphocytes in a migration inhibition type of assay. He finds that incubation with thyroid extract results in inhibition of the migration of T cells taken from patients with Hashimoto's or Graves' disease. This effect can be reversed by adding a small percentage of T cells from normal individuals, but not from other patients with these conditions. His concept is that *specific* suppressor T cells are lacking in Hashimoto's and Graves' diseases. Is this concept generally accepted?

Bottazzo: The concept of antigen-specific helper and suppressor factors is receiving a great deal of attention at present. Volpé's latest experiments suggest that if a thyroid patient has defective T suppressors in response to thyroid antigen this can be restored by adding not only normal T cells but also diabetic T cells which are incapable of restoring Migration Inhibitor Factor production when tested against pancreatic islet antigens (Topliss et al 1981).

Newsom-Davis: Was there HLA matching in those studies?

Roitt: He has not done the HLA-matched controls.

Drachman: Has anybody else studied general or specific suppressor cells, in autoimmune thyroid disorders? Is there a deficiency of these suppressors?

Rees Smith: Sandy McLachlan in our group (McLachlan et al 1980) and also Beall & Kruger (1979) have done analogous experiments in which, instead of looking at migration inhibition, they have studied thyroid autoantibody or IgG synthesis. Peripheral blood B cells taken from Hashimoto's disease patients (which make very little IgG or thyroid autoantibody on their own) were cultured with normal T cells or Hashimoto T cells. Similar amounts of thyroid autoantibodies were synthesized in the two situations.

McLachlan: We had to use pokeweed mitogen, because at that time we were measuring thyroid autoantibodies by haemagglutination; in the absence of the mitogen it was usually not possible to detect microsomal or thyroglobulin antibody synthesis in culture (McGregor et al 1979). However, it is possible that the mitogen may mask the suppressive effect of normal T cells.

Mitchison: To go back to Professor Drachman's question, it is going to be difficult to see what initiates these diseases, because that would need prospective studies. A more approachable question might be to ask whether one can analyse the fluctuations that occur during the course of such diseases. Can one relate remission to any parameter of the regulatory lymphocyte population?

Hall: Until recently, nobody has had material for looking at specific T cell subsets in the different phases of Graves' disease. To extend Professor Drachman's other point, we have on the one side Volpé's theory of a specific suppressor T cell defect. Then there is Dr L. de Groot's work on the other side. He thinks there is a general defect in suppressor T cells; whereas Volpé says this is because the hyperthyroidism itself causes a general defect in suppressor T cell function. There are thus two groups of workers with slightly different results. Further studies are required before we can reconcile these possibilities.

Roitt: It may not be necessary to reconcile them. There may be defects in more than one type of suppressor cell, and they may both be right, as I suggested in my paper.

Knight: If there were a defect in suppressor cells in such autoimmune conditions, when you have clones of cells producing anti-thyroglobulin antibodies, for instance, these would progress into a plasma cell tumour. That doesn't happen often; these immune responses wax and wane, just like any other immune response. This indicates that there are suppressor T cells present that turn these responses off.

Hall: If so, do these immune responses in fact ever go out of control? The answer is that they do; a few patients with Hashimoto's disease develop lymphoma of the thyroid; and a small proportion of patients with Sjögren's syndrome develop lymphoma of the parotid gland.

Vincent: Do those lymphomas actually make the anti-receptor antibody? In our experience, lymphomas from thymomas don't make anti-acetylcholine receptor antibodies in culture (Scadding et al 1981).

Hall: The antibody-producing capability of thyroid lymphomas remains uncertain.

Bottazzo: We tested some 200 myeloma sera by immunofluorescence on endocrine tissue secretions and obtained no positive results, suggesting that autoantibody specificities are rare. However, we know of at least three myelomas that synthesized thyroglobulin antibodies, and one myeloma produced parietal cell antibodies.

Hall: Professor Deborah Doniach has demonstrated myelomas producing rheumatoid factor and thyroglobulin autoantibodies, though this is a rare occurrence.

Roitt: Many patients with Waldenström's macroglobulinaemia have monoclonal rheumatoid factors, but this is not really relevant to our discussion.

Rees Smith: Surely, a shift in the control or restriction of autoantibody synthesis seems a reasonable step in the development of thyroid autoimmunity.

Knight: If there were no suppressor cells I think that progression is exactly what you would expect; this is evidence that a defect in suppressor cells is *not* the explanation for these conditions.

Rees Smith: I agree. I don't think there is good evidence for suppressor cells having a singularly important role.

McLachlan: There is one point that we can make: it does not appear that a polyclonal activation underlies the initiation of thyroid autoimmune disease— for example, an Epstein-Barr virus infection. This does not seem to be a sufficient trigger for the autoimmune disease process by itself (Sutton et al 1974, McLachlan et al 1981).

REFERENCES

Beall GN, Kruger SR 1979 Antithyroglobulin (ATG) production by peripheral blood leukocytes in vitro. J Clin Endocrinol Metab 48:712-714

Dean BM, McNally JM, Doniach D 1980 IgG subclass distribution in islet-cell and other organ-specific autoantibodies. Diabetologia 19:268 (abstr)

Drexhage HA, Chayen J, Bitensky L, Bottazzo GF, Doniach D 1982 Application of cytochemical bioassay techniques to the study of thyrotropin-receptor antibodies. In: Chayen J, Bitensky L (eds) Cytochemical bioassay techniques and applications. Dekker, New York, in press

Kanellopoulos JM, Beverley PCL, Landers E, Crumpton MJ 1982 Characterization of the antigen recognized by the mitogenic human T lymphocyte monoclonal antibody UCH-T1. Biochem Soc Trans 10:101-102

Khoury EL 1982 Re-expression of blood group ABH antigens on the surface of human thyroid cells in culture. J Cell Biol, in press

McGregor A, McLachlan S, Clark F, Rees Smith B, Hall R 1979 Thyroglobulin and microsomal autoantibody production by cultures of Hashimoto peripheral blood lymphocytes. Immunology 36:81-85

McLachlan SM, Wee SL, McGregor AM, Smith BR, Hall R 1980 In vitro studies on the control of thyroid autoantibody synthesis. J Clin Lab Immunol 3:15-21

McLachlan SM, Bird AG, Weetman AP, Rees Smith B, Hall R 1981 Use of plaque assays to study thyroglobulin autoantibody synthesis by human peripheral blood lymphocytes. Scand J Immunol 14:233-242

Maino VC, Hayman MJ, Crumpton MJ 1975 Relationship between enhanced turnover of phosphatidylinositol and lymphocyte activation by mitogens. Biochem J 146:247-252

Okita N, Kidd A, Row VV; Volpé R 1980 Sensitization of T-lymphocytes in Graves' and Hashimoto's diseases. J Clin Endocrinol Metab 51:316-320

Okita N, Row VV, Volpé R 1981 Suppressor T-lymphocyte deficiency in Graves' disease and Hashimoto's thyroiditis. J Clin Endocrinol Metab 52:529-533

Owen MJ, Crumpton MJ 1981 In: Knox P (ed) Biochemistry of cellular regulation. CRC Press Inc, Boca Raton, vol 4:21-47

Report 1981 Human hybridomas: further progress. Immunol Today 2(7):ii

Rodriguez Boulan E, Sabatini DD 1978 Asymmetric budding of viruses in epithelial monolayers: a model system for study of epithelial polarity. Proc Natl Acad Sci USA 75:5071-5075

Rozengurt E 1980 Curr Top Cell Regul 17:59-88

Scadding GK, Vincent A, Newsom-Davis J, Henry K 1981 Acetylcholine receptor antibody synthesis by thymic lymphocytes: correlation with thymic histology. Neurology 31:935-943

Sutton RNP, Edmond RTD, Thomas DM, Doniach D 1974 The occurrence of autoantibodies in infectious mononucleosis. Clin Exp Immunol 17:427-436

Symington T 1969 Functional pathology of the human adrenal gland. Livingstone, Edinburgh

Topliss DJ, How J, Lewis M, Row VV, Volpé R 1981 Evidence for a specific suppressor lymphocyte defect in Graves' disease. Proceedings of the annual meeting of the American Thyroid Association (16–18 September, Minneapolis, Minnesota)

Tzartos SJ, Seybold ME, Lindstrom JM 1982 Specificities of antibodies to acetylcholine receptors in sera from myasthenia gravis patients measured by monoclonal antibodies. Proc Natl Acad Sci USA 79:188-192

Structure of the acetylcholine receptor and specificities of antibodies to it in myasthenia gravis

JON M. LINDSTROM

The Salk Institute for Biological Studies, P.O. Box 85800, San Diego, California 92138, USA

Abstract Acetylcholine receptors in skeletal muscle and fish electric organs are intrinsic membrane proteins whose function is to bind acetylcholine released from the nerve ending and trigger the opening of a cation-specific channel in the postsynaptic membrane, thereby facilitating transmission of the nerve signal to the muscle. Investigations from several laboratories indicate that acetylcholine receptors from fish electric organs are composed of four homologous glycoprotein subunits of apparent relative molecular masses (M_r) approximating 40, 50, 57 and 64 $\times$ 10^3 designated, respectively, α, β, γ and δ. These subunits are present in receptor monomers in the mole ratio $\alpha_2\beta\gamma\delta$. Receptor purified from skeletal muscle appears to have a similar structure. The α subunits compose part or all of the acetylcholine-binding sites, but the functions of the other subunits are unknown. It is known that the cation channel regulated by acetylcholine binding is located within the receptor monomer.

Experimental autoimmune myasthenia gravis (EAMG) is induced by immunizing animals with purified receptor. The mechanisms by which neuromuscular transmission is impaired in this model are very similar to those in myasthenia gravis (MG). Although there are many immunogenic determinants on receptors, and EAMG can be induced in rats by any of the denatured subunits, there is a main immunogenic region at which most of the antibodies to native receptors are directed. The main immunogenic region is a conformationally dependent part of the external surface of α subunits other than the acetylcholine-binding site or the attached carbohydrate. Antisera from MG patients are also directed primarily at this region. No correlation was detected between the specificities of antibodies to receptor in patients' sera and the severity of their weakness.

The structure of acetylcholine (ACh) receptors purified from fish electric organs is better defined than is the structure of this receptor from mammalian skeletal muscle because large amounts of receptor can be purified from the modified muscle tissue which forms electric organs (reviewed in Karlin 1980,

1982 Receptors, antibodies and disease. Pitman, London (Ciba Foundation symposium 90) p 178-196

Changeux 1981), but there is increasing evidence that the structure of ACh receptors from the two sources is quite similar. The first evidence for structural similarity between receptors from fish electric organs and mammalian muscle was that rabbits immunized with receptor purified from electric organ tissue developed antibodies which cross-reacted slightly with receptors in skeletal muscle, causing impaired neuromuscular transmission and, consequently, muscular fatigue and weakness (Patrick & Lindstrom 1973). This was termed 'experimental autoimmune myasthenia gravis' (EAMG). Subsequently it became clear that the muscular weakness and fatigability characteristic of human myasthenia gravis (MG) is caused by an autoimmune response to ACh receptors in skeletal muscle (reviewed in Lindstrom 1979, Lindstrom & Engel 1981, Vincent 1980).

In both MG and its animal model the immune assault on ACh receptors is mediated by antibodies. Most of these antibodies are directed at sites on the receptor other than the ACh-binding site and do not competitively or allosterically inhibit receptor function (Lindstrom et al 1976, Cull-Candy et al 1979). Instead, the primary mechanism by which these antibodies impair transmission is a reduction in the amount of receptor. This is achieved by an increase in the normal rate of receptor destruction induced by antibody cross-linking of receptors (antigenic modulation) (Drachman et al 1978, Lindstrom & Einarson 1979) and by antibody-targeted, complement-induced focal lysis of the postsynaptic membrane (Engel et al 1976, 1979). Probably as a result of this lysis, the normal complex, folded morphology of the postsynaptic membrane is simplified, thereby altering the normal orientation of presynaptic sites of ACh release and postsynaptic concentrations of receptor, and no doubt further compromising transmission (Engel et al 1976, 1979).

In MG patients the absolute concentration of antibodies to receptor in serum varies widely and is not closely correlated with the severity of muscular weakness (Lindstrom et al 1976, Compston et al 1980). It is true, however, that the most mildly affected patients, who show obvious weakness only in the extra-ocular muscles, have lower antibody concentrations than do patients with generalized weakness (Lindstrom et al 1976, Compston et al 1980). It is also true that relative decreases in antibody concentration in excess of 50% brought about by plasmapheresis, immunosuppressive therapy, or spontaneous remissions are associated with decreased muscular weakness (Dau et al 1977, Newsom-Davis et al 1978, Seybold & Lindstrom 1981). Finally, one cannot expect a simple linear correlation between serum antibody concentration and efficacy of neuromuscular transmission, since at each neuromuscular junction there is a large 'safety factor' to ensure effective transmission (ACh and its receptor are both present in large excess to ensure that enough receptors will be activated to trigger an action potential in the muscle fibre) and only when this threshold is exceeded will transmission fail. However, it is appealing to think that antibodies of some specificities would be more pathogenic than others. For example, it is possible to make monoclonal antibodies to the ACh-binding site (James et al 1980), and antibodies of this specificity would be expected to be highly pathogenic. It is also possible to make monoclonal antibodies to determinants which are not exposed when the receptor is in the membrane (Gullick et al 1981), and these would not be expected to be pathogenic. Also, monoclonal antibodies to some determinants on the receptor can cross-link receptors and induce antigenic modulation, while others cannot (Conti-Tronconi et al 1981). If only a very limited and defined fraction of antibodies to the ACh receptor were pathologically significant, it would have interesting therapeutic implications. Another reason for wanting to know the specificities of the autoantibodies to receptor in MG patients is that this pattern of specificities is potentially a fossil record of the immunogen which initiated the autoimmune response. If the immunogen were a peculiar cross-reacting determinant on a virus, the range of specificities of antibodies to receptor in MG patients might be quite limited and different from animals with EAMG, whereas if the immunogen were human muscle ACh receptor and MG patients recognized the same structures as immunogenic as animals do, the pattern of antibody specificities in MG and EAMG might be quite similar.

In order to study the specificities of antibodies to receptor in MG patients we have taken the following approach. First, we have tried to define the structure of the receptor molecule as well as possible. Then we have studied the specificities in antisera to native receptor and its denatured subunits. In order to obtain more defined immunological reagents, we have developed a large library of monoclonal antibodies to the ACh receptor. We are now mapping their binding specificities and determining their functional effects. These mapped monoclonal antibodies are proving useful as probes of receptor structure and function, as model autoantibodies, and as probes for the specificities of autoantibodies in the sera of MG patients.

Structure of the ACh receptor from fish electric organs

The electric organ tissue of marine rays like *Torpedo californica* contains about 1 nanomole per gram of receptor, since there are many thousands of synapses on each large electrocyte. We routinely solubilize this receptor in cholate and purify it on affinity columns of cobra toxin-agarose, from which it is eluted by a high affinity antagonist at yields in excess of 75 mg/kg (Lindstrom et al 1981a). As a consequence of the large amounts of receptor available and the availability of snake venom toxins with high affinity and specificity for the ACh-binding sites, the structure of these receptors is becoming known.

Acetylcholine receptors are intrinsic membrane glycoproteins containing four kinds of subunits designated α ($M_r \simeq 38\,000$), β ($M_r \simeq 49\,000$), γ ($M_r \simeq 57\,000$) and δ ($M_r \simeq 64\,000$) (Fig. 1) (Karlin 1980, Changeux 1981). Receptor

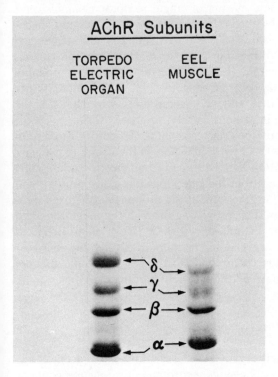

AChR Subunits

TORPEDO
ELECTRIC
ORGAN

EEL
MUSCLE

FIG. 1. Subunits of acetylcholine receptors affinity-purified from the electric organ of the ray, *Torpedo californica*, and the muscle of the electric eel, *Electrophorus electricus*, were separated by electrophoresis on acrylamide gels containing sodium dodecylsulphate (SDS), then stained with Coomassie brilliant blue. The subunits of receptor from eel muscle appear identical to the subunits of receptor purified from eel electric organ (Lindstrom et al 1980c).

monomers have the subunit composition $\alpha_2\beta\gamma\delta$ and a relative molecular mass (M_r) of about 250 000 (Lindstrom et al 1979a, Raftery et al 1980, Karlin 1980). From affinity labelling experiments (Karlin 1980) it is known that the α subunits comprise part or all of two similar but distinct (Neubig & Cohen 1979) ACh-binding sites per monomer. If receptor is solubilized in cholate–lipid mixtures, denaturation of the cation channel whose opening is regulated by ACh binding is prevented, and purified monomers can be reconstituted into lipid vesicles by dialysis of the cholate (Lindstrom et al 1980a, Anholt et al 1980, 1981). The ability of agonists to specifically induce cation permeability in these reconstituted vesicles shows that the cation channel as well as the ligand-binding sites which regulate it are integral parts of the receptor monomer, but which subunits form the channel is unknown. Receptor can also be reconstituted into planar bilayers where its activity can be monitored electrically, and the opening and closing of single receptor channels on a millisecond time scale can be observed (Nelson et al 1980). From immunochemical studies (Tzartos & Lindstrom 1980) and partial amino acid sequencing (Raftery et al 1980) it is known that the receptor subunits are homologous peptides. All contain carbohydrate (Lindstrom et al 1979a) and probably traverse the membrane (Karlin 1980, Changeux 1981). The subunits are strongly non-covalently associated, and we know of no way to dissociate the subunits short of denaturation in sodium dodecyl sulphate (SDS).

High resolution electron microscopy suggests that the receptor viewed from above looks like a doughnut with a hydrophilic hole in the centre (Changeux 1981, Kistler & Stroud 1981). Both X-ray diffraction and electron microscopy suggest that the receptor viewed from the side looks like a mushroom, with the button of the mushroom (i.e., the bulk of the protein) on the extracytoplasmic surface and the narrow stem projecting through the membrane and extending only slightly on the cytoplasmic surface (Ross et al 1977). A hydrophilic channel appears to traverse the membrane through the centre of the molecule, and this probably corresponds to the cation-specific channel whose transient opening is caused by the transient binding of ACh.

Structure of muscle ACh receptors

Normal skeletal muscle contains very little ACh receptor (~ 0.3 picomoles/g) because each muscle fibre has only a single neuromuscular junction containing about 2×10^7 receptors (Fambrough et al 1973). Denervated and fetal muscles have extrajunctional receptors, which increases receptor content from these sources to around 8 picomoles/g. Small amounts of ^{125}I-labelled receptor with a subunit structure resembling electric organ receptor have been purified from normal and denervated rat muscle (Nathanson & Hall 1979). We have been able to purify near-milligram amounts from fetal bovine muscle. Not only is the amount of muscle receptor a serious problem, but proteolysis, especially of the higher M_r subunits, is extremely difficult to avoid. Proteolysis of high M_r subunits was a problem in some laboratories until recently even with electric organ receptor, and this produced a controversy over the subunit structure of the receptor because these laboratories observed only α subunits (Changeux 1981). It is now recognized that despite proteolysis of some or all of the receptor subunits, the subunits remain strongly non-covalently associated and even retain agonist-induced cation flux (Lindstrom et al 1980b).

Recently we have observed that the muscles of the electric eel are very densely innervated and contain large amounts of receptor (25 picomoles/g) (unpublished). We have purified near-milligram amounts from this source and observed a four-subunit structure identical to that of receptor from eel electric organ (see Fig. 1). The apparent molecular weights (M_r) of receptor subunits from eel muscle closely resemble those of receptor purified from bovine muscle, but there is less proteolysis of γ and δ. Using antisera and monoclonal antibodies to receptor subunits from *Torpedo* we have shown that each of the subunits of eel electric organ receptor corresponds immunochemically to a *Torpedo* subunit (Lindstrom et al 1980c). We have identified antigens corresponding to all four receptor subunits from *Torpedo* in receptor from both bovine and human muscle (Lindstrom et al 1978a, 1979b, Tzartos et al 1982). Antibodies to the main immunogenic region (a region on α subunits which will be described below), when added in excess, form complexes with receptors from both electric organ and muscle of the size of two antibody molecules and one receptor. This suggests that there are two α subunits in receptor monomers from eel electric organ and mammalian muscle as well as in receptor from *Torpedo* electric organ. Further similarities between receptors from electric organs and mammalian muscle include the same apparent size on sucrose gradients, and the same doughnut-shaped appearance of negatively stained purified receptor by electron microscopy (B. Conti-Tronconi & J. Lindstrom, unpublished). Thus, it seems likely that receptors from electric organ and muscle have a very similar $\alpha_2\beta\gamma\delta$ subunit structure.

Specificities of antibodies to receptor in EAMG

Immunization with electric organ receptor of all species tested has produced EAMG (reviewed in Lindstrom 1979), but in fact the antibodies produced are highly species-specific with usually much less than 5% which cross-react with receptor from muscle. The ACh receptor is a strong immunogen, and less than 10 µg in complete Freund's adjuvant injected into a rat will produce serum antibody concentrations in excess of 1 micromolar. Thus, even with a low degree of cross-reaction, the absolute amount of antibody is large in relation to the amount of receptor in muscle.

Rat antisera to receptor react preferentially with native receptor, but detectably with all four receptor subunits (Lindstrom et al 1979b). Correspondingly, native receptor is a much stronger immunogen than are SDS-denatured receptor subunits, but prolonged immunization of rats with large amounts (250 μg total) of any of the purified subunits produces substantial anti-receptor antibody concentrations in serum, and EAMG (Lindstrom et al 1978a, 1979b). Interspecies cross-reaction is most pronounced with α subunits.

We have prepared a large library of monoclonal antibodies to receptors and receptor subunits from several species, and now have more than 200 such antibodies. About half of the monoclonal antibodies raised to native receptor react detectably with denatured subunits, and most of these react with α (Tzartos & Lindstrom 1980, 1981, Tzartos et al 1981, 1982, Gullick et al 1981, Conti-Tronconi et al 1981, Lindstrom et al 1981b). In competition experiments for binding to native receptor we could define regions within subunits at which the binding of one monoclonal antibody could prevent the binding of others. Most of these regions probably correspond to single antigenic determinants, but we use the term 'region' because a bound antibody occludes an area significantly larger than the six or seven amino acid residues which form the actual determinant to which it binds. Most of the monoclonal antibodies to native receptors from *Torpedo* or eel electric organ (approximately 60%) fell into one mutually competitive group. Correspondingly, any of these could prevent the binding of a large fraction (60–80%) of the antibodies in an antiserum. For this reason, we termed this the 'main immunogenic region'. The second two columns of Fig. 2 show the prominence of this region in inducing rat antibodies to receptors purified from human or fetal calf muscle. Several antibodies can bind to receptor simultaneously, but antibodies (M_r 150 000) are large in relation to the receptor (M_r 250 000) and the total percentage inhibition of serum antibodies by several different monoclonal antibodies exceeds 100%. Atassi studied the antigenic determinants on small (M_r 13 000–15 000) soluble proteins like lysozyme and myoglobin. He observed about one determinant per 3000–4000 M_r and noted that four out of five determinants on a 15 300 M_r myoglobin could be bound simultaneously by antibody (Atassi 1975, 1978). At this rate we might expect 60 different determinants on a receptor monomer, but subunit interactions and lipid interactions probably substantially reduce the surface available to form determinants in a multi-subunit membrane protein like the receptor, as compared to small soluble proteins.

All the monoclonal antibodies to the main immunogenic region which reacted detectably with denatured subunits reacted with α; thus the main immunogenic region is on α (Tzartos & Lindstrom 1980, Tzartos et al 1981). These antibodies can bind to receptor in intact membrane vesicles, so this region is on the extracellular surface (Gullick et al 1981). This region is oriented so that antibodies bound to it can cross-link the α subunits of one monomer to another, whereas cross-linking of the two α subunits within a monomer is prevented. Other antibodies to α apparently cross-link the two α

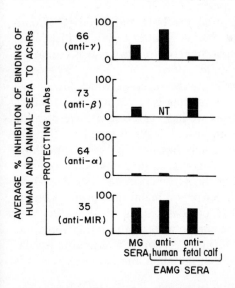

FIG. 2. Specificities of antibodies in the sera of rats with EAMG and of MG patients. Rat monoclonal antibodies 35 (to the main immunogenic region, MIR), 64 (to another region on α), 73 (to the β subunit) and 66 (to the γ subunit) were used to protect receptor from human muscle or fetal calf muscle against the binding of antibodies in MG sera or antisera to receptors purified from these sources. Column one shows the average values for sera from 86 MG patients. Columns two and three show values for rat antiserum pools to receptors purified from human muscle and fetal calf muscle, respectively. The methods used have been previously described (Tzartos & Lindstrom 1980, Tzartos et al 1981, 1982). (Reproduced from Tzartos et al 1982.)

subunits within a monomer, and so when added in excess bind at only one antibody per receptor instead of two. These studies were done using sucrose density gradient centrifugation to resolve the complexes formed between mixtures of ^{125}I-toxin-labelled receptors with various ratios of monoclonal antibodies (Conti-Tronconi et al 1981). The main immunogenic region is not the ACh-binding site, since binding of ^{125}I-α-bungarotoxin to receptor does not impair antibody binding. This is consistent with previous results showing that very few if any of the antibodies in a serum are directed at this site (Lindstrom 1976). The two sites for binding ACh (M_r 146) are undoubtedly a very small part of the receptor monomer (M_r 250 000). Antibodies to the main immunogenic region bind to two characteristic peptides generated by proteolysis of α with V8 (Gullick et al 1981). One of these (19 000 M_r) contains the binding site for the affinity-labelling reagent 4-(N-maleimido) benzyl-trimethylammonium chloride (MBTA) and the other (17 000 M_r) contains most or all of the carbohydrate. From this we conclude that the main immunogenic region is not carbohydrate and that the main immunogenic region is not very far from the ACh-binding site. We know that the 19 000 M_r

fragment begins on the 47th residue from the N-terminal end (B. Conti-Tronconi, M. Hunkapiller, L. Hood, M. A. Raftery, W. Gullick & J. Lindstrom, unpublished). From this and other constraints we suspect that the main immunogenic region is near the middle of α.

Most of the monoclonal antibodies to native receptor which cross-react between species are directed at the main immunogenic region (Tzartos et al 1981). This observation, and the fact that we have detected a corresponding antigen and immunogen on every receptor tested, leads us to believe that this region is structurally conserved because it is functionally important. Antibodies bound to this region do not impair agonist binding or channel opening (Lindstrom et al 1981b). What then might its function be? It is becoming evident that the receptor interacts with peripheral membrane proteins on the cytoplasmic surface such as the 43 000 M_r protein (Changeux 1981, Froehner et al 1981) and that basement membrane components on the extracytoplasmic surface are very important in the localizing of receptors and neuromuscular junctions (Sanes et al 1978). It may be that the main immunogenic region is involved in such interactions.

Antibodies to the main immunogenic region can passively transfer the complement- and phagocyte-dependent acute form of EAMG (Tzartos & Lindstrom 1980, and unpublished). Such antibodies are also capable of causing antigenic modulation, as expected from their ability to cross-link receptors (Conti-Tronconi et al 1981). What will be at least as interesting will be to determine which monoclonal antibodies cannot cause EAMG. Many in our library cannot for the trivial reason that they do not cross-react between species, but many remain to be tested.

Antisera to receptor have small effects on the opening time and single-channel conductance of receptor (Heinemann et al 1977) and antisera can block the function of receptors in electrocytes without significantly inhibiting toxin binding (Lindstrom et al 1977). These results suggest that antibody specificities are present at least infrequently which can non-competitively inhibit receptor function. Only a few of our monoclonal antibodies have been tested, and most do not block function. However, some do block function non-competitively (Lindstrom et al 1981b). One of these, no. 13, is to *Torpedo* α subunit, while another, no. 10, was raised to β subunits, but cross-reacts somewhat with α.

Specificities of antibodies to receptor in MG

Antibodies from MG patients, like those from animals with EAMG, are highly species-specific and cross-react very little with fish electric organ receptors, on the average 16% with fetal calf muscle receptor and 49% with squirrel monkey muscle receptor (Lindstrom et al 1978b). Like antibodies from animals with EAMG, they are directed primarily at determinants other than the ACh-binding site (Lindstrom et al 1976). Also like antibodies from rats with EAMG, most of the antibodies from patients are directed at conformationally dependent determinants and their reaction with ^{125}I-labelled, SDS-denatured receptor subunits is quite limited. Such reaction is detectable, but can be especially capricious when going across species lines. For example, one patient whose antibodies are directed primarily at the main immunogenic region on α also has antibodies that react very specifically with β subunits of ^{125}I-labelled fetal calf muscle receptor and others which react very specifically with δ subunits of ^{125}I-labelled *Torpedo* receptor.

In order to map the specificities of antibodies to receptor in sera from MG patients we took monoclonal antibodies known to be specific for particular determinants on electric organ receptors and used them in protection experiments to determine the fraction of serum antibodies against these determinants (Tzartos et al 1982). Rat monoclonal antibodies were added in large excess to ^{125}I-toxin-labelled human receptor. Then limiting amounts of human anti-receptor antibodies were added, and after a short time (4 h, during which the monoclonals behaved as if they were irreversibly bound), goat anti-human IgG was added to precipitate any receptor to which the MG patient antibodies were bound. Some monoclonal antibodies, like nos. 35 or 42, which bind to the main immunogenic region, could prevent the binding of more than half of the antibodies in most sera. Another monoclonal antibody, like no. 64, which is to a different determinant on α, bound very well to human receptor and was not displaced by antibodies from MG patients, but prevented binding of a substantial fraction of the antibodies in only a few patients (Figs. 2 and 3).

These studies on 87 MG patients showed that most of these patients, like rats with EAMG, make the major portion of their antibodies to the main immunogenic region. This result is consistent with the observation that most antibodies in the MG patients whom we have tested are capable of cross-linking receptors (Lindstrom et al 1981b). This result, and the overall pattern of specificities produced (Fig. 2 and Lindstrom et al 1978b), suggests that the immunogen in MG is the receptor. These results also suggest that although one region is particularly immunogenic, several determinants are involved. We found that the pattern of anti-receptor specificities produced by individual patients was remarkably constant over periods as long as seven years, despite changes in titre and the use of immunosuppressive therapy. We detected no correlation between the pattern of antibody specificity and antibody concentration, severity of muscular weakness, or the presence of thymoma (Tzartos et al 1982). Thus we could detect no especially pathogenic specificity of anti-receptor antibody whose concentration pre-

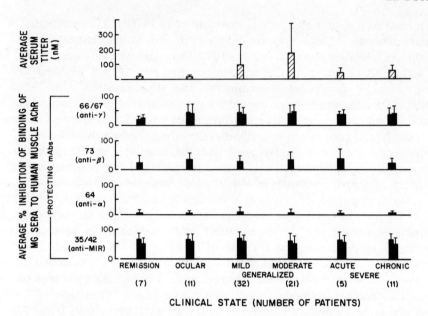

FIG. 3. Specificities of antibodies to ACh receptors averaged for 87 MG patients and grouped according to severity of muscular weakness. Specificities were determined by competition with monoclonal antibodies for binding to human receptor. The top segment of the figure shows the average total anti-receptor titre in each group. (Reproduced from Tzartos et al 1982.)

dicted the severity of muscular weakness better than did the total anti-receptor concentration. Even patients with extremely high titres had mostly antibodies to the main immunogenic region that are known to be able to bind to receptor *in vivo* and can cause antigenic modulation and passively transfer EAMG.

What then accounts for the loose correlation between anti-receptor antibody concentration and muscle weakness? One might invoke an especially pathogenic specificity which we did not detect but, against this, there is every reason to believe that the predominant specificity, namely antibodies to the main immunogenic region, is pathogenetically important. Also, of course, isotypes as well as idiotypes are important. Another fact to bear in mind is that the average MG patient with a serum titre of 5×10^{-8} M is in antibody excess. If antibody is in excess, and if antigenic modulation of receptor, for example, is proceeding at its maximal rate of two- or three-fold greater than normal, then other endogenous factors at the neuromuscular junction must be rate limiting. These might include hormonally and genetically variable rates of receptor synthesis or destruction, or amount of ACh release.

Simple explanations for pathological mechanisms in MG have proved elusive. For example, antibodies to receptor don't act primarily as simple competitive antagonists, but impair transmission by several mechanisms, primarily involving receptor loss. The burden of evidence seems to suggest that most aspects of the pathology are multivariant.

Acknowledgements

This research was supported by grants from the National Institutes of Health (NS 11323), the Muscular Dystrophy Association, and the Los Angeles Chapter of the Myasthenia Gravis Foundation.

REFERENCES

Anholt R, Lindstrom J, Montal M 1980 Functional equivalence of monomeric and dimeric forms of purified acetylcholine receptor from *Torpedo californica* in reconstituted lipid vesicles. Eur J Biochem 109: 481-487

Anholt R, Lindstrom, J, Montal M 1981 Stabilization of acetylcholine receptor channels by lipids in cholate solution and during reconstitution in vesicles. J Biol Chem 256:4377-4387

Atassi MZ 1975 Antigenic structure of myoglobin: the complete immunochemical anatomy of a protein and conclusions relating to antigenic structures of proteins. Immunochemistry 12:423-438

Atassi MZ 1978 Precise determination of the entire antigenic structure of lysozyme. Immunochemistry 15:909-936

Changeux J-P 1981 The acetylcholine receptor: an allosteric membrane protein. Harvey Lect 75:85-254

Compston D, Vincent A, Newsom-Davis J, Batchelor J 1981 Clinical, pathological, HLA antigen and immunological evidence for disease heterogeneity in myasthenia gravis. Brain 103:579-601

Conti-Tronconi B, Tzartos S, Lindstrom J 1981 Monoclonal antibodies as probes of acetylcholine receptor structure. II. Binding to native receptor. Biochemistry 20:2181-2191

Cull-Candy SG, Miledi R, Trautmann A 1979 End-plate currents and acetylcholine noise at normal and myasthenic human end-plates. J Physiol (Lond) 287:247-265

Dau PC, Lindstrom JM, Cassel CK, Denys EH, Shev E, Spitler LE 1977 Plasmapheresis and immunosuppressive drug therapy in myasthenia gravis. N Engl J Med 297:1134-1140

Drachman DB, Angus CW, Adams RN, Michelson JD, Hoffman GJ 1978 Myasthenic antibodies crosslink acetylcholine receptors to accelerate degradation. N Engl J Med 298:1116-1122

Engel A, Tsujihata M, Lambert E, Lindstrom J, Lennon V 1976 Experimental autoimmune myasthenia gravis: a sequential and quantitative study of the neuromuscular junction ultrastructure and electrophysiologic correlation. J Neuropathol Exp Neurol 35:569-587

Engel A, Sahashi K, Lambert E, Howard F 1979 The ultrastructural localization of the acetylcholine receptor, immunoglobulin G, and the third and ninth complement components at the motor endplate and the implications for the pathogenesis of myasthenia gravis. In: Aguayo AJ, Karpati G (eds) Current topics in nerve and muscle research. Excerpta Medica, Amsterdam. (Int Congr Series 455), p 111-122

Fambrough DM, Drachman DB, Satyamurti S 1973 Neuromuscular junction in myasthenia gravis: decreased acetylcholine receptors. Science (Wash DC) 182:293-295

Froehner SC, Gulbrandsen V, Hyman C, Jung AY, Neubig RR, Cohen JB 1981 Immuno-fluorescence localization at the mammalian neuromuscular junction of the M_r 43 000 protein of *Torpedo* postsynaptic membranes. Proc Natl Acad Sci USA 78:5230-5234

Gullick W, Tzartos S, Lindstrom J 1981 Monoclonal antibodies as probes of acetylcholine receptor structure. I. Peptide mapping. Biochemistry 20:2173-2180

Heinemann S, Bevan S, Kullberg R, Lindstrom J, Rice J 1977 Modulation of the acetylcholine receptor by anti-receptor antibody. Proc Natl Acad Sci USA 74:3090-3094

James R, Kato A, Rey M, Fulpius B 1980 Monoclonal antibodies directed against the neurotransmitter binding site of nicotinic acetylcholine receptor. FEBS (Fed Eur Biochem Soc) Lett 120:145-148

Karlin A 1980 Molecular properties of nicotinic acetylcholine receptors. In: Cotman CW et al (eds) The cell surface and neuronal function. Elsevier/North-Holland Biomedical Press, Amsterdam (Cell Surface Reviews 6) p 191-260

Kistler J, Stroud RM 1981 Crystalline arrays of membrane-bound acetylcholine receptor. Proc Natl Acad Sci USA 78:3678-3682

Lindstrom J 1976 Immunological studies of acetylcholine receptors. J Supramol Struct 4:389-403

Lindstrom J 1979 Autoimmune response to acetylcholine receptors in myasthenia gravis and its animal model. Adv Immunol 27:1-50

Lindstrom J, Einarson B 1979 Antigenic modulation and receptor loss in EAMG. Muscle & Nerve 2:173-179

Lindstrom J, Engel A 1981 Myasthenia gravis and the nicotinic cholinergic receptor. In: Lefkowitz RJ (ed) Receptor regulation. Chapman & Hall, London (Receptors and recognition, Series B vol 13) p 161-214

Lindstrom JM, Seybold ME, Lennon VA, Whittingham S, Duane DD 1976 Antibody to acetylcholine receptor in myasthenia gravis: prevalence, clinical correlates and diagnostic value. Neurology 26:1054-1059

Lindstrom J, Einarson B, Francy M 1977 Acetylcholine receptors and myasthenia gravis: the effect of antibodies to eel acetylcholine receptors on eel electric organ cells. In: Hall Z et al (eds) Cellular neurobiology. Alan R. Liss, New York, p 119-130

Lindstrom J, Einarson B, Merlie J 1978a Immunization of rats with polypeptide chains from torpedo acetylcholine receptor causes an autoimmune response to receptors in rat muscle. Proc Natl Acad Sci USA 75:769-773

Lindstrom J, Campbell M, Nave B 1978b Specificities of antibodies to acetylcholine receptors. Muscle & Nerve 1:140-145

Lindstrom J, Merlie J, Yogeeswaran G 1979a Biochemical properties of acetylcholine receptor subunits from *Torpedo californica*. Biochemistry 18:4465-4470

Lindstrom J, Walter (Nave) B, Einarson B 1979b Immunochemical similarities between subunits of acetylcholine receptors from *Torpedo, Electrophorus*, and mammalian muscle. Biochemistry 18:4470-4480

Lindstrom J, Anholt R, Einarson B, Engel A, Osame M, Montal M 1980a Purification of acetylcholine receptors with functional cation channels and reconstitution into lipid vesicles. J Biol Chem 255:8340-8350

Lindstrom J, Gullick W, Conti-Tronconi B, Ellisman M 1980b Proteolytic nicking of the acetylcholine receptor. Biochemistry 19:4791-4795

Lindstrom J, Cooper J, Tzartos S 1980c Acetylcholine receptors from *Torpedo* and *Electrophorus* have similar subunit structures. Biochemistry 19:1454-1458

Lindstrom J, Einarson B, Tzartos S 1981a Production and assay of antibodies to acetylcholine receptors. Methods Enzymol 74:452-460

Lindstrom J, Tzartos S, Gullick B 1981b Structure and function of acetylcholine receptors studied using monoclonal antibodies. Ann NY Acad Sci 377:1-19

Nathanson N, Hall Z 1979 Subunit structure and peptide mapping of junctional and extrajunctional acetylcholine receptors from rat muscle. Biochemistry 18:3392-3401

Nelson, N, Anholt R, Lindstrom J, Montal M 1980 Reconstitution of purified acetylcholine receptors with functional ion channels in planar lipid bilayers. Proc Natl Acad Sci USA 77: 3057-3061

Neubig RR, Cohen JB 1979 Equilibrium binding of [3H]tubocurarine and [3H]acetylcholine by *Torpedo* postsynaptic membranes: stoichiometry and ligand interactions. Biochemistry 18:5464-5475

Newsom-Davis J, Pinching AJ, Vincent A, Wilson S 1978 Function of circulating antibody to acetylcholine receptor in myasthenia gravis investigated by plasma exchange. Neurology 28:266-272

Patrick J, Lindstrom J 1973 Autoimmune response to acetylcholine receptor. Science (Wash DC) 180:871-872

Raftery M, Hunkapiller MW, Strader CD, Hood LE 1980 Acetylcholine receptor: complex of homologous subunits. Science (Wash DC) 208: 1454-1456

Ross MJ, Klymkowsky MW, Agard DA, Stroud RM 1977 Structural studies of a membrane-bound acetylcholine receptor from *Torpedo californica*. J Mol Biol 116:635-659

Sanes J, Marshall L, McMahan J 1978 Reinnervation of muscle fiber basal lamina after removal of myofibers. Differentiation of regenerating axons at original synaptic sites. J Cell Biol 78:176-198

Seybold M, Lindstrom J 1981 Patterns of acetylcholine receptor antibody fluctuation in myasthenia gravis. Ann NY Acad Sci 377:292-306

Tzartos SJ, Lindstrom JM 1980 Monoclonal antibodies used to probe acetylcholine receptor structure: localization of the main immunogenic region and detection of similarities between subunits. Proc Natl Acad Sci USA 77: 755-759

Tzartos S, Lindstrom J 1981 Production and characterization of monoclonal antibodies for use as probes of acetylcholine receptors. In: Fellows R, Eisenbarth G (eds) Monoclonal antibodies in endocrine research. Raven Press, New York, p 69-86

Tzartos SJ, Rand DE, Einarson BL, Lindstrom JM 1981 Mapping of surface structures of *Electrophorus* acetylcholine receptor using monoclonal antibodies. J Biol Chem 256:8635-8645

Tzartos SJ, Seybold ME, Lindstrom JM 1982 Specificities of antibodies to acetylcholine receptors in sera from myasthenia gravis patients measured by monoclonal antibodies. Proc Natl Acad Sci USA 79:188-192

Vincent A 1980 Immunology of acetylcholine receptors in relation to myasthenia gravis. Physiol Rev 60:757-824.

DISCUSSION

Vincent: Have you used monoclonal antibodies to look at the antigenic specificities of the anti-ACh receptor very early on in the disease? We have some evidence that antibodies change their characteristics during the course of the disease (Vincent & Newsom-Davis 1982). Perhaps early on there may be particular specificities which could be related to the initial antigenic stimulation.

Lindstrom: We haven't looked early on. However, the pattern of antibody specificity in patients with ocular as against generalized symptoms appears to be essentially the same. That is the only instance we have studied in which there appears to be a significant difference in anti-receptor titre between groups of patients differing in severity. Many patients who present with ocular signs later have more generalized weakness. That is the nearest we have come to comparing early and late stages.

Newsom-Davis: You say that your patients with ocular symptoms went on to develop weakness in other muscle groups. One can, however, distinguish a different group of 'ocular' patients in which the disorder remains restricted to the eye muscles, during observation over many years. Most patients whose symptoms from their onset have been confined to the eye muscles for two years will fall into this group. As we shall discuss in our paper, we have found in these ocular cases some differences in anti-ACh receptor characteristics from those in patients with generalized myasthenia.

Vincent: Can you tell whether the response in myasthenia gravis is directed against the whole receptor molecules, as it presumably is in EAMG, or against only the external, exposed surface of the receptor? Do monoclonals that bind to the C-terminal end of the α subunit inhibit the binding of MG antibodies?

Lindstrom: The overall pattern of antibody specificities in EAMG and MG is very similar. In both cases most antibodies are directed at the main immunogenic region, which is on the external surface of the receptor. The antibodies which we used for mapping determinants on the α subunits of *Torpedo* do not cross-react sufficiently with human receptor to be useful in studies of antibody specificity in MG patients.

Kahn: In your model of the α subunit, one end is carbohydrate, which we presume is on the external surface of the cell; but there are other receptor proteins, such as the visual receptor proteins, which fold back on themselves so that both the C-terminal and the N-terminal ends are exposed on the external surface of the cell. The ACh-binding site appears to be somewhere in the middle of the protein and yet is presumably also on the external surface of the cell. Have you done studies with surface labelling, which could tell you which antigenic determinants are exposed on the outer surface of the cell?

Lindstrom: We know that the main immunogenic region is exposed on the external surface, not only because it's near the ACh-binding site, but also because antibodies to this region can bind to receptors in native membrane vesicles and to receptors in intact muscle. Of the antibodies to the terminal end, which I attribute to the C-terminal end, we find two closely spaced determinants. Antibodies to what we believe is the more N-terminal of those two determinants (e.g., monoclonal antibody no. 5) can bind to the external surface of reconstituted membrane vesicles in which we know that most of the receptors are oriented outwards. Antibodies to what we think is the more C-terminal of the two determinants (e.g., monoclonal antibody no. 8) can bind when the receptor is solubilized in cholate, but bind less well when solubilized in cholate-lipid. When the cholate is dialysed away, lipid and receptor reassociate leaving the antibody free in solution. So this antibody-binding site is close to the protein–lipid interface, but we can't say whether it dips below it.

Crumpton: How close is 'close', in terms of the number of amino acid residues?

Lindstrom: I can't really say.

Raftery: The identification of the anti-α or anti-β binding antibodies is based on the use of denatured subunits; how sure can you be that, say, antibody no. 10, which blocks receptor function, actually binds to the β subunit in the intact molecule?

Lindstrom: Antibody. no. 10 is a good example of the limits of our certainty, beause it is a relatively low affinity antibody. It was raised against the β subunit but it weakly cross-reacts with α as a result of the amino acid sequence homology between the two subunits. It binds at one antibody molecule per receptor, independent of the amount of antibody added, so we suspect that in the native molecule it probably cross-links β and α. As a consquence, we can't say, by binding, which site is critical to the inhibition of function. We need higher affinity monospecific antibodies for that purpose.

Raftery: This may be a general problem for any protein that is made up of several subunits, when one is using monoclonal antibodies as specific reagents.

Fuchs: It may be even more complicated, because about half of the monoclonal anti-ACh receptor antibodies are directed against conformation-al antigenic determinants on the receptor molecule, and react only with the native intact receptor. Such antibodies would not recognize any of the isolated subunits which have been denatured during their isolation and purification. Only monoclonal antibodies which also bind the denatured receptor, and are defined as antibodies against non-structural (or sequential) determinants, can react with the isolated subunits. Thus, we actually do not have appropriate monoclonal antibody reagents with which we can analyse conformation-dependent antigenic determinants in the individual subunit as they are expressed in the intact receptor. Nevertheless, antibodies of such specificities may exist and play an important role in myasthenic patients.

Lindstrom: This is not a great problem. Most of the monoclonal antibodies are directed against the main immunogenic region. These are antibodies which can passively transfer EAMG and cause antigenic modulation. Most of the antibodies in MG patients are also against the main immunogenic region. It is true that mapping monoclonal antibodies is tricky, in particular because the rarer specificities are the most interesting ones. The ion channel is the Holy Grail here, and we should like to be able to plug it up. However, it's difficult to define, for the reasons that Dr Raftery and Dr Fuchs point out. So although we have monoclonal antibodies that inhibit function in ways consistent with blocking the ion channel, they could, alternatively, be affecting some linkage between the binding site and the channel. We can't distinguish those possibilities yet. We hope to be able to distinguish them in the planar lipid bilayer, where we can see single channels.

Fuchs: I believe you have monoclonal antibodies that have no effect on sodium influx, but do affect some other features?

Lindstrom: We have monoclonal antibodies to the main immunogenic region that do not inhibit carbamylcholine-induced sodium influx. However, antibodies to some other determinants on the α-subunit, or lying somewhere between α and β, inhibit this influx. From studies of antisera and their ability to inhibit carbamylcholine-induced sodium influx in eel electroplax out of proportion to their ability to inhibit α-bungarotoxin binding (Lindstrom et al 1977), we knew that antibodies with these interesting specificities were present in sera. We also knew they were rare, because to see that blockage of sodium influx we needed large excesses of antibody, and all the receptors in the electroplax became labelled with some antibodies before we managed to get antibodies to the critical sites which impair function.

Mitchison: Do I gather that you do not see many 'conformational' antibodies—that is, antibodies which react only with the native subunit molecules?

Lindstrom: About half of our monoclonal antibodies react only with the native molecule. Of the other half, which react with denatured subunits, many are conformation-dependent in that they react with denatured subunits with much lower affinities than with the intact molecule.

Raftery: So you don't know in the native molecule where the antibodies are binding? You could have a three-dimensional determinant on a subunit made up of given amino acids but just by bad luck you might find that sequence, or part of it, in another subunit in the denatured state.

Lindstrom: That is possible. However, all the monoclonal antibodies which fall in a group by peptide mapping fall in the same groups by the competition studies. This suggests that they recognize the same determinants on the denatured fragments as they do on the intact subunit molecule. Nonetheless, the potential problem that you point out is important, and we shall continue to bear it in mind in future studies.

Mitchison: Does the ratio of about half and half of the monoclonal antibodies depend on the screen used to pick up the monoclonals?

Lindstrom: It depends how the monoclonal antibodies are raised. I am speaking in terms of monoclonals raised against virtually native (Triton-solubilized) subunits and screened for using Triton-solubilized receptor. We have also raised antibodies against purified denatured subunits and screened for them using Triton-solubilized receptor. Such antibodies react with both native and denatured receptor, but denaturation of the immunogen destroys the immunogenicity of some regions, for example the main immunogenic region.

Harrison: You said that the concentration of antibody wasn't limiting because it was always present in excess, but you showed results that indicated that when antibody is in excess, when it gets past equivalence, the ability to modulate antigenically could be impaired. Is that so?

Lindstrom: For monoclonal antibodies, that may be true. For polyclonal antibodies, however, it may not be. For the monoclonals, I showed that when we went into antibody excess on sucrose gradients we went from antibody-cross-linked receptors to complexes of antibody and receptor. *In vivo,* immunizing with receptor, there are many antigenic determinants present, so you always probably end up with a meshwork of antibody-cross-linked receptors. We have looked at the interaction of limiting amounts of sera from MG patients with receptor. Virtually all the antibodies seem to cross-link receptors, which is not surprising since most of them are directed against the main immunogenic region, which has that property. Also, other antibodies against a single subunit would also be expected to cross-link receptors.

Bottazzo: In the anti-thyroglobulin system the human antibodies are directed against a very small number of epitopes whereas antibodies produced in animals are far less restricted. Is the same difference observed in the anti-ACh receptor system?

Lindstrom: There is a range of specificities. However, patients with thymoma, for example, produce the same range of specificities, predominantly against the main immunogenic region, as those with no thymoma. Thus, there are probably no large differences in the specificities of antibodies produced, depending on the origin of the immune response. Also, the pattern of antibody specificities in MG patients is basically what we see in animals (which is the same whether we immunize with receptors from *Torpedo*, the electric eel, humans or cows). The inherently immunogenic parts of the receptor molecule preferentially stimulate an immune response in MG patients. I think that's what we are seeing reflected in the specificities of antibodies produced.

Kahn: Have you used your monoclonal antibodies to screen other tissues, to see whether the same antigenic determinants are present in other mammalian tissues, apart from skeletal muscle?

Lindstrom: We have tried to use them to localize ACh receptors in brain tissues, but without success yet. We have not looked at the thymus.

REFERENCES

Lindstrom J, Einarson B, Francy M 1977 Acetylcholine receptors and myasthenia gravis: the effect of antibodies to eel acetylcholine receptors on eel electric organ cells. In: Hall Z et al (eds) Cellular neurobiology. Alan R. Liss, New York, p 119-130

Vincent A, Newsom-Davis J 1982 Acetylcholine receptor antibody characteristics in myasthenia gravis. II. Patients with penicillamine-induced myasthenia or idiopathic myasthenia of recent onset. Clin Exp Immunol, in press

Mechanisms of acetylcholine receptor loss from the neuromuscular junction

ANDREW G. ENGEL and GUIDO FUMAGALLI

Neuromuscular Research Laboratory and Department of Neurology, Mayo Clinic and Mayo Foundation, Rochester, Minnesota 55905, USA

Abstract At the normal mammalian neuromuscular junction the half-life of the acetylcholine receptor (AChR) ranges from 6 to 13 days (estimates from seven different laboratories). Indirect evidence suggests that the internalized receptor is degraded by a lysosomal mechanism. We have now traced the fate of the AChR labelled *in vivo* with peroxidase-α-bungarotoxin. Segments of junctional folds bearing AChRs are internalized by endocytosis. The endocytosed vesicles are engulfed by tubules and larger vesicles which, by electron cytochemical criteria, represent secondary lysosomes.

Pathological mechanisms increase AChR loss from the end-plate. These include destruction of junctional folds, formation of immature junctions with few or no junctional folds, accelerated internalization of AChR, impaired membrane insertion of new AChR and, possibly, decreased AChR synthesis. The common mechanism for destruction of the junctional folds is an altered subsynaptic ionic milieu, and especially focal calcium excess. This can be induced by antibody and complement, too frequent or prolonged openings of the acetylcholine (ACh)-induced ion channel, and other membrane defects.

In acquired autoimmune myasthenia gravis there is (a) antibody-dependent complement-mediated lysis of the junctional folds, (b) accelerated internalization of AChR cross-linked by antibody and (c) decreased insertion of AChR into the postsynaptic membrane. The last mechanism is attributed to lack of membrane patches available for tight packing and secure anchoring of the receptor. In acute, but not in chronic, experimental autoimmune myasthenia gravis, and infrequently in human myasthenia gravis, macrophages destroy junctional folds opsonized by antibody and C3. In a recently recognized congenital syndrome attributed to a prolonged open time of the ACh-induced ion channel, and to a lesser extent in congenital end-plate acetylcholinesterase deficiency, AChR is lost with degradation of junctional folds. In other, less well-defined, congenital syndromes there is deficiency or abnormal function of AChR. This could arise from decreased synthesis or membrane insertion or accelerated degradation of AChR, or from a structurally abnormal AChR with reduced affinity for ACh or with a diminished conductance or open time of its ion channel.

1982 Receptors, antibodies and disease. Pitman, London (Ciba Foundation symposium 90)
p 197-224

The nicotinic acetylcholine receptor (AChR) occurs on the postsynaptic membrane of the neuromuscular junction, and extrajunctionally on non-innervated or denervated muscle fibres *in vivo* and on aneurally cultured myotubes *in vitro*. Junctional and extrajunctional AChRs differ in several respects. In particular, the junctional AChrR has greater metabolic stability, higher packing density and a shorter ion channel open time than the extrajunctional AChR (reviewed by Fambrough 1979).

At the mature end-plate the postsynaptic membrane lines complicated junctional folds. Ultrastructural morphometric analysis of human intercostal muscle end-plates indicates that the postsynaptic membrane represents a 10-fold amplification of the presynaptic membrane (Engel & Santa 1971). The distribution of the junctional AChR is clearly visualized with peroxidase-labelled α-bungarotoxin. This shows AChRs on the terminal expansions of the junctional folds, where these face the presynaptic membrane, and on the stalks of some of the folds (Fig. 1). Only 30% of the postsynaptic membrane

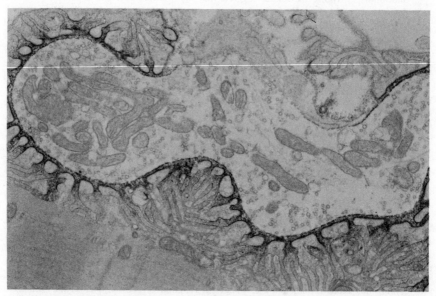

FIG. 1. Ultrastructural localization of AChR with peroxidase-α-bungarotoxin. Normal rat end-plate ×13 100. (From Engel et al 1977a, with permission. © 1977 by Harcourt Brace Jovanovich Inc.)

bears AChRs, but this fraction of the postsynaptic membrane is still three times larger than the presynaptic membrane (Engel et al 1977a). Thus, one result of having junctional folds at the end-plate is to increase the number of AChRs that can be present under a given nerve terminal. The ratio of the postsynaptic membrane area containing AChRs to the presynaptic membrane area is referred to as the AChR index.

Newly formed end-plates are small in size and lack junctional folds. During development, junctional folds appear and increase in complexity; and the entire end-plate occupies a larger area of the muscle fibre. These changes are associated with a progressive increase in the number of AChRs per end-plate (Steinbach 1981).

The packing density of AChR on the junctional folds is estimated at 22 000 to 30 000 α-bungarotoxin binding sites per μm^2 (Fertuck & Salpeter 1976). Freeze-fracture electron microscopy reveals putative AChR macromolecules, or aggregates of macromolecules arranged in double parallel rows on the junctional folds (Rash & Ellisman 1974) (Fig. 2). One can infer that the

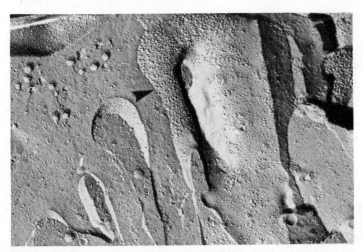

FIG. 2. Freeze-fractured human end-plate. Receptor particles, exposed on protoplasmic (P) fracture faces of two junctional folds, are packed in double parallel rows. The fold in the centre displays particles on its terminal expansion and its stalk (arrow). The particles have the same packing density at each site. ×50 000.

maintenance of a constant number of precisely arrayed and densely packed AChRs at predetermined loci on the junctional folds requires cytoskeletal anchors and close regulation of the insertion and removal of AChRs.

Degradation of extrajunctional AChR labelled with ^{125}I-α-bungarotoxin has been studied in cultured myotubes. It has been presumed, but not demonstrated, that the labelled receptor is internalized by endocytosis. The internalized label is found in structures resembling lysosomes by auto-radiography (Devreotes & Fambrough 1976, Fambrough 1979). Degradation of the internalized receptor is inhibited by chloroquine and leupeptin, which is also consistent with a lysosomal mechanism of degradation (Libby et al

1980). Recent cytochemical studies of the degradation of the junctional AChR are described below.

The half-life of extrajunctional AChR on cultured myotubes can be estimated by monitoring the release of radioactivity into the culture medium after labelling AChR on the cell surface with ^{125}I-α-bungarotoxin. The radioactivity released into the medium is derived from degraded toxin. This technique yields AChR half-lives that range from six to 35 hours. The release of radioactivity is a monoexponential function of time, indicating that recently and less recently synthesized receptor molecules have the same probability of degradation (Fambrough 1979).

The half-life of end-plate AChR has been estimated by several investigators (Table 1). Two different methods have been used. In one method

TABLE 1 Estimates of half-life of end-plate AChR

Investigators	Method[a]	AChR half-life (days)	
		Free	Cross-linked by anti-AChR antibody
Berg & Hall 1975	A	6	—
Chang & Huang 1975	A	7.5	—
Heinemann et al 1978	B	7.9	3.7
Stanley & Drachman 1978	A	5.7	1.6–2.9
Reiness et al 1978	B	6.0	3.8
	B	10.9[b]	6.6[b]
Linden & Fambrough 1979	B	13.0[b]	—
This investigation 1981	A	9.8	3.7
	C	8.4	3.7

[a] Methods A, B and C are described in the text.
[b] Half-life corrected for dissociation of the labelled toxin from the end-plate *in vivo*.

(Method A, Table 1) end-plate receptors are labelled *in vivo* (as, for example, by labelling AChRs in diaphragm by injecting ^{125}I-α-bungarotoxin into the pleural cavity). After a fixed interval, the labelled muscle is removed and the radioactivity remaining per end-plate estimated. In the second method (Method B, Table 1) muscle strips labelled *in vivo* are placed in organ culture and the release of radioactivity into the culture medium is monitored *in vitro*. We recently devised a third method (Method C, Table 1). A selected limb muscle is labelled with an intramuscular injection of a suitable dose of ^{125}I-α-bungarotoxin *in vivo* and the loss of radioactivity from that muscle is then monitored daily, or more frequently, with an externally placed γ-counter of fixed geometry (Fig. 3). This method determines AChR half-life in the living animal, allows close evaluation of experimental modifications of AChR

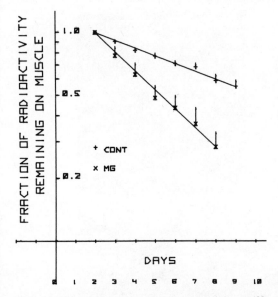

FIG. 3. Estimation *in vivo* of the degradation of ^{125}I-α-bungarotoxin-labelled AChR in rat forelimb muscle with an externally placed γ-counter of fixed geometry. Each point represents the mean of observations in 11 control or myasthenic rats. Vertical lines indicate standard deviation.

turnover and clinical state, and makes it possible to correlate the morphology, cytochemistry and AChR turnover rate *in vivo* at end-plates of a single muscle.

Ultrastructural study of the internalization and degradation of the junctional AChR in normal muscle

This was investigated *in vivo* by labelling of junctional AChR with peroxidase-α-bungarotoxin (Fumagalli et al 1981). A small dose of the tracer was injected into the forelimb toe extensor muscle of the rat with a fine needle. Injected muscles were removed 2–120 hours after labelling, fixed in 2% glutaraldehyde, reacted with the diaminobenzidine medium for peroxidase localization and then processed for electron microscopy. This approach enabled us to trace the intracellular fate of the receptor *in vivo* with excellent preservation of fine structure. Specificity controls included blocking of the binding of the labelled toxin with unlabelled toxin, and the incubation of unlabelled tissues in the diaminobenzidine medium.

Two to six hours after the injection of the marker, the label was present on the surface of the junctional folds where AChR is usually found after *in vitro*

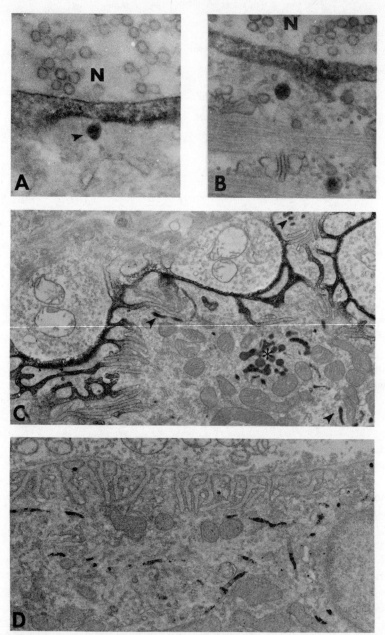

FIG. 4. Ultrastructural study of the internalization of peroxidase-α-bungarotoxin-labelled AChR at the normal rat end-plate. Two hours after labelling, the reaction for peroxidase is on the surface of the postsynaptic membrane, in endocytotic invaginations of this membrane (arrow-

labelling. In addition, the label was also present in endocytotic invaginations of the postsynaptic membrane (Fig. 4A), in small, membrane-bound spaces under the postsynaptic membrane (Fig. 4B), and in large tubulovesicular structures within the junctional folds and in the nearby junctional sarcoplasm (Fig. 4C). The internalized label was most abundant at 24 hours when it was also observed in deeper layers of the junctional sarcoplasm. Between 24 and 120 hours the surface label gradually decreased with a parallel decrease in the abundance of the internalized label. The tubulovesicular structures that engulfed the internalized AChR were identified as lysosomes by the acid phosphatase reaction (Fig. 4D). These studies clearly show that degradation of the junctional AChR is initiated by endocytosis and completed by a lysosomal mechanism.

General comments on mechanisms that can decrease end-plate AChR

Table 2 lists the mechanisms that can cause end-plate AChR deficiency and the associated clinical conditions. In some disorders multiple mechanisms determine the AChR deficiency and, conversely, some mechanisms can operate in more than one disorder.

Destruction of the folds, or of those segments of the folds that bear AChR, represents a very obvious mechanism of AChR loss. The folds cannot be adequately resolved by light microscopy and electron microscopic study is required to show this change. Proof that complement destroys junctional folds in myasthenia gravis (MG) rests on the immunoelectron microscopic demonstration of the lytic ninth complement component (C9) on disintegrating fragments of the folds (Sahashi et al 1980). Phagocytosis of junctional folds opsonized by IgG and C3 was demonstrated by ultrastructural and cytochemical methods (Engel et al 1976, 1979) in the acute form of experimental autoimmune MG (EAMG).

Activation of the lytic phase of the complement reaction sequence results in the formation of transmembrane ion channels made up of the C5b–9 membrane attack complex. The insertion of such channels into the postsynaptic membrane is likely to cause an uncontrolled influx of extracellular ions, focal calcium excess (Campbell et al 1979), protease activation and disruption of cytoskeletal elements within the folds. The subsquent shedding of injured

---

head) (A) and in more deeply situated vesicles (B). At six hours (C) the reaction is also present in tubules and vesicles in the junctional sarcoplasm (arrowheads). Small osmiophilic granules in C (asterisk) represent lipofuscin. D shows reaction for lysosomal acid phosphatase in subsynaptic structures that are similar in size, shape and distribution to those that react for peroxidase. N, nerve terminal. A, ×67 000; B, ×51 000; C, ×12 100; D, ×15 000. (C and D are reproduced from Engel et al 1982a, by permission of the New York Academy of Sciences.)

TABLE 2 Mechanisms that can decrease end-plate AChR[a]

Mechanism	Clinical condition
Destruction of junctional folds	
Antibody-dependent complement-mediated lysis of junctional folds	MG, chronic EAMG
Macrophage invasion of junctional folds opsonized by antibody and complement	Acute and passively transferred EAMG; seldom in human MG
Abnormal subsynaptic ionic milieu	Congenitally prolonged open time of the ACh-induced ion channel ('slow-channel syndrome') Congenital end-plate AChE deficiency Experimental myopathies induced by anti-AChE drugs ?Muscular dystrophies
Immature junctions with few or no junctional folds	
Regenerating muscle fibres	Any myopathy
Newly formed end-plate regions on pre-existing muscle fibres	MG; chronic EAMG; recovery phase of acute EAMG
Accelerated internalization and destruction of AChR not balanced by insertion of new AChR	
AChR cross-linked by antibody	MG, chronic EAMG
AChR not cross-linked by antibody	?Congenital end-plate AChR deficiency
Impaired insertion of new AChR	
Abnormal and/or reduced postsynaptic membrane and/or cytoskeleton	MG, chronic EAMG ?Congenital end-plate AChR deficiency
Decreased AChR synthesis	
	?Exposure to anti-AChE drugs ?Congenital end-plate AChE deficiency ?Slow-channel syndrome ?Congenital end-plate AChR deficiency General failure of protein synthesis

[a] More than one pathogenetic mechanism can be associated with a given clinical condition. Query indicates putative association. ACh, acetylcholine; AChR, acetylcholine receptor; AChE, acetylcholinesterase; MG, human autoimmune myasthenia gravis; EAMG, experimental autoimmune myasthenia gravis.

segments of the folds which bear AChR, IgG and the membrane attack complex may be the outcome of disturbed membrane dynamics and impaired cytoskeletal support. The postsynaptic membrane reseals itself over the junctional folds which are now shorter and bear fewer AChRs than the pre-existing folds.

An abnormal subsynaptic ionic milieu in itself can cause disintegration of the junctional folds, loss of AChR and morphological alterations in the junctional sarcoplasm. This type of end-plate myopathy can be induced experimentally by acetylcholinesterase inhibitors (Engel et al 1973, Salpeter et al 1979) and cholinergic agonists (Leonard & Salpeter 1979). Similar morphological changes occur in the congenital myasthenic syndrome attributed to a prolonged open time of the ACh-induced ion channel ('slow-channel syndrome') (Engel et al 1982b). Intracellular calcium accumulation has been implicated in the pathogenesis of these disorders. The experimentally induced end-plate myopathy is calcium-dependent (Leonard & Salpeter 1979) and abnormal calcium deposits can be demonstrated at the end-plate in some cases of the slow-channel syndrome (Engel et al 1982b). That focal calcium excess in the junctional folds can result from either unduly frequent or prolonged openings of the ACh-induced ion channel is consistent with the observation that a fraction of the end-plate current is carried by calcium (Miledi et al 1980).

Focal degeneration of the junctional folds also occurs in Duchenne dystrophy and occasionally in other dystrophies (Engel et al 1975). Once again, this may be a calcium-dependent phenomenon. Abnormal calcium deposits occur in non-necrotic fibres in dystrophic muscle (Bodensteiner & Engel 1975). When such deposits accumulate at or near the postsynaptic region, they could affect the structural integrity of the junctional folds. Thus, shedding of fragments of the junctional folds can be viewed as a basic pathological reaction to diverse stimuli which perturb the microenvironment of the folds.

Accelerated internalization and destruction of AChR cross-linked by myasthenic immunoglobulin has been demonstrated in cultured myotubes (reviewed by Vincent 1980) and, more importantly, at the motor end-plate (Table 1 and Fig. 3). Marked acceleration of AChR internalization also occurs at the denervated motor end-plate at a time when the number and packing density of junctional AChRs remain constant (Levitt & Salpeter 1981). Thus, factors in addition to accelerated loss must operate in decreasing the number of AChRs at the myasthenic end-plate. Evidence that AChR insertion into the myasthenic end-plate is decreased is presented in the next section.

AChR synthesis is reduced in cultured myotubes exposed to cholinergic agonists (Noble et al 1978, Gardner & Fambrough 1979). An analogous mechanism might down-regulate end-plate AChR synthesis in myasthenic patients treated with acetylcholinesterase inhibitors, in congenital end-plate acetylcholinesterase deficiency, and in the slow-channel syndrome. Direct evidence that this mechanism operates in any of these conditions is not available. AChR synthesis may also decrease with a general failure of protein synthesis in terminal states. This could contribute to AChR depletion in severe EAMG in starving, dehydrated and moribund animals.

Disorders in which end-plate AChR is decreased

Acquired autoimmune myasthenia gravis and chronic experimental auto-immune myasthenia gravis

The amount of AChR which remains at the end-plate, evaluated morphometrically with peroxidase-α-bungarotoxin (Engel et al 1977a) or radiochemically with ^{125}I-α-bungarotoxin (Ito et al 1978, Lindstrom & Lambert 1978), correlates linearly with the amplitude of the miniature end-plate potential. This indicates that the AChR deficiency can account for the defect in neuromuscular transmission.

In addition to the AChR deficiency, blocking by antibody of the binding of ACh to the receptor, or interference by antibody with the opening of the ACh-induced ion channel, could contribute to the decrease of the end-plate current in MG. Blocking antibodies are present in at least some myasthenic sera but single-channel conductance and open time are not affected in MG (reviewed by Vincent 1980). Three major mechanisms are responsible for the AChR loss in MG and chronic EAMG: (1) antibody-dependent complement-mediated lysis of segments of the junctional folds; (2) accelerated internalization of AChR cross-linked by antibody; (3) reduced insertion of AChR into the postsynaptic membrane.

Antibody-dependent complement-mediated lysis of the junctional folds. IgG deposits at the end-plate have been demonstrated in MG (Engel et al 1977b) and chronic EAMG (Sahashi et al 1978) with peroxidase-labelled protein A as the primary or secondary immunoreagent. The abundance of antibody on the junctional folds was proportional to the amount of AChR remaining on the folds. In less severe cases, IgG was localized on terminal expansions of well-preserved folds (Fig. 5A). In more severe cases, with less well-preserved folds, less IgG was present on the postsynaptic membrane (Figs. 5B,C) but IgG was detected on degenerated remnants of the folds in the synaptic space (Fig. 5C). Infrequently, moderately severe MG was associated with well-preserved junctional folds which bound abundant IgG. It can be inferred that (1) in most cases of MG, the transmission defect is determined by the loss of AChR rather than because IgG is bound to AChR; (2) in most cases of MG,

---

FIG.5. IgG localization at the MG end-plate with peroxidase–protein A. IgG is detected on terminal expansions of well-preserved junctional folds (A), on short segments of the simplified postsynaptic membrane (B and C) and on degenerated fragments of the folds shed into the synaptic space (asterisk) (C). Presynaptic staining in this and other figures is reciprocal to the postsynaptic reaction and represents diffusion artifact. A, ×15 300; B, ×25 200; C, ×29 700. (From Engel et al 1977b, by permission of *Mayo Clinic Proceedings*.)

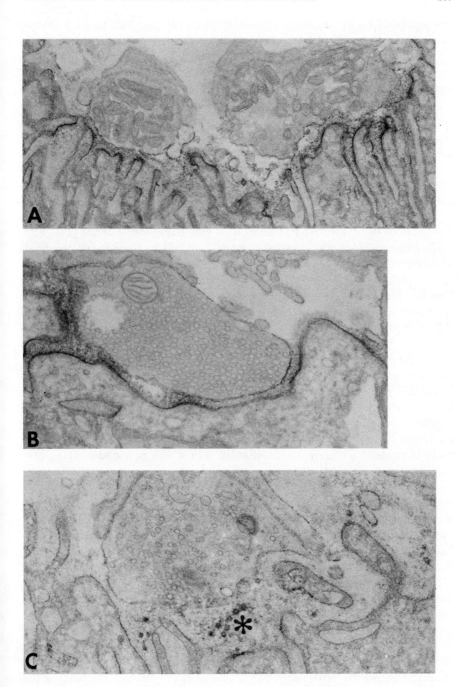

antibodies to AChR do not significantly block the response to ACh, but in occasional patients antibodies do have a significant blocking effect.

The ultrastructural localization of C3 in MG and chronic EAMG is identical with that of IgG (Engel et al 1977b, Sahashi et al 1978). This indicates that anti-AChR antibodies fix complement *in situ* and that the assembly phase of the complement reaction sequence goes to completion (Müller-Eberhard 1975). The C3 localization, however, does not prove that there is activation of lytic complement components. Unambiguous evidence for the latter was obtained by the localization of C9 at the MG end-plate (Sahashi et al 1980). At end-plates where the architecture of the postsynaptic region was well preserved, C9 was localized on short segments of the junctional folds and on sparse debris in the synaptic space (Fig. 6A). At abnormal end-plate regions there was intense reaction for C9 on degenerated remnants of the folds that had been shed into the synaptic space (Fig. 6B). Highly degenerated postsynaptic regions denuded of their nerve terminals also bound abundant C9. In places the debris reacting for C9 was arranged in the shape of pre-existing folds that were still surrounded by traces of basal lamina. Whereas IgG and C3 were localized on the intact postsynaptic membrane as well as on debris, most of the reaction for C9 was associated with debris. From this we concluded that (1) the postsynaptic membrane is not injured directly by IgG or C3; (2) lytic complement components are not formed at all sites that bind C3; (3) once formed, the C5b–9 membrane attack complex is more stable than the membrane that it attacks; (4) segments of the junctional folds attacked by the C5b–9 complex are shed into the synaptic space where they further degenerate; (5) repeated cycles of destruction and regeneration of postsynaptic regions result in progressive separation of end-plate regions on the surface of the muscle fibre as nerve sprouts move away from destroyed regions to adjacent sites where new end-plate regions can develop.

Accelerated internalization and destruction of AChR cross-linked by antibody. We recently investigated ultrastructural aspects of this process in EAMG by monitoring the internalization *in vivo* of AChR labelled with peroxidase-α-bungarotoxin (Fumagalli et al 1981, Engel et al 1982a). The results were compared with those obtained in normal muscle (described in a preceding section). In chronic EAMG, as at the normal end-plate, AChR was internalized by endocytosis and then taken up by tubulovesicular lysosomes. In subclinical and mild EAMG, initially there was abundant AChR on the postsynaptic membrane and internalized label was readily observed during the study (Fig. 7A). In more severe EAMG, only sparse AChR was present on the postsynaptic membrane at the outset and much less internalized label appeared during the experiment. At 120 hours after labelling, the label on the

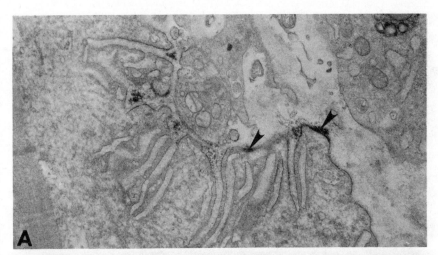

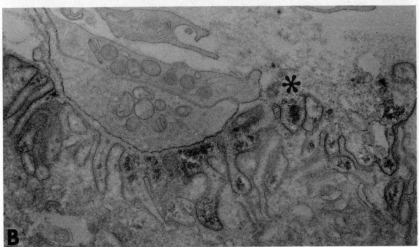

FIG. 6. Ultrastructural localization of C9 at the end-plate in myasthenia gravis. In A the postsynaptic region is well preserved. Reaction for C9 is confined to short segments of the folds (arrowheads) and sparse debris in the synaptic space. In B the junctional folds are degenerating at the right and there is abundant reaction for C9 on nearby debris (asterisk). The folds are well preserved at the left and here there are only traces of C9-positive material. A, ×16 200; B, ×16 000. (From Sahashi et al 1980, by permission of the *Journal of Neuropathology and Experimental Neurology*.)

postsynaptic membrane was very faint or not discernible in rats with subclinical, mild (Fig. 7B) or more severe EAMG, but was still abundant in control animals (Fig. 7C). At this time peroxidase-α-bungarotoxin was again injected into an adjacent forelimb extensor muscle. A few hours after the

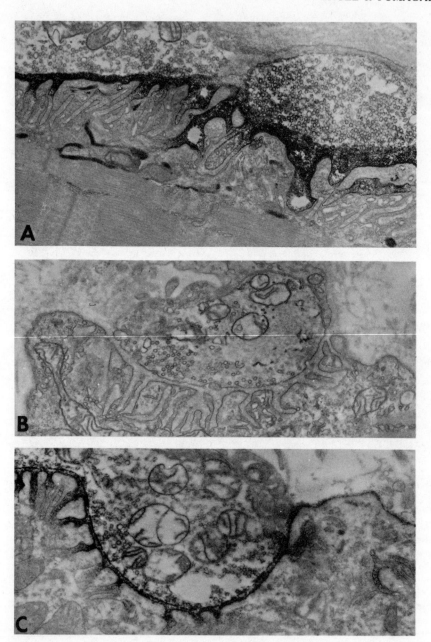

FIG. 7. Localization of AChR labelled *in vivo* in a rat with mild EAMG (A,B) and a control rat (C) 12 hours (A) and 120 hours (B,C) after labelling. Myasthenic rat shows abundant label on the postsynaptic membrane and in subsynaptic tubulobvesicular structures at 12 hours (A) but has no

second injection, the label on the postsynaptic membrane in a given animal was as abundant as a few hours after the first injection, and this was confirmed by morphometric analysis. These experiments indicate that (1) the fractional rate of end-plate AChR internalization is accelerated in chronic EAMG; (2) the absolute amount of electron microscopically detectable internalized AChR is reduced when the amount of AChR on the postsynaptic membrane is reduced; (3) removal and insertion of end-plate AChR are in balance in EAMG by morphometric criteria.

In a parallel study, we used an externally placed γ-counter to monitor *in vivo* the loss of ^{125}I-α-bungarotoxin-labelled AChR from forelimb digit extensor muscles (Fig. 3). This again showed accelerated degradation of end-plate AChR in EAMG, as noted in previous studies (Table 1). In both control and EAMG muscles radioactivity decreased as a single exponential function of time, indicating an equal probability of degradation for recently and less recently synthesized AChR.

Reduced insertion of AChR into the postsynaptic membrane. Neither complement attack on the postsynaptic membrane nor accelerated internalization of AChR causes depletion of AChR if the loss is balanced by increased insertion of new receptor. Therefore, it was of interest to assess the insertion of new AChR into the myasthenic end-plate. Left and right forelimb toe extensor muscles were used in EAMG and control rats. On Day 0 ^{125}I-α-bungarotoxin binding sites per end-plate were determined in the left muscle *in vitro*. The right muscle was then saturated *in vivo* with the labelled toxin and the loss of radioactivity was monitored daily with an externally placed γ-counter. Three to 10 (X) days later the right muscle was removed and toxin-binding sites per end-plate were determined before and after relabelling *in vitro*. This study provided the following information: (1) The mean number of AChRs per end-plate on Days 0 and X; (2) estimates of end-plate AChR half-life and fractional degradation rate by two separate methods; (3) the number of AChRs removed from the end-plate per day; (4) the number of new AChRs inserted into the end-plate per day (Table 3 and Fig. 8). In addition, clinical status and AChR degradation rate were compared in each animal (Fig. 8), and cytochemical and quantitative ultrastructural studies were done on aliquots of the excised muscles.

The mean fractional end-plate AChR turnover rate was approximately 2.5 times higher in the EAMG than in the control rats. The mean number of AChRs at the EAMG end-plate was only 28% of the control mean. However,

label at the end-plate at 120 hours (B). Control rat has abundant label on the postsynaptic membrane, and some in the junctional sarcoplasm, even at 120 hours (C). A, B, C, ×17900. (From Engel et al 1982a, by permission of the New York Academy of Sciences.)

TABLE 3 Balance of end-plate AChR removal and insertion

	Controls	EAMG animals
AChRs/end-plate, $\times 10^6$		
Day 0	22.16 ± 3.12^e ⎫	6.17 ± 1.88^e ⎫
Day X[b]	22.66 ± 2.05 ⎭	6.19 ± 1.49 ⎭
AChR half-life, days[c]		
Method A	9.8 ± 1.6	3.7 ± 0.7
Method C	8.4 ± 1.3	3.7 ± 1.1
Percentage of end-plate AChR degraded/day[d]	7.2 ± 1.1	19.4 ± 3.6
AChRs removed/end-plate per day, $\times 10^6$	1.57 ± 0.12^e ⎫	1.18 ± 0.26^e ⎫
AChRs inserted/end-plate per day, $\times 10^6$	1.67 ± 0.23 ⎭	1.14 ± 0.34 ⎭

[a] All values indicate mean ± SD based on observations in six control and six EAMG rats except for the determination of AChR half-life by method C, for which 11 control and 11 EAMG animals were used.

[b] All control rats were studied for nine days. Four EAMG rats were studied for 8–10 days, one for three days, and one for four days. Two animals studied for the shortest periods were moribund when killed.

[c] Methods A and C are described in the text.

[d] Values shown were calculated from measurements obtained by method A. The fraction of end-plate AChR degraded per day (k) is derived from the expression $Y(t) = Y_0 e^{-kt}$, where Y_0 and $Y(t)$ represent radioactivity at the end-plate at 0 time and on Day t, respectively. AChR half-life equals $(\ln 2)/k$. The product $k \times$ (AChRs/end-plate) provides an estimate of AChRs removed/end-plate per day.

[e] Comparison of bracketed values by paired t-test shows no significant difference.

in both control and EAMG rats, the mean number of AChRs remained essentially unchanged during the course of the study. Therefore, the end-plate AChR was at a steady state in both groups of animals, and, for each animal, the number of AChRs removed from and inserted into the end-plate was the same. On the average, this number was 30% lower in rats with EAMG than in the controls ($P < 0.005$).

AChR degradation rate showed no consistent correlation with the clinical status, or with a change in clinical status, in the EAMG animals during the study (Figs. 8B,C,D). Complement C9 was present at all EAMG end-plates. Morphometric analysis of end-plate ultrastructure revealed more marked destructive changes in the weakest rats.

The results clearly indicate that the myasthenic muscle fibre is unable to compensate for the accelerated loss of end-plate AChR. A 2.5-fold increase in fractional degradation rate would be compensated by a 2.5-fold increase in insertion rate. Such a response is well within the capability of muscle fibre, because a constant AChR level is maintained at denervated end-plates in which the fractional turnover rate of the newly inserted AChR is increased 10-fold (Levitt & Salpeter 1981). Instead of a compensatory increase, there is a 30% decrease in the insertion of new receptor into the myasthenic

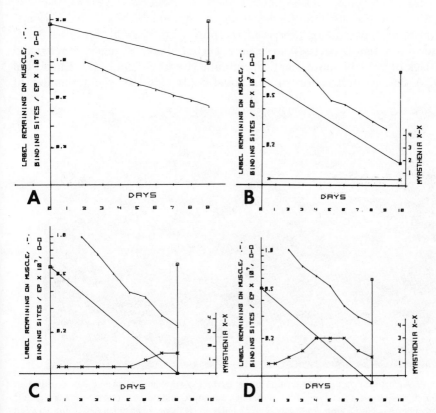

FIG. 8. Correlation of clinical status (x—x), AChR degradation rate monitored *in vivo* (.—.) and mean number of α-bungarotoxin binding sites per end-plate (o—o) shown in one control (A) and three EAMG (B, C, D) rats. The clinical scale ranges from weak grip and easy fatigability (1) to moribund (3). *In vivo* degradation of AChR is normalized for radioactivity detected on muscle on Day 2. One animal had subclinical disease (B), one became mildly affected near the end of the study (C), and one became severely ill during the middle of the study and then improved (D). There is no correlation between the clinical state and the rate of AChR degradation monitored *in vivo*. For a given animal, the slope of the line which connects the number of labelled sites per end-plate on Day 0 with the number of sites that remain labelled on the last day of the study is not significantly different from the slope of the line which indicates the rate of AChR degradation *in vivo*. For a given animal, the number of toxin-binding sites per end-plate after relabelling the muscle at the end of the study *in vitro* does not significantly differ from the mean number of toxin-binding sites in the corresponding contralateral muscle determined on Day 0 *in vitro*.

end-plate. In the absence of other factors lowering the number of end-plate AChRs, this decrease in itself would reduce the count per end-plate from 22 to 15.4×10^6.

A decreased insertion of new receptors into the myasthenic end-plate could be due to a decrease in receptor synthesis or impaired insertion of newly synthesized receptor into the postsynaptic membrane, or both. No reason is at present apparent for decreased receptor synthesis. On the other hand, insertion of tightly packed and securely anchored AChRs might be restricted by lack of available postsynaptic membrane (Engel & Santa 1971, Engel et al 1976) due to destruction of junctional folds (Fig. 9), the formation of

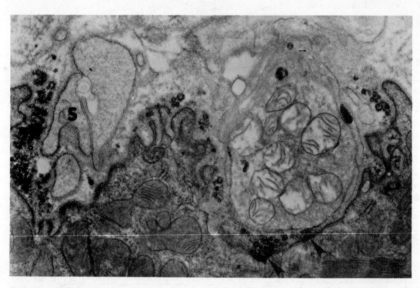

FIG. 9. AChR localization in a rat with chronic EAMG. Two regions of an end-plate are imaged. At both regions most junctional folds have been destroyed and postsynaptic membrane length is markedly reduced. Region at left has been abandoned by its nerve terminal and is now covered by a Schwann cell (S). Reaction for AChR is detected on remnants of junctional folds that had been shed into the synaptic cleft, and on very short segments of the simplified postsynaptic membrane (arrows). Loss of junctional folds, shortening of the postsynaptic membrane and lack of appropriate cytoskeletal anchorage may restrict sites available for AChR insertion. ×16 600.

immature end-plates lacking junctional folds, and by disorganization of cytoskeletal elements in injured junctional folds. AChR synthesis could be normal or even increased. If so, AChRs not inserted into the postsynaptic membrane would either accumulate subsynaptically or undergo lysosomal destruction, or both.

Acute and passively transferred experimental autoimmune myasthenia gravis

An acute phase of EAMG is observed in some, but not all, animals after immunization with AChR plus adjuvants. In female Lewis rats this can occur 7–11 days after the inoculation. At this time both antibody and complement

C3 and C9 are present on the junctional folds and the initial ultrastructural change is lysis of the tips of the junctional folds. Shortly thereafter, end-plate regions are split away from the underlying muscle fibre and the separating, degenerating and opsonized junctional folds are invaded and destroyed by macrophages (Engel et al 1976). A similar sequence of events takes place within 48 hours after passive transfer of immunoglobulin from rats with chronic EAMG to normal recipients (Engel et al 1979). For unknown reasons, macrophages do not invade junctional folds in chronic EAMG and only seldom do so in human MG.

Congenital myasthenic syndromes

Congenital myasthenic syndrome attributed to a prolonged open time of the ACh-induced ion channel (slow-channel syndrome). This is a dominantly inherited disorder with symptoms presenting in infancy or later life and with a selective distribution of the clinically affected muscles (Engel et al 1982b). In all muscles there is a repetitive muscle action potential response to a single nerve stimulus and end-plate currents are markedly prolonged. There is abundant AChE at the end-plate and the prolonged end-plate current is therefore attributed to a prolonged open time of the ACh-induced ion channel. In clinically affected muscles there is degeneration of junctional folds with concomitant loss of AChR (Fig. 10), and the amplitude of the miniature end-plate potential is reduced. Complement does not participate in the lysis of the folds. The injury to the folds and other structural alterations occurring near the end-plate are attributed to the altered ionic milieu caused by the prolonged openings of end-plate ion channels. Hypothetically, insertion of AChR into the end-plate could also be reduced, due to lack of available postsynaptic membrane, and synthesis of AChR might be down-regulated, as it is in cultured muscle cells exposed to cholinergic agonists (Noble et al 1978, Gardner & Fambrough 1979). Direct evidence for these additional mechanisms is not available.

Congenital myasthenic syndrome associated with end-plate acetylcholinesterase deficiency. This disorder is transmitted by recessive, or autosomal recessive, inheritance and severely disabling symptoms appear at birth (Engel et al 1977c). As in the slow-channel syndrome, there is a repetitive muscle action potential response to a single nerve stimulus and the end-plate currents are prolonged. The number of ACh quanta released by nerve impulse, and the number of quanta readily available for release from the nerve terminal, are reduced. The amplitude of the miniature end-plate potential is normal or slightly reduced. There is total absence of acetylcholinesterase from every

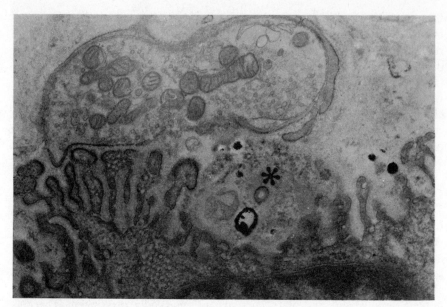

FIG. 10. AChR localization in a congenital myasthenic syndrome attributed to a prolonged open time of the ACh-induced ion channel. AChR is lost where the junctional folds have degenerated (asterisk). Circular, dense, calcific deposits occur in remnants of the folds. ×20 000.

end-plate, and this adequately explains the prolonged end-plate current. Nerve terminals are small on the average and this accounts for the decrease of readily releasable quanta. At some end-plates there is degeneration of the junctional folds with concomitant loss of AChR (Engel et al 1977c). As in the slow-channel syndrome, the focal degeneration of the junctional folds is attributed to an abnormal subsynaptic ionic milieu caused by the prolonged end-plate currents. However, this is less marked than in the slow-channel syndrome because ACh release is also reduced. By hypothesis, down-regulation of AChR synthesis might also occur and contribute to the AChR deficiency.

Congenital end-plate AChR deficiency. Myasthenic symptoms present in early life but autoantibodies to AChR are lacking. End-plate acetylcholinesterase is preserved and end-plate currents are not abnormally long. The number of α-bungarotoxin binding sites per end-plate is reduced. In some cases end-plate remodelling is indicated by increased spatial dispersion of end-plate regions on the surface of the muscle fibre (Vincent et al 1981). Ultrastructural studies are not available.

The AChR deficiency in this disorder could be due to decreased synthesis or membrane insertion or accelerated degradation of AChR, or a combination of these. Structural abnormalities in the receptor could accelerate AChR degradation (Prives & Olden 1980), or decrease the affinity for ACh, as in the case studied by Morgan-Hughes et al (1981). Other structural mutations might diminish the conductance or open time of the ACh-induced ion channel and cause myasthenic symptoms without decreasing the number of AChRs per end-plate. A recessively inherited syndrome in dogs is associated with end-plate AChR deficiency (Lennon et al 1981). The aetiology of the canine disorder is also undefined.

Duchenne dystrophy

Focal degeneration of the junctional folds has been noted in Duchenne dystrophy, and also occasionally in other dystrophies (Engel et al 1975). However, the clinical features of myasthenia are lacking, there is no net decrease in end-plate AChR by ultrastructural morphometric criteria, and the amplitude of the miniature end-plate potential is normal (Sakakibara et al 1977). Therefore, the increased loss of AChR must be balanced by increased synthesis and insertion of new AChR, or the AChR loss is too small to compromise the safety margin of neuromuscular transmission.

Acknowledgements

Work in our laboratory was supported in part by NIH Research Grant NS 6277 and by a Research Center Grant from the Muscular Dystrophy Association. Dr Fumagalli was the recipient of a research fellowship from the Muscular Dystrophy Association. Mrs Linda McConahey assisted in the preparation of the manuscript.

REFERENCES

Berg DK, Hall ZW 1975 Loss of α-bungarotoxin from junctional and extrajunctional acetycholine receptors in rat diaphragm muscle *in vivo* and in organ culture. J Physiol (Lond) 252:771–789
Bodensteiner J, Engel AG 1975 Intracellular calcium accumulation in Duchenne dystrophy and other myopathies. Neurology 28:439-446
Campbell AK, Daw RA, Luzio JP 1979 Rapid increase in intracellular free Ca^{2+} induced by antibody plus complement. FEBS (Fed Eur Biochem Soc) Lett 107:55-60
Chang CC, Huang MC 1975 Turnover of junctional and extrajunctional acetylcholine receptors of rat diaphragm. Nature (Lond) 253:643-644
Devreotes PN, Fambrough DM 1976 Turnover of acetylcholine receptors in skeletal muscle. Cold Spring Harbor Symp Quant Biol 40:237-251
Engel AG, Santa T 1971 Histometric analysis of the ultrastructure of the neuromuscular junction in myasthenia gravis and the myasthenic syndrome. Ann NY Acad Sci 183:46-63
Engel AG, Lambert EH, Santa T 1973 Study of long-term anticholinesterase therapy. Effects on neuromuscular transmission and on motor end-plate fine structure. Neurology 23:1273-1281

Engel AG, Jerusalem F, Tsujihata M, Gomez MR 1975 The neuromuscular junction in myopathies. A quantitative ultrastructural study. In: Bradley WG et al (eds) Recent advances in myology. Excerpta Medica, Amsterdam. (International Congress Series 360) p 132-143

Engel AG, Tsujihata M, Lambert EH, Lindstrom J, Lennon VA 1976 Experimental autoimmune myasthenia gravis. A sequential and quantitative study of the neuromuscular junction ultrastructure and electrophysiologic correlations. J Neuropathol Exp Neurol 35:569-587

Engel AG, Lindstrom J, Lambert EH, Lennon VA 1977a Ultrastructure localization of the acetylcholine receptor in myasthenia gravis and in its experimental autoimmune model. Neurology 27:307-315

Engel AG, Lambert EH, Howard FM 1977b Immune complexes (IgG and C3) at the motor end-plate in myasthenia gravis. Ultrastructural and light microscopic localization and electrophysiologic correlations. Mayo Clin Proc 52:267-280

Engel AG, Lambert EH, Gomez MR 1977c A new myasthenic syndrome with end-plate acetylcholinesterase deficiency, small nerve terminals, and reduced acetylcholine release. Ann Neurol 1:315-330

Engel AG, Sakakibara H, Sahashi K, Lindstrom J, Lambert EH, Lennon VA 1979 Passively transferred experimental autoimmune myasthenia gravis. Sequential and quantitative study of the motor end-plate fine structure and ultrastructural localization of immune complexes (IgG and C3), and of the acetylcholine receptor. Neurology 29:179-188

Engel AG, Sahashi K, Fumagalli G 1982a The immunopathology of acquired myasthenia gravis. Ann NY Acad Sci 377:158-174

Engel AG, Lambert EH, Mulder DM et al 1982b A newly recognized congenital myasthenic syndrome attributed to a prolonged open time of the acetylcholine induced ion channel. Ann Neurol, in press

Fambrough DM 1979 Control of acetylcholine receptors in skeletal muscle. Physiol Rev 59:165-227

Fertuck HC, Salpeter MM 1976 Quantitation of junctional and extrajunctional acetylcholine receptor by electron microscope autoradiography after ^{125}I-α-bungarotoxin binding at mouse neuromuscular junctions. J Cell Biol 69:144-158

Fumagalli G, Engel AG, Lindstrom J 1981 Ultrastructural aspects of acetylcholine receptor turnover at the normal and myasthenic motor end-plate. J Neuropathol Exp Neurol 40:301

Gardner JM, Fambrough DM 1979 Acetylcholine receptor degradation measured by density labeling: effects of cholinergic ligands and evidence against recycling. Cell 16:661-674

Heinemann S, Merlie J, Lindstrom J 1978 Modulation of acetylcholine receptor in rat diaphragm by anti-receptor sera. Nature (Lond) 274:65-68

Ito Y, Miledi R, Vincent A, Newsom-Davis J 1978 Acetylcholine receptors and end-plate electrophysiology in myasthenia gravis. Brain 101:345-368

Lennon VA, Lambert EH, Palmer AC, Cunningham JG, Christie TR 1981 Acquired and congenital myasthenia gravis in dogs—a study of 20 cases. In: Japanese Medical Research Foundation (ed) Myasthenia gravis. Pathogenesis and treatment. University of Tokyo Press, Tokyo, p 41-54

Leonard JP, Salpeter MM 1979 Agonist-induced myopathy at the neuromuscular junction is mediated by calcium. J Cell Biol 82:811-819

Levitt TA, Salpeter MM 1981 Denervated end-plates have a dual population of junctional acetylcholine receptors. Nature (Lond) 291:239-241

Libby P, Bursztajn S, Goldberg AL 1980 Degradation of the acetylcholine receptor in cultured muscle cells: selective inhibitors and the fate of undegraded receptors. Cell 19:481-491

Linden DC, Fambrough DM 1979 Biosynthesis and degradation of acetylcholine receptors in rat skeletal muscles. Effects of electrical stimulation. Neuroscience 4:527-538

Lindstrom JM, Lambert EH 1978 Content of acetylcholine receptor and antibodies bound to receptor in myasthenia gravis, experimental autoimmune myasthenia gravis, and Eaton-Lambert syndrome. Neurology 28:130-138

Miledi R, Parker I, Schalow G 1980 Transmitter induced calcium entry across the post-synaptic membrane at frog end-plates measured using arsenazo III. J Physiol (Lond) 300:197-212

Morgan-Hughes JA, Lecky BRF, Landon DN, Murray NMF 1981 Alterations in the number and affinity of junctional acetylcholine receptors in a myopathy with tubular aggregates. A newly recognized receptor defect. Brain 104:279-295

Müller-Eberhard HJ 1975 Complement. Annu Rev Biochem 44:697-724

Noble MD, Brown TH, Peacock JH 1978 Regulation of acetylcholine levels by a cholinergic agonist in mouse muscle cell cultures. Proc Natl Acad Sci USA 75:3488-3492

Prives MP, Olden K 1980 Carbohydrate requirement for expression and stability of acetylcholine receptor on the surface of embryonic muscle cells in culture. Proc Natl Acad Sci USA 77:5263-5267

Rash JE, Ellisman MH 1974 Studies of excitable membranes. I. Macromolecular specializations of the neuromuscular junction and the nonjunctional sarcolemma. J Cell Biol 63:567-586

Reiness CG, Weinberg CB, Hall ZW 1978 Antibody to acetylcholine receptor increases degradation of junctional and extrajunctional receptors in adult muscle. Nature (Lond) 274:68-70

Sakakibara H, Engel AG, Lambert EH 1977 Duchenne dystrophy: Ultrastructural localization of the acetylcholine receptor and intracellular microelectrode studies of neuromuscular transmission. Neurology 27:741-745

Sahashi K, Engel AG, Lindstrom JM, Lambert EH, Lennon VA 1978 Ultrastructural localization of immune complexes (IgG and C3) at the end-plate in experimental autoimmune myasthenia gravis. J Neuropathol Exp Neurol 37:212-223

Sahashi K, Engel AG, Lambert EH, Howard FM 1980 Ultrastructural localization of the terminal and lytic ninth complement (C9) component at the motor end-plate in myasthenia gravis. J Neuropathol Exp Neurol 39:160-172

Salpeter MM, Kasprzak H, Feng H, Fertuck H 1979 End-plates after esterase inactivation in vivo: correlations between esterase concentration, functional response and fine structure. J Neurocytol 8:95-115

Stanley EF, Drachman DB 1978 Effect of myasthenic immunoglobulin on acetylcholine receptors of intact mammalian neuromuscular junctions. Science (Wash DC) 200:1285-1287

Steinbach JH 1981 Developmental changes in acetylcholine receptor aggregates at rat skeletal neuromuscular junctions. Dev Biol 84:267-276

Vincent A 1980 Immunology of acetylcholine receptors in relation to myasthenia gravis. Physiol Rev 60:756-824

Vincent A, Cull-Candy SG, Newsom-Davis J, Trautmann A, Molenaar PC, Polak RL 1981 Congenital myasthenia: end-plate acetylcholine receptors and electrophysiology in five cases. Muscle & Nerve 4:306-318

DISCUSSION

Kahn: What is the explanation for the selectivity in myasthenia gravis, where some muscle groups are affected more than others, such as the ocular muscles, or variants of the disease where certain muscle groups are affected? *Engel:* First, there is some evidence from studies by Angela Vincent that the acetylcholine receptor on ocular muscles, which are typically affected in myasthenia gravis, may be antigenically different from the receptor on other muscles. Second, the safety margin of neuromuscular transmission may be lower in those muscles that are more readily affected, either because they have a lesser number of ACh receptors underlying the nerve terminal, or a lower number of quanta are released from the terminal by nerve impulse. Finally, we do not understand clearly why there is selective involvement of muscles in almost any muscle disease.

Vincent: We have compared the binding of anti-AChR to innervated ocular and denervated leg muscle AChR. Most patients' antibodies react better with leg muscle receptor, but some, almost always those from ocular cases, react better with receptor from extraocular muscle. This suggests that not only are the two sources of AChR antigenically different in some respect(s) but also that patients with disease restricted to ocular muscle have anti-ACh receptors which differ from those in patients with generalized disease (Vincent & Newsom-Davis 1982, Newsom-Davis et al, this volume).

This is not, however, the whole story. In most skeletal muscle the postsynaptic response, the end-plate potential, has to be reduced by more than 60% before the depolarization is insufficient to rise above the firing threshold and activate the action potential. About 20% of the fibres in extraocular muscle are 'slow' fibres, similar to those found in avian muscle, which have multiple end-plates and do not propagate an action potential. These fibres show a graded response to stimulation rather than the all-or-none response of most skeletal muscle. This means that there is no safety margin as such and weakness may be evident even when there is a relatively small decrease in the number of functioning receptors.

Knight: Is there always bilateral involvement in ocular myasthenia?

Newsom-Davis: No. Patients frequently get ptosis on one side only.

Knight: How does one explain that localization, then?

Vincent: We really don't know. There must be other factors involved at any end-plate, such as accessibility of the end-plates to circulating antibodies. I agree that that doesn't explain why involvement should be unilateral.

Drachman: The question of why some myasthenic patients are weaker than others has not been well explained in the past. Anti-ACh receptor antibody titres in different patients correspond poorly with their clinical status. We therefore examined certain *functional* activities of antibodies, to determine whether these properties might influence the clinical status. We first examined the antibody affinities in a series of myasthenic patients with a broad range of disease severity (Bray & Drachman 1982). We selected patients to include at least some with high antibody titres who were not severely affected, and some with rather low titres who were quite weak. One might expect that the higher affinity antibodies would produce more severe manifestations of myasthenia gravis. Our findings showed that the antibody affinities were very high in all sera tested, of the order of 10^{10} M^{-1}. There was only a six-fold variation in different patients. Thus, the antibody affinity failed to correlate with the clinical severity of the disease.

However, we also examined two of the known functional effects of the antibodies that are thought to reduce the number of available ACh receptors, namely the ability to accelerate the normal degradation rate of the receptor, and blockade of the receptor. We used a rat skeletal tissue culture system, and adjusted the experimental conditions to optimize the effects of the antibodies.

We found that the antibodies' ability to accelerate receptor degradation and to block receptors corresponded closely with the severity of clinical involvement. The effects were additive, and when they were examined by regression analysis the combined effects of accelerated degradation and blockade were very closely associated with the clinical status.

These cannot be the only factors related to the clinical severity of myasthenia gravis. For example, a given patient may express different degrees of weakness in different muscles despite the systemic circulation of the same population of antibodies. We believe that additional properties of antibodies, as well as factors intrinsic to the patient, may also be important in determining myasthenic weakness.

Mitchison: If you were to use those sera to do the kind of analysis which we heard about from Jon Lindstrom, using blocking by monoclonal antibodies, would you be able to make the kind of analysis that he makes?

Drachman: If one could accurately determine the site of binding to the intact human ACh receptor, this ought to be related to the clinical effects of accelerated degradation and blockade of ACh receptors. Since there is such poor cross-reactivity between human myasthenic antibodies and *Torpedo* receptor, I would expect that it would take a library of antibodies derived from *human patients* to analyse this question appropriately.

Engel: You measured the ability of myasthenic serum to accelerate the internalization of the extrajunctional receptor on myotubes, but could this ability be simply a reflection of the antibody titre? It is conceivable that you are looking not at a cause-and-effect relationship but at a concomitant variation.

Drachman: Our analysis showed that the abilities to induce accelerated degradation and blockade of ACh receptors were associated far more closely with the patient's clinical class than was the antibody titre. While antibody titre influences accelerated degradation ($P < 0.5$), this was shown statistically to represent only a small part of the functional abilities of the antibody to decrease the number of available receptors.

Bottazzo: Dr Engel, you did not mention class and subclass specificities. Is it possible that complement-fixing ability, together with affinity binding to the receptor, may influence some of the clinical features?

Engel: That is a possibility. Different subclasses of IgG do not fix complement equally. Incidentally, I'm not sure whether the ability of anti-AChR antibodies to cross-link AChR and to accelerate its internalization is subclass-dependent.

Vincent: In our experience, virtually every patient with myasthenia has antibodies in IgG subclasses 1 and 2 and very few in 3 (and subclasses 1 and 3 are those that bind complement). We certainly see IgG1 anti-receptor antibodies in almost every myasthenia patient (Vincent & Bilkhu 1982).

Mitchison: Dr Engel, you have beautiful micrographs localizing complement components. Have studies been made of the turnover of complement components in serum, or decrements in C levels in serum, in myasthenia?

Engel: One of the two early studies suggesting that myasthenia gravis was an autoimmune disease was by Nastuk et al (1960), who noted a correlation between serum complement levels and changes in clinical status. On the basis of that rather indirect evidence, they correctly inferred that myasthenia was an autoimmune disease. However, the total amount of the ACh receptor in the body is exceedingly low and the amount of circulating complement is relatively high (e.g. 1 mg/ml of C3 and 0.1 mg/ml of C9). Also, one cannot make much of serum complement levels unless one knows the rate of complement synthesis by mononuclear cells, which may well be accelerated in this disease. So total and individual serum complement levels are probably not very sensitive indicators of disease activity.

Rodbell: There is apparently a protein molecule of M_r 43 000 in the membrane that is hooked on to the ACh receptor and is not involved in its function (Changeux 1981, Froehner et al 1981). Could such a protein be involved in degradation of the receptor, or the rate of degradation? Dr Engel appeared to suggest some linkage between the rate of degradation and the rate of re-incorporation of fresh receptors into the cell membrane. There is obviously an antibody-induced, or perhaps a complement-induced change in the receptor. Perhaps this releases the 43 000 M_r protein, which results in a greater rate of internalization and somehow also a slipping into the cell membrane, so that you could have a synchronous affair, changing the dynamics of the entire complex?

Engel: I am not sure that one needs to postulate something that increases the propensity of AChR to become internalized other than its being cross-linked by IgG. We know that this occurs quite readily even at end-plates that show no structural change. The important questions are: (1) Can the muscle fibre respond with accelerated synthesis of AChR? (2) Can the newly synthesized receptor be inserted into the postsynaptic membrane? (3) What are the relative contributions of (a) accelerated internalization (due to cross-linking) of AChR, (b) repeated destruction of junctional folds (due to complement-mediated lysis), and (c) reduced insertion of the receptor into the postsynaptic membrane (due to cytoarchitectonic alterations) in causing the deficiency of AChR at the end-plate?

Our studies, presented here, show that: (1) The total number of AChRs at the end-plate is reduced. (2) Despite the accelerated turnover rate, the number of these receptors removed per day from the end-plate is about one-third less than the number removed from the normal end-plate. (3) The number of AChRs inserted into the myasthenic end-plate equals the number removed, and is again about one-third lower than normal. An inevitable conclusion is that the muscle fibre cannot restore to normal the number of ACh receptors at its end-plate, because of a hindrance in either the synthesis of the receptor or its insertion into the postsynaptic membrane.

The insertion of densely packed and regularly arrayed ACh receptors into the postsynaptic membrane must be a highly ordered process, with each receptor occupying a locus defined by cytoarchitectonic restraints. When the architecture of the postsynaptic membrane is not disturbed, accelerated degradation of the receptor is readily balanced by accelerated reinsertion of newly synthesized receptor, as beautifully exemplified by what happens to the end-plate AChR after denervation (Levitt & Salpeter 1981). By contrast, in myasthenia gravis the architecture of the postsynaptic folds is greatly disturbed by complement-mediated lysis and by the repeated cycles of degeneration and regeneration. It is very likely that these changes hinder the reinsertion of AChR into the postsynaptic membrane.

Drachman: The rates of degradation and synthesis of the receptor are independent. However, after loss of the motor nerve supply, the rate of synthesis of ACh receptors increases, and these receptors turn over more rapidly. The pre-existing ACh receptors at the neuromuscular junction are degraded at a rate about 40% faster than normal (Stanley & Drachman 1981); the newly inserted ACh receptors turn over very rapidly, at a rate comparable to that of extrajunctional receptors. There is a complex system of controls by which the ACh receptor turnover is regulated by the nerve supply to the muscle.

Mitchison: And that must be something to do with the cytoskeleton underneath the receptor, presumably?

Raftery: Actin is a known component of the subsynaptic density. In the preparations we have made of mammalian ACh receptor, actin is a constant component, as well as very high molecular weight polypeptides. So there may be a connection of the receptor to the cytoskeleton.

Lindstrom: The protein vinculin has also been implicated in these structures.

REFERENCES

Bray JJ, Drachman DB 1982 Neurotrophic regulation of two properties of skeletal muscle by impulse-dependent and spontaneous ACh transmission. J Immunol, in press

Changeux J-P 1981 The acetylcholine receptor: an allosteric membrane protein. Harvey Lect 75:85-254

Froehner SC, Gulbrandsen V, Hyman C, Jung AY, Neubig RR, Cohen JB 1981 Immunofluorescence localization at the mammalian neuromuscular junction of the M_r 43 000 protein of Torpedo postsynaptic membranes. Proc Natl Acad Sci USA 78:5230-5234

Levitt TA, Salpeter MM 1981 Denervated end-plates have a dual population of junctional acetylcholine receptors. Nature (Lond) 291:239-241

Nastuk WL, Plescia O, Osserman KE 1960 Changes in serum complement activity in myasthenia gravis. Proc Soc Exp Biol Med 105:177-184

Newsom-Davis J, Vincent A, Willcox N 1982 Acetylcholine receptor antibody: clinical and experimental aspects. This volume, p 225-238

Stanley EF, Drachman DB 1981 Denervation accelerates degradation of junctional acetylcholine receptors. Exp Neurol 73:390-396

Vincent A, Bilkhu M 1982 Anti-acetylcholine receptor antibody. Use of polyethylene glycol as an aid to precipitation of antibody receptor complexes in determination of light chain and subclass. J Immunol Methods, in press

Vincent A, Newsom-Davis J 1982 Acetylcholine receptor antibody characteristics in myasthenia gravis. I. Patients with generalised myasthenia or disease restricted to ocular muscles. Clin Exp Immunol, in press

Acetylcholine receptor antibody: clinical and experimental aspects

JOHN NEWSOM-DAVIS, ANGELA VINCENT and NICK WILLCOX

Department of Neurological Science, The Royal Free Hospital School of Medicine, Pond Street, London NW3 2QG, and Institute of Neurology, National Hospital for Nervous Diseases, Queen Square, London WC1N 3BG, UK

Abstract Anti-acetylcholine (ACh) receptor antibody is the specific antibody in myasthenia gravis (MG). Groups of patients distinguished by thymic pathology and age of onset have shown differences in sex and HLA antigen incidence and in anti-ACh receptor antibody levels. Group differences in the characteristics of this antibody, including the percentage of $\varkappa$ and λ light chains, IgG subclass and reactivity with other ACh receptor preparations, were detected only in patients with ocular MG. This group alone showed a possible association with Gm allotype in Caucasians; the anti-ACh receptor antibody had a greater proportion of $\varkappa$ light chain and better reactivity with human ocular ACh receptor than did generalized MG. The results indicate heterogeneity of this disease.

Thymic cells from myasthenic patients with thymic hyperplasia spontaneously synthesize anti-ACh receptor antibody in culture and, after irradiation to abrogate antibody production and any suppressor effects, can selectively enhance the synthesis of anti-ACh receptor antibody by autologous blood lymphocytes in co-culture. The cell types that underlie these responses have been investigated by depleting cell subsets by complement-mediated lysis using monoclonal antibodies. Neither cortical (NA1/34+) thymocytes nor mature T cells (MBG6+) are essential for antibody production *in vitro* by thymic cells. The enhancement of antibody production by irradiated thymic cells may depend on antigen-presenting cells not expressing the HLA-DR surface marker, or possibly antigen-specific helper T cells, or both.

This paper will focus on two aspects of anti-acetylcholine (ACh) receptor antibody, the specific antibody in myasthenia gravis (MG). The first concerns the specificities and properties of the antibody. Taken together with the clinical and pathological features of myasthenia and the genetically determined immunological constitution of individuals with MG, these suggest clinical heterogeneity in the disease which may have implications for both its causation and its management.

1982 Receptors, antibodies and disease. Pitman, London (Ciba Foundation symposium 90) p 225-247

The second aspect relates to the cellular mechanisms underlying the production of anti-ACh receptor antibody, which we have studied in cultured thymic and peripheral blood cells obtained from patients undergoing thymectomy. The pathological changes in the myasthenic thymus and the clinical response to its removal have led to the view that the thymus plays a part in the disease process. The fact that these changes occur in the site where developing T lymphocytes acquire tolerance to self antigens suggests that the disease process may even be initiated there. Similar mechanisms may play a part in other autoimmune disorders such as thyrotoxicosis and systemic lupus erythematosus, in which thymic pathology resembling that in myasthenia has occasionally been reported (Barnes & Irvine 1973).

The weakness and excessive fatigability of striated muscle in MG arises from a postsynaptic defect in neuromuscular transmission, characterized by a reduction in the number of functional ACh receptors (Fambrough et al 1973). This reduction is sufficient to account for the decreased amplitudes of the end-plate potentials and miniature end-plate potentials that have been demonstrated in biopsied myasthenic muscle *in vitro* (Elmqvist et al 1964, Ito et al 1978). It now seems clear that anti-ACh receptor antibody is implicated in the loss of ACh receptors from the membrane, and possible mechanisms by which this occurs have already been discussed.

The observation that rabbits immunized with ACh receptors from electric fish developed striking muscle weakness similar to that in MG (Patrick & Lindstrom 1973), and the presence in these immunized rabbits of anti-ACh receptor antibody, stimulated the search for these antibodies in MG patients. Many groups have demonstrated an IgG anti-ACh receptor antibody in MG patients, and most have used the immunoprecipitation method developed by Lindstrom et al (1976), based on ^{125}I-α-bungarotoxin-labelled human ACh receptors extracted from amputated calf muscle. The toxin binds with high affinity and specificity to the acetylcholine-binding site on the receptor. With this method, serum anti-ACh receptor titres in control subjects, including those with other neurological disorders or with rheumatoid arthritis, are <0.2 nmol/l, while about 90% of MG patients have values above this (Compston et al 1980). An elevated titre thus appears highly specific for MG. Anti-ACh receptor antibody can be detected in the serum of babies born to myasthenic mothers for a few weeks after birth, and may be associated with transient myasthenic symptoms (neonatal MG). It is not detectable, however, in congenital myasthenia (Vincent et al 1981). This latter disorder needs to be distinguished from MG; it appears to be primarily hereditary rather than acquired and immunological in origin.

The fact that anti-ACh receptor antibody appears to be specific for MG makes its measurement a useful diagnostic test. In addition, the serum level of anti-ACh receptor antibody *within* an individual seems to correlate with the extent of his muscle weakness. When the antibody concentration is lowered by a procedure such as plasma exchange or by steroid treatment, improvement in symptoms occurs; conversely, a rise in the antibody level is associated with clinical deterioration (Newsom-Davis et al 1978). It has become clear, however, that *between* individuals the absolute serum titre of antibody does not correlate with disease severity. Thus some patients with severe disease may have a low titre while the titre may be very high in others in remission. A possible explanation for this is the variability that exists in the antibody characteristics between individuals with MG (Vincent & Newsom-Davis 1980).

Clinical heterogeneity in myasthenia gravis

Several clinical features of MG seem to suggest the possibility of heterogeneity of this disease. The most striking of these is the differing thymic pathology. About 10% of patients with generalized MG have a thymoma, and in this group the sex incidence is equal and the age of onset typically in the fourth or fifth decade. Among non-thymomatous cases, two types of thymic histology are encountered, namely hyperplasia and atrophy (normal or involuted). In hyperplasia, the thymic medulla contains lymphoid follicles with germinal centres which may be very numerous. Females considerably exceed males in this group (3:1 in our series of 85 patients) and the age of onset is usually less than 40 years. When the illness starts after the age of 40, the sex incidence is reversed (M:F = 3:1) and the thymus, if examined, is usually atrophic (Table 1).

We analysed the immunological and HLA characteristics in 68 Caucasian patients with MG and found significant associations within these three groups (Compston et al 1980). For example, highly significant differences were observed in the mean anti-ACh receptor antibody titre, values being highest in those with thymoma and lowest in the late onset group. Anti-striated muscle antibody was present in over 90% of thymoma cases and much less frequent in the other two groups. The incidences of other autoantibodies and of other autoimmune disorders also differed between the groups, and were highest in the older patients. When we examined the HLA frequencies, no associations were found in those with thymoma with the possible exception that DRw7 was increased with respect to the other groups. Other studies have also failed to show strong HLA associations with thymoma. In patients with thymic hyperplasia, there was a significant increase in HLA-B8, as Pirskanen (1976) has described, and also in A1 and DR3, while in the late-onset group there were significant associations with A3, B7 and DR2. Interestingly, in Japanese the associations are different, being with B12 for the thymic

TABLE 1 Clinical heterogeneity of myasthenia gravis

	Thymoma	Thymus hyperplasia Onset <40 years	Thymus involution Onset >40 years	Ocular
Sex incidence (M:F)	1:1	1:3	3:1	3:1
Anti-ACh receptor antibody titre	High	Intermediate	Low	Very low
HLA antigen associations				
Caucasian	DR7?	A1,B8,DR3	A3,B7,DR2	n/a
Japanese[a]	None	B12	A10	B12
Gm allotype associations				
Caucasian	None	None	None	zaxgfnb
Japanese[b]	axg		axg	?none

[a]Yoshida et al (1977).
[b]Nakao et al (1980).
n/a, not available.

hyperplasia group and with A10 for the late-onset patients (Yoshida et al 1977; Table 1).

Gm allotypes have been investigated in Japanese by Nakao et al (1980), who have reported a highly significant increase in the axg haplotype in all myasthenic patients, the association being strongest in those with thymoma. In a study of 64 Caucasians, we have been unable to demonstrate an association between any Gm phenotype and any of the three myasthenic groups referred to above (E. van Loghem, J. Newsom-Davis, A. Vincent & N. Willcox, unpublished observations) (Table 1).

We have recently investigated the anti-ACh receptor antibody characteristics in these three groups of patients to see whether the clinical and immunological distinctions were associated with antibody differences (Vincent & Newsom-Davis 1982). Several different features have been examined, including the percentage of $\varkappa$ and λ light chains, the representation of IgG subclasses, the proportion of anti-α-bungarotoxin binding-site antibody and the reactivity with different ACh receptor preparations. No major differences were observed between the groups, suggesting similarity in the nature of the humoral response.

Differences in the anti-ACh receptor antibody characteristics were, however, observed when patients with symptoms that had been restricted to the ocular muscles for two years or more (ocular MG) were considered separately. There are good grounds for making this distinction. Such patients rarely develop generalized disease and, as among those with MG of late onset, males exceed females by about 3:1 (Table 1). The age of onset, on the other hand, has a wide range. This form of MG is usually incompletely responsive to treatment with anti-cholinesterase drugs but remits with steroid treatment, even at quite low dosage.

No adequate information appears to be available on HLA antigen associations with ocular MG, but we have found an increase in the Gm phenotype zaxgfnb in this group (7 of 18; expected frequency, 0.091). This increase, although significant at the 5% level, requires confirmation with larger numbers (E. van Loghem et al, unpublished observations).

Anti-ACh receptor antibody in ocular MG also differs from that in the other groups in the greater proportion of $\varkappa$ light chain (Fig. 1). The mean percentage $\varkappa$ for ocular MG was 91.4% ± 6.7 (SD) ($n = 9$), significantly greater than that for generalized MG (78.5% ± 21.1 (SD) ($n = 35$; $P < 0.05$). Anti-ACh receptor antibody in ocular MG also reacts relatively better with human ocular than denervated ACh receptors (Fig. 1), the percentage ratio being 107.1% ± 47.0 (SD) ($n = 9$), compared to 54.0% ± 20.6 (SD) ($n = 21$; $P < 0.05$) in generalized MG (Vincent & Newsom-Davis 1982).

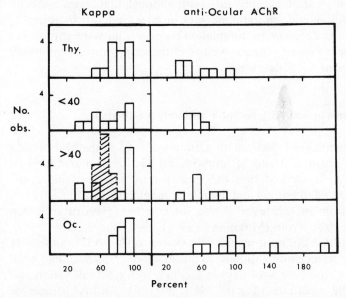

FIG. 1. Properties of anti-ACh receptor antibody in four groups of myasthenic patients: (1) thymoma (Thy); (2) non-thymoma, age of onset <40 years (<40); (3) non-thymoma, age of onset >40 years (>40); and (4) ocular (Oc.). Note that the percentage of $\varkappa$ light chain is on average greater in ocular than non-ocular cases. (Values for normal IgG are hatched.) Anti-(human) ocular ACh receptor antibody is expressed as a percentage of anti-(human) denervated ACh receptor antibody. In generalized MG, all values were <100%, in contrast to those in the ocular group.

There is thus reasonable evidence to support the concept of at least four types of acquired MG, which show differences in clinical features, thymus pathology, immunological characteristics and HLA associations, and, in the case of ocular MG, in antibody properties and Gm associations as well. Some of these are summarized in Table 1. These differences can also be reflected in the response to treatment. The myasthenic weakness in patients with thymic hyperplasia typically improves after thymectomy, in contrast to thymoma cases.

These observations raise the possibility that there may be more than one mechanism leading to the breakdown in tolerance to the ACh receptor and that the events that trigger this may be diverse. An individual's inherited immunological characteristics might then predispose to a particular form of the disease.

The finding of Gm associations in Japanese myasthenic patients is interesting. Their absence in Caucasians (except possibly in ocular MG) may be because the susceptibility genes are more widespread in Caucasians, and are not in linkage disequilibrium with the markers tested. Alternatively, it could be because the disease itself is subtly different, although that seems unlikely. Interestingly, experimental autoimmune MG in mice, induced by injecting ACh receptor from *Torpedo* in complete Freund's adjuvant, also shows influences of Ig heavy chain genes as well as of the major histocompatibility locus (*H–2*) (Berman & Patrick 1980).

Cellular mechanisms in anti-ACh receptor antibody production

The presence of lymphoid follicles with germinal centres in the MG thymus implies that this organ is a site of antibody production. Enumeration of thymic B and T cells showed that the former were increased in thymic hyperplasia, compared to normal and thymomatous glands (Lisak et al 1978). Thymic extracts from such cases may also show higher levels of anti-ACh receptor antibody than serum (Mittag et al 1976).

We have shown that cultured myasthenic thymic cells can spontaneously synthesize anti-ACh receptor antibody (Vincent et al 1978, Scadding et al 1981). Cells are cultured for 8–14 days in medium with fetal calf serum and antibiotics, and the supernatant is sampled at intervals. Anti-ACh receptor antibody is detectable from as early as Day 4 of culture, but is virtually absent if the cells are cultured with cycloheximide, indicating spontaneous synthesis of the antibody during the culture period. In most cases, the addition of pokeweed mitogen in optimal amounts did not further enhance antibody production, suggesting that the cells were already maximally stimulated *in vivo*.

   Production of anti-ACh receptor antibody was related to thymic histology, which was assessed without knowledge of the culture result. Anti-ACh receptor antibody synthesis rates exceeding 1 fmol/10⁶ cells per 24 hours occurred almost exclusively in patients with hyperplasia but did not appear to correlate with the degree of this change. We have now undertaken thymic culture studies in 64 patients. Of those with thymic hyperplasia, 68% have shown significant antibody production at rates up to $100\,\text{fmol}/10^6$ cells per 24 hours (Fig. 2). The amount of antibody produced correlates positively with

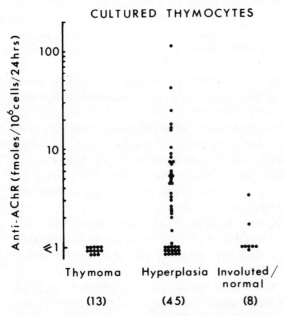

FIG. 2. Rate of anti-ACh receptor antibody production by cultured human thymocytes. Note the generally higher rates of production in thymic hyperplasia.

the duration of the disease. Most of the non-responders had serum anti-ACh receptor antibody titres below 20 nmol/l. Thymic cells from only two of eight patients with involuted or normal thymus synthesized antibody in culture; two of the negative cases were receiving immunosuppressive therapy at the time of surgery. None of the 13 thymoma patients produced appreciable amounts, even though several had very high serum titres of this antibody. However, supernatant from thymoma cases sometimes has a greater specific activity than serum, suggesting that small amounts of antibody may be synthesized or concentrated there *in vivo*.

   These differences in thymus antibody production, even if quantitative rather than qualitative, provide a further indication of heterogeneity in the clinical expression of MG. An estimate of the total ACh receptor antibody production in patients showing high rates of synthesis in culture indicates that the thymus produces only a small proportion of the total (probably < 5%). This is consistent with the observation that anti-ACh receptor antibody levels do not fall sharply after thymectomy, although a slow decline is evident in many patients over the first postoperative year. These long-term effects of thymectomy suggested that the thymus might in some way be aiding the production of antibody elsewhere, and we therefore explored this possibility by co-culturing autologous thymic and blood lymphocytes.

Thymic and peripheral blood cell co-cultures

Blood lymphocytes from myasthenic patients usually make little or no anti-ACh receptor antibody spontaneously in culture, although cells from a proportion of cases can be stimulated to do so by pokeweed mitogen. However, the addition of autologous thymic cells (irradiated with 1000–1500 rad [10–15 Gy] to abrogate their own antibody production and possible suppressor effects) can enhance anti-ACh receptor antibody production by blood lymphocytes up to 10-fold, in the absence of pokeweed (Newsom-Davis et al 1981). This response is as great as that produced by pokeweed mitogen stimulation of blood lymphocytes cultured alone, but occurs earlier and is more consistent. The effect appears to depend on viable thymic cells, since cells that were sonicated, or heated to 46 °C for 20 minutes, or repeatedly frozen and thawed, did not evoke any response. The ability of irradiated thymic cells to enhance the production of anti-ACh receptor antibody by blood lymphocytes seems to be selective for this antibody. Neither total IgG nor a different specific antibody, anti-influenza A (X31) antibody, was increased, although pokeweed mitogen could stimulate the production of both by blood lymphocytes cultured alone. Interestingly, pokeweed also stimulated the production of anti-influenza antibody by unirradiated thymic cells, indicating that the myasthenic thymus often contains influenza A-reactive B cells.

Thymic cells enhancing anti-ACh receptor antibody production

The thymic cells responsible for the selective enhancement of anti-ACh receptor antibody production would seem likely to be either antigen-presenting cells or helper T cells specific for the ACh receptor. Several studies have indicated that the thymus contains ACh receptor-like material on various cell types including myoid (muscle-like) cells, which have been shown to express the ACh receptor in culture (Kao & Drachman 1977). Wekerle & Ketelsen (1977) have suggested that an alteration in myoid cell receptor could lead to a breakdown in tolerance. Our finding that in generalized myasthenia, anti-ACh receptor antibody reacts better with receptor from denervated muscle than with normal ACh receptor is consistent with this hypothesis, since myoid cells are not innervated and their ACh receptors would be expected to be of the denervated (non-junctional) type. Other evidence for ACh receptors in the thymus exists: components of calf thymus appear to cross-react with *Torpedo* ACh receptor, and ACh receptor-like material has been precipitated from rat thymus using experimentally raised anti-ACh receptor antibody (see Vincent 1980). In addition, about 80% of mouse thymocytes have been reported to express ACh receptor-like material on their surface, as shown by indirect immunofluorescence using experimentally raised anti-ACh receptor antibody (Fuchs et al 1980). The only cell subset likely to constitute such a high proportion of thymic cells is the cortical (immature) thymocyte.

Whatever the cell types responsible for the presence of ACh receptor-like material in the thymus, there are also specialized antigen-presenting cells in large numbers in the medulla—the interdigitating reticular cells which possess large amounts of Ia (HLA-DR) antigens—which could take up the ACh receptor and present it to the lymphocytes in a very stimulating form.

We have done some preliminary experiments in which the contribution of these different cells types has been investigated using monoclonal antibodies to deplete certain cell subpopulations by complement-mediated lysis. The results of such an experiment are illustrated in Fig. 3 (left panel). Each vertical bar is the titre at eight days for supernatants pooled from triplicate culture wells. Thymic cells cultured alone made moderate amounts of anti-ACh receptor antibody and production was not appreciably enhanced by pokeweed mitogen. Rabbit complement alone produced a non-specific reduction in spontaneous anti-ACh receptor antibody synthesis, but the pokeweed response was unchanged. Depletion of cortical (T34$^+$) thymocytes, using the monoclonal antibody NA1/34(T34) which identifies this subset, considerably and consistently enhanced the spontaneous and pokeweed-stimulated responses (see also Fig 4), roughly in proportion to the enrichment of the thymic responder B cells.

Adherence-depletion of T34$^+$-depleted thymocytes, which would be expected to reduce the number of macrophages, did not substantially alter the spontaneous production of anti-ACh receptor antibody. Killing of Ia$^+$ cells, on the other hand, abolished antibody production, as would be expected, since B cells as well as antigen-presenting cells express the Ia antigen (Fig. 3).

To test whether T lymphocytes are necessary for the production of anti-ACh receptor antibodies by thymic cells we used a highly lytic IgM

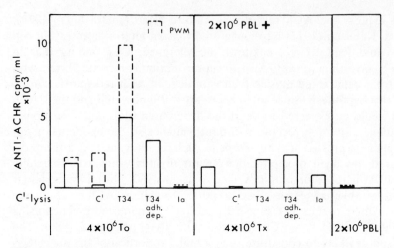

FIG. 3. Anti-ACh receptor antibody production (pool of triplicate 2 ml wells) in a patient with thymic hyperplasia, by (*left panel*) cultured thymic cells (To; 4 × 10⁶/well); (*centre panel*) blood lymphocytes (PBL; 2 × 10⁶/well) co-cultured with autologous irradiated thymic cells (Tx, 1250 rad [12.5 Gy]; 4 × 10⁶/well); and (*right panel*) PBL cultured alone (2 × 10⁶/well). Cell populations were depleted by complement (C′)-mediated lysis using the monoclonal antibody NA1/34 (T34) that identifies cortical thymocytes, without and with adherence depletion (adh.dep.), or an anti-Ia (HLA-DR) antibody. Results with pokeweed mitogen (PWM) at 10 μl/ml are shown by broken lines.

monoclonal antibody, MBG6, that identifies mature T cells, a major fraction of the medullary lymphocytes. Combined killing with this antibody plus NA1/34 enriched antibody production much more than did NA1/34 alone, again in proportion to the roughly 10-fold enrichment of B cells (Fig. 4). This suggests that T lymphocytes are not essential for these responses, though they might nevertheless be driven by accessory cells that have already adsorbed T cell factors *in vivo*. Alternatively, the T cells may exert their effects at some much earlier stage: we cannot therefore conclude that the anti-ACh receptor antibody response is T cell-independent.

In a parallel experiment to that described in Fig. 3 (left panel), thymic cells were irradiated (1250 rad [12.5 Gy]), subjected to a similar depletion of defined cell populations, and co-cultured with autologous peripheral blood lymphocytes (Fig. 3, centre panel). The irradiated thymic cells made negligible antibody when cultured alone, and this value has in any case been subtracted from the values plotted. Peripheral blood lymphocytes cultured alone or with pokeweed mitogen produced no anti-ACh receptor antibody (Fig. 3, right panel). The addition of irradiated thymocytes enhanced antibody production, as previously reported. This effect was lost when the irradiated thymic cells were treated with complement alone. Depletion of

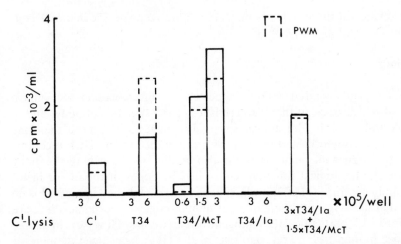

FIG. 4. Anti-ACh receptor antibody production (pool of triplicate microtitre wells) by cultured human thymic cells (0.6–6 × 10^5/well). Cell depletion was by complement (C')-mediated lysis using monoclonal antibody NA1/34 (T34) alone, or plus MBG6 (McT), which identifies mature T cells, or plus an anti-Ia monoclonal antibody. The response with pokeweed mitogen (PWM, at 10 μl/ml) is shown by broken lines.

T34+-irradiated thymic cells again re-enriched the enhancing activity and the relevant cells were non-adherent. These results, where blood lymphocytes were the responder cells (Fig. 3, centre), were broadly similar to those with unirradiated thymic cells cultured alone (Fig. 3, left). However, killing irradiated thymic cells with monoclonal anti-Ia (HLA-DR) antibody and complement clearly did not eliminate the enhancing effect but appeared rather to augment it; a similar result has been observed in another individual. This suggests that if antigen-presenting cells are responsible for the antibody response observed in these experiments, then either they are Ia⁻, or they are not readily killed by anti-Ia antibody. The effectiveness of the selective complement killing was indicated by the abrogation of antibody production, as shown in Fig. 3 (left).

An alternative cell type that might underlie this enhancement of antibody production would be an ACh receptor-specific helper T cell. Calculating the ratio of helper to suppressor cells in the thymus appeared to support this. We enumerated 'helper-inducer' and 'suppressor-cytotoxic' T cells by indirect immunofluorescence using the monoclonal antibodies OKT4 and OKT8, respectively, after removing the immature cortical thymocytes (T34+) that carry both the OKT4 and the OKT8 markers. The helper:suppressor (OKT4+: OKT8+) ratio in the thymus appeared to correlate significantly with the ability of the irradiated thymic cells to enhance anti-ACh receptor antibody production by autologous blood lymphocytes, raising the possibility that the thymus in these patients may contain antigen-specific helper T cells (Newsom-Davis et al 1981).

Conclusions

Heterogeneity in acquired MG is suggested by differences in the clinical features of the disease, in the characteristics of the specific antibody, and in the HLA and possibly Gm associations. This suggests that more than one mechanism may underlie the breakdown in tolerance to the ACh receptor, and that the trigger mechanisms might also be diverse. In view of the many important immunological functions controlled by genes of the major histo-compatibility complexes (MHC) which have been established in mice, it is no surprise that in MG—and in many other immunological disorders—there are associations with particular HLA antigens or haplotypes. However, in almost no instance in man has the relevant part of the HLA locus been defined, or the role of the MHC been clarified, even in general terms. We have previously suggested that the role of the HLA system in MG appears to be concerned more with determining the susceptibility of the individual to particular mechanisms causing breakdown in tolerance to ACh receptors than with determining the characteristics of the resulting immune response (Compston et al 1980).

The association of generalized (and thymomatous) MG with Gm allotype in Japanese patients (and possibly in ocular MG in Caucasians) suggests a role for inherited heavy chain variable (V_H) regions, which could be encoding part of a particular antibody against one crucial site on the ACh receptor. However, the heterogeneity of anti-ACh receptor antibodies that we have observed suggests that, at least in Caucasians with generalized MG, there is no single crucial antibody species. Alternatively, the V_H gene product may contribute to the structure of the helper T cell receptor for antigen, although it is still uncertain whether V_H regions are included in these receptors.

Longstanding clinical evidence implicating the thymus in MG, together with the experimental cell culture studies described here, establish that the thymus has an important role in the disease process. The non-thymomatous thymus contains not only ACh receptor-specific B cells but also cells that can selectively enhance anti-ACh receptor antibody production by autologous blood lymphocytes. We have not yet resolved the question of whether these cells are helper T cells or antigen-presenting cells (or both). If they are antigen-presenting cells, they appear not to express Ia, raising the possibility that they might be follicular dendritic cells. Could the thymus be the primary site of development of the autoimmune response, as has been suggested (Wekerle & Ketelsen 1977)? If one assumes that most autoantibody re-sponses are governed by T lymphocytes (not yet proven in man), the evidence that developing T cells learn to become tolerent to self antigens in the thymus lends some support to this view. So also does the presence in thymus of antigen and antigen-presenting cells. However, other possibilities have not yet been excluded, and we remain ignorant about the mechanisms that underlie the initiation of the autoimmune response.

Acknowledgements

We thank Ms Linda Calder for her help, Mr M. Sturridge and Dr L. Loh for assistance in obtaining thymus, Dr A. McMichael, Dr H. O. McDevitt and Professor W. Bodmer for the gift of monoclonal antibodies, and Dr G. Janossy for help and advice. This work was supported by the Medical Research Council.

REFERENCES

Barnes EW, Irvine WJ 1973 Clinical syndromes associated with thymic disorders. Proc R Soc Med 66:151-154

Berman PW, Patrick J 1980 Linkage between the frequency of muscular weakness and loci that regulate immune responsiveness in murine experimental myasthenia gravis. J Exp Med 152:507-520

Compston DAS, Vincent A, Newsom-Davis J, Batchelor JR 1980 Clinical, pathological, HLA antigen and immunological evidence for disease heterogeneity in myasthenia gravis. Brain 103:579-601

Elmqvist D, Hofmann WM, Kugelberg J, Quastel DMJ 1964 An electrophysiological investigation of neuromuscular transmission in myasthenia gravis. J Physiol (Lond) 174:417-434

Fambrough D, Drachman DB, Satyamurti S 1973 Neuromuscular junction in myasthenia gravis. Decreased acetylcholine receptors. Science (Wash DC) 182:293-295

Fuchs S, Schmidt-Hopfeld I, Tridente G, Tarrab-Hazdai R 1980 Thymic lymphocytes bear a surface antigen which cross-reacts with acetylcholine receptor. Nature (Lond) 287:162-164

Ito Y, Miledi R, Vincent A, Newsom-Davis J 1978 Acetylcholine receptors and end-plate electrophysiology in myasthenia gravis. Brain 101:345-368

Kao I, Drachman DB 1977 Thymic muscle cells bear acetylcholine receptors: possible relation to myasthenia gravis. Science (Wash DC) 195:74-75

Lindstrom JM, Seybold ME, Lennon VA, Whittingham S, Duane DD 1976 Antibody to acetylcholine receptor in myasthenia gravis. Prevalence, clinical correlates, and diagnostic value. Neurology 26:1054-1059

Lisak RP, Zweiman B, Phillips SM 1978 Thymic and peripheral blood T- and B-cell levels in myasthenia gravis. Neurology 28:1298-1301

Mittag T, Kornfeld P, Tormay A, Woo C 1976 Detection of anti-acetylcholine receptor factors in serum and thymus from patients with myasthenia gravis. N Engl J Med 294:691-694

Nakao Y, Miyazaki T, Ota K, Matsumoto H, Nishitani H, Fujita T, Tsuji K 1980 Gm allotypes in myasthenia gravis. Lancet 1:677-680

Newsom-Davis J, Pinching AJ, Vincent A, Wilson SG 1978 Function of circulating antibody to acetylcholine receptor in myasthenia gravis investigated by plasma exchange. Neurology 28:266-272

Newsom-Davis J, Willcox N, Calder L 1981 Thymus cells in myasthenia gravis selectively enhance production of anti-acetylcholine receptor antibody by autologous blood lymphocytes. N Engl J Med 305:1313-1318

Patrick J, Lindstrom JM 1973 Autoimmune response to acetylcholine receptor. Science (Wash DC) 180:871-872

Pirskanen R 1976 Genetic associations between myasthenia gravis and the HL-A system. J Neurol Neurosurg Psychiatry 39:23-33

Scadding GK, Vincent A, Newsom-Davis J, Henry K 1981 Acetylcholine receptor antibody synthesis by thymic lymphocytes: correlation with thymic histology. Neurology 31:935-43

Vincent A 1980 Immunology of acetylcholine receptors in relation to myasthenia gravis. Physiol Rev 60:756-824

Vincent A, Newsom-Davis J 1980 Anti-acetylcholine receptor antibodies. J Neurol Neurosurg Psychiatry 43:590-600

Vincent A, Newsom-Davis J 1982 Acetylcholine receptor antibody characteristics in myasthenia gravis. I. Patients with generalised myasthenia or disease restricted to ocular muscles. Clin Exp Immunol, in press

Vincent A, Scadding GK, Thomas HC, Newsom-Davis J 1978 In vitro synthesis of anti-acetylcholine receptor antibody by thymic lymphocytes in myasthenia gravis. Lancet 1:305-307

Vincent A, Cull-Candy SG, Newsom-Davis J, Trautmann A, Molenaar PC, Polak RL 1981 Congenital myasthenia: end-plate acetylcholine receptors and electrophysiology in five cases. Muscle & Nerve 4:306-318

Wekerle H, Ketelsen U-P 1977 Intrathymic pathogenesis and dual genetic control of myasthenia gravis. Lancet 1:678-680

Yoshida T, Tsuchiya M, Ono A, Yoshimatsu H, Satoyoshi E, Tsuji K 1977 HLA antigens and myasthenia in Japan. J Neurol Sci 32:195-201

DISCUSSION

Knight: You say that an antigen in the thymus seems to be analogous to the ACh receptor. Is it possible that as a result of somatic mutation, clones of ACh receptor-specific plasma cells are produced elsewhere in the body and, because the antigen is in the thymus, some of those plasma cells migrate there? The antigen-presenting effect that you describe may then be solely due to, say, thymic epithelial cells that have this antigen on their surface. To test this perhaps you could co-culture plasma cells from the thymus of a patient with myasthenia gravis with thymic cells from a normal subject, and test for ACh receptor antibodies.

Newsom-Davis: That ACh receptor-reactive B cells might migrate to the thymus cannot be excluded, and we have previously suggested this possibility to account for our finding that the rate of production of anti-ACh receptor antibody by cultured thymic cells correlates with the duration of the illness at the time of thymectomy (Scadding et al 1981). The mixed-culture study that you suggest is likely to be invalidated unless undertaken with HLA-matched material, however.

Rees Smith: I would like to pin the myasthenologists down on the effects of thymectomy. We have wide experience of looking at changes in anti-receptor antibody levels during treatment for Graves' disease. In our studies, we took blood samples from patients every two weeks or so, over a period of many months. We stored the sera and assayed them in the same assay against the same standards. Have you looked sequentially at 10 or 12 patients and assayed them individually in the same assay?

Newsom-Davis: We have studied 25 cases in this way, assaying serial serum samples, taken over periods ranging from one year to $4\frac{1}{2}$ years after thymectomy, for anti-ACh receptor antibody. In myasthenia, thymectomy is total, so we have a slightly cleaner effect than you do with partial thyroidectomy. At the end of the period of study, 25% of our patients were in remission and showed a fall in anti-receptor antibody to 75–27% of the pre-thymectomy value. Those who improved but still had symptoms showed as a group a less pronounced fall in antibody. Antibody did not generally show a sharp and sustained fall postoperatively but rather a slow decline. We have also cultured lymph node cells from patients of this type and find that they synthesize anti-receptor antibody. Thus there are other sites where the antibody might be produced and it is not therefore so surprising that thymectomy does not totally eliminate the antibody response.

Mitchison: In your cell separation studies, my impression is that cell depletion experiments tend to give spotty results. Are you thinking of switching over to positive cell selection? In particular, are you going to try stimulating T cells with the antigen and raising cell lines?

Newsom-Davis: Cell depletion is a sensible technique to use initially, when one is trying to define the active cell type, before we go on to confirm the results by positive selection.

Mitchison: Panning seems to be a cheap and effective method of selecting lymphocytes.

Knight: Why do you suggest cloning T cells, when T cells are apparently not involved?

Newsom-Davis: We don't think our findings should be taken as evidence that production of thymic anti-ACh receptor antibody is T cell-independent.

Mitchison: What about making cell lines of those T cells?

Newsom-Davis: We are already making plans to do that.

McLachlan: To return to your original thymic cultures, you were unable to increase ACh receptor antibody production using pokeweed mitogen; these results are in contrast to our own detailed studies (McLachlan et al 1981a). In your experiments, did pokeweed mitogen not increase the level of total IgG synthesized?

Newsom-Davis: Typically, total IgG production did increase, whereas anti-ACh receptor antibody levels did not.

McLachlan: Perhaps the T cells in the thymus of myasthenic patients are different from other T cells, if they are unable to respond to pokeweed. Your peripheral blood lymphocytes from those patients *do* respond.

Newsom-Davis: An alternative explanation is that B cells are already maximally activated *in vivo*. They certainly make antibody very early in culture, in contrast to the pokeweed response.

McLachlan: Did you try different concentrations of pokeweed?

Newsom-Davis: Yes. The optimal concentration seems to be 10 μl/ml.

McLachlan: If you infect thymic lymphocytes with Epstein-Barr virus, can you also stimulate ACh receptor antibody synthesis, as we have done for thyroid autoantibodies using peripheral blood lymphocytes from patients with Hashimoto's disease (McLachlan et al 1981b)?

Newsom-Davis: Yes; we found that infection of myasthenic thymic lymphocytes by Epstein-Barr virus enhanced the production of anti-ACh receptor antibody.

McLachlan: How does the specific activity of that increase in antibody compare with the pokeweed-stimulated response? It seems that EB virus tends to trigger a different (perhaps less mature) cell population than does pokeweed in the peripheral blood (Pasquali et al 1981). It would be interesting to know whether large amounts of total IgG are produced and whether you are triggering thymic B cells other than those producing autoantibody early in culture.

Newsom-Davis: We have not yet looked at that.

McLachlan: What happened to the levels of total IgG synthesized after adding irradiated thymic lymphocytes to peripheral blood lymphocytes in the *absence* of pokeweed?

Newsom-Davis: The anti-receptor antibody activity was much enhanced but the effects on total IgG were minimal.

Kahn: Your subdivision of myasthenia by thymus pathology is reminiscent of a pattern that one might make for diabetes mellitus. That is to say, one can divide diabetics into early-onset and late-onset. In the latter patients, the islet cells are maintained, whereas in early-onset diabetes they are depleted. There are anti-islet cell antibodies in early-onset diabetes and not in the late-onset disease. Also, the HLA associations are different in the two forms. We believe that these are diseases of different aetiology even though they have the same final manifestation. Does the thymic pathology suggest that myasthenia gravis is a disease of several different aetiologies? If so, what are the aetiologies? We have heard some elegant studies of myasthenia but nobody has addressed the question of the inciting factor in this disease.

Newsom-Davis: Our evidence for heterogeneity in myasthenia suggests to us that the mechanisms for autommunity may differ in the several forms of MG, as may the putative triggering factor(s).

Drachman: We have searched for a recoverable virus in thymus glands of patients with myasthenia gravis. Thymus glands from nine myasthenic patients, some with recent onset of the disease, were studied in the laboratory of Dr C. Gibbs, in collaboration with Dr Aoki. This material was studied by tissue culture, co-cultivation with a variety of cell lines, inoculation of animals, and the use of fluorescence antibody techniques. All these studies have been negative. This does not prove that a virus could not be present, but only that it could not be revealed or 'rescued' by these techniques. Moreover, a viral infection at some site other than the thymus gland remains a possibility.

Newsom-Davis: We have investigated serum antibody levels against a number of common viruses, including rubella, cytomegalovirus, herpes simplex type 1, varicella zoster, influenza A and measles, and have found no significant differences from controls (L. Klavinskis, J. Oxford, N. Willcox & J. Newsom-Davis, unpublished observations). The virological findings in a young patient of ours are of interest in this context. She developed symptoms of myasthenia gravis at 15 years and had had juvenile rheumatoid arthritis since early childhood. The serum anti-rubella antibody titre was very high in samples taken in 1974 and 1978 (kindly made available to us by Dr Barbara Ansell) and in 1981. Anti-ACh receptor antibody, however, was not detected in the two early samples, but was present at high titre in 1981. One wonders whether the persistent and extraordinarily high levels of anti-rubella antibody, and the development of antibodies to the ACh receptor, might reflect a common feature of disordered immune regulation.

Harrison: Did she receive penicillamine?

Newsom-Davis: No.

Mitchison: Should we consider antibody heterogeneity in this disease? The evidence on ϰ and λ light chains is evidence of heterogeneity. What about heterogeneity in isoelectric point? We heard earlier that anti-thyroid receptor antibodies are heterogeneous in this respect. Could you perhaps examine their spectrotype?

Vincent: Bethan Lang and I have tried isoelectric focusing of MG sera but haven't been very successful in demonstrating clear bands of anti-ACh receptor activity. Ann-Kari Lefvert (Lefvert & Bergström 1978) also found rather broad regions of anti-ACh receptor antibody on preparative focusing.

Lindstrom: The isoelectric focusing pattern of anti-receptor antibodies is also very heterogeneous in EAMG. Dr Mark De Baetes, working with Dr Ari Theofilopoulos, has done these experiments.

Mitchison: So the antibody is heterogeneous in charge but remarkably confined in what it recognizes. What is the likely mechanism for confining a multiclonal response so that it is directed at, perhaps, a single epitope?

Knight: Perhaps there are shared idiotypes on the precursors of multiple clones with similar paratopes.

Newsom-Davis: Or on the T cell receptor?

Lindstrom: I don't think that the antibodies to the main immunogenic region are likely to be identical in idiotype. We can't even say that a single antigenic determinant is involved in the main immunogenic region of the receptor. Vanda Lennon (Lennon & Lambert 1981) has raised high titres of anti-idiotype antibody in rats immunized with monoclonal antibodies to receptor which were probably directed against the main immunogenic region. This antibody didn't suppress the initiation of EAMG subsequently in these rats. So even in this particularly immunogenic part of the receptor molecule, a range of antibodies could be produced. I think this is simply what happens as a result of the structural properties of the receptor molecule. Most patients in our study make most of their antibodies against the main immunogenic region of the α subunit, but even patients making a high proportion of their antibodies to this region also make antibodies to determinants on β and γ subunits, and some also make antibodies to other determinants on the α subunits that we can detect. In addition they may also make other antibodies that we don't detect with the monoclonals we have used for screening. There are rare patients (six out of 87) who make a large proportion of their antibodies to a determinant on the α subunit other than the main immunogenic region.

Mitchison: What is going on in those few patients?

Lindstrom: I suppose this may reflect their immune response gene repertoire, in that this other structure, which is present on all these receptors, happens to provoke a response in these rare patients.

Mitchison: Isn't that unlikely, if the antibodies are heterogeneous?

Crumpton: Some years ago, various workers including myself studied the nature of protein antigenic determinants using a variety of model globular proteins (Crumpton 1974). The collective results of these studies suggest that proteins possess 'antigenic regions' (an immunogenic region, as Jon Lindstrom would call it), the size of each region being larger than the combining site on an individual antibody molecule. In this case it is possible to generate a variety of antibodies against the same region that see overlapping (i.e. different) portions of the region; the antibodies conceivably also recognize different immunodominant groups. If these interpretations are correct, then it is even possible to generate a heterogeneous antibody response against an individual immunogenic region.

Roitt: The situation here, with myasthenia, is exactly the same as with antibodies to thyroglobulin in Hashimoto's disease. There are perhaps only two different regions on this very large molecule. All patients make antibodies to the same two epitopes. The response is poly-disperse in that it is poly-spectrotypic and poly-idiotypic. One can only argue that certain parts of the antigen are particularly vulnerable to *not* suppressing the potential response.

Kahn: To further complicate the issue, consider the antigen with which the

T cell is presented by the macrophage. The T cell may not be recognizing the same region of that antigen to which the final antibody is produced. Certainly for insulin there is a discordance between the part of the molecule that causes the T cell to proliferate and the site to which the immunoglobulin binds (Rosenthal 1978). If this is correct, does the fact that a patient has an antibody directed to a certain antigenic site necessarily mean that that was the antigen which was initially recognized? It could have been the whole molecule, or a different domain which included, or didn't include entirely, all of that site. Is that correct?

Crumpton: Yes, the T cell does not necessarily recognize the same structure as is recognized by the B cell. Further, if antigen processing, including possibly degradation and/or presentation in association with class II histocompatibility antigens, is a prerequisite for T cell recognition, then what the T cell sees could be very different from what interacts with the B cell.

Mitchison: This is true, but there is another phenomenon that myasthenia patients show, namely the propensity of individuals to *narrow* their response to a protein to one particular region, or even a single epitope. They then go on making antibody against that region when other individuals make other antibodies.

Crumpton: That is an interesting point; but I was trying to suggest that monoclonality is not the way in which we shall recognize antibody against a particular antigenic region.

Mitchison: That is exactly the point, that these restricted-determinant responses are not monoclonal; they can be 'monoregional', but polyclonal. So, therefore, restriction is not something to do with the combining site of the antibody.

Lindstrom: I think that there are structures on the ACh receptor which are inherently immunogenic, but would not lead to a monoclonal antibody response. The main immunogenic region happens to be a part of the molecule which, although conformationally dependent, is very resistant to proteases, whereas proteolysis destroys several of the determinants on the α subunit. Perhaps the main immunogenic region is immunogenic in part because it survives 'antigen processing' by macrophages.

MG antibodies are highly species-specific for human receptors, although we see some slight cross-reaction with the *Torpedo* receptor. We (M. De Baetes et al, unpublished) looked at stimulation of the proliferation of peripheral blood lymphocytes from MG patients by purified receptor (presumably a T cell response). Using receptor from *Torpedo* electric organ we obtained very small responses. Surprisingly, the response was no better with receptor from human muscle. This suggests that the specificities of the receptor-specific T helper cells are fundamentally different from the specificities of anti-receptor antibody-producing B cells in myasthenia gravis patients.

Venter: Has anyone looked at cooperativity in the binding of multiple antibody molecules to the receptor or other antigens in a situation such as this where you have multiple determinants and a polyclonal response? The heterogeneity of charge was discussed. There may be different charge interactions between cooperating IgG molecules. Ron Kahn commented earlier on the multiplicities of binding affinities (p 72). It is possible that you obtain cooperating complexes?

Lindstrom: Mark De Baetes (unpublished) has done isoelectric focusing on EAMG sera, as I mentioned. He sees a number of discrete bands of anti-receptor antibody. He tried doing competitions with monoclonal antibodies, to try to take out particular specificities at specific isoelectric points. There was no correlation between isoelectric point and specificity.

Roitt: The problem with the poly-spectrotypic isoelectric focusing is that you may have identical V_H regions giving multiple spectrotypes, because of differences in isotype in the heavy chain, and differences in the light chains. A variety of light chains will still give specific antigen binding.

Rodbell: Thinking of the presentation and processing of antigen, could we suppose that the receptor for acetylcholine is initially a very large molecule which has to be cut up into small pieces before it is inserted in the membrane, and that the processing by which it is normally put into the membrane, as a five-part segment which makes a channel, doesn't happen with some cells? Instead it passes out of the cell and is now a ligand (antigen) for those cells which can process it in a different way. This might be only a small amount of material, but enough to trigger off the antigen-presenting cells, to make the whole process unique for that particular form of the receptor that came out of the cell instead of staying in the membrane. One could mimic this, perhaps, by extracting receptor components from the membrane.

Lindstrom: In fact, the receptor subunits are normally synthesized individually rather than synthesized as a large piece (Anderson & Blobel 1981, Merlie et al 1981).

Vincent: What do you think of the possibility that the response is directed against isolated α subunits, which we know can be made in soluble form in cell-free systems (Merlie et al 1981) and which don't bind bungarotoxin (Mendez et al 1980)? Most of the anti-ACh receptor antibodies don't inhibit the binding of bungarotoxin to the receptor, which suggests that the binding site may not be intact in the autoantigen. Moreover, this would explain why it is apparently not possible to find circulating ACh receptor by using bungarotoxin binding (unpublished results). Perhaps the autoimmune response is directed against nascent subunits before they associate to form the fully functional, α-bungarotoxin-binding ACh receptor.

Lindstrom: Newly synthesized α chains not only cannot bind toxin, they do not bind antibodies to the main immunogenic region (J. P. Merlie et al, unpublished). Therefore I think it unlikely that isolated α subunits provoke the autoimmune response. The second most prominent specificity that we saw, after the main immunogenic region, was the γ subunit unit, so a number of subunits appear to be involved in the immune response. Also, the pattern of specificities of antibodies produced by MG patients closely resembles that produced by rats immunized with intact receptor.

Drachman: Another argument against isolated ACh receptor being the primary antigen is that 50% of myasthenic patients have anti-skeletal *muscle* antibody as well as anti-ACh receptor antibody; almost 100% of the patients with thymoma have anti-muscle antibody. This could mean that ACh receptor *as a component of skeletal muscle* serves as the antigen.

Vincent: These muscle proteins are intracellular, and one would find nascent chains intracellularly. I don't know if anyone has looked for them in the circulation. Since we don't think that the thymus is the main source of anti-ACh receptor antibodies, there must be antibody synthesis elsewhere, and circulating antigens could be responsible for stimulating the response in the peripheral immune system.

Lindstrom: Dr John Merlie has shown (Merlie et al 1982) that antibodies specific for denatured α chains react quite well with nascent α chains in muscle, but that antibodies to native receptor (i.e., antibodies mainly directed against the main immunogenic region) don't react until a maturation process has taken place over about 15 minutes, involving subunit interaction and the maturity to be able to bind toxin. So I don't think the α subunit exists in this way you suggest, or that the main immunogenic region would exist in a free α subunit.

Mitchison: If one is thinking about antibodies against muscle proteins, Dr Engel showed a micrograph of a macrophage running underneath an end-plate and exposed to muscle on its other side (not reproduced). That macrophage might act as an antigen-presenting cell seeing muscle.

Roitt: Is there any information on the use of the antisera or monoclonal antibodies to investigate the presence of receptor-like material in the human circulation? We really have no idea of what the concentrations are. Myelin basic protein-like material can apparently be detected in the circulation, even though myelin basic protein was thought to be entirely restricted to the brain. There may be many proteins circulating that we haven't had the right methods to test for.

Kahn: Probably every protein is circulating in some small concentration, yet we don't have an autoimmune disease to every known protein. The most common serum proteins are not those commonly associated with autoimmune responses. If we knew that ACh receptor was present in the circulation, would this help us in deciding anything about the pathogenesis of the disease?

Roitt: It might depend on the circulating concentration. If you looked at the unaffected relatives of patients with myasthenia gravis and you found, for example, that they had a very different level of circulating acetylcholine receptor-like material, that might be a clue to a genetic influence on the level of this (hypothetical) circulating material.

Kahn: But consider thyroglobulin, where you know that a small amount is present normally in the circulation; has that helped to unravel the pathogenesis of Hashimoto's thyroiditis, in which there is an anti-thyroglobulin antibody?

Roitt: Noel Rose is now looking at the effects of changing the circulating level of thyroglobulin (by giving TRH to change the activity of the thyroid) on the induction of experimental allergic encephalitis. But from the point of view of pathogenesis, the thyroglobulin coming from the thyroid acini into the extra-acinar space provides the focus for the agents of the immune response to initiate an inflammatory focus.

Friesen: For the record, would Jon Lindstrom answer Ron Kahn's assertion that we will learn nothing new using monoclonal antibodies?

Kahn: He has already proved me wrong! He has shown that using monoclonal antibodies you can determine antigen-binding sites with a fair degree of specificity. My point was, however, that we have not really learned anything about the fundamental mechanism of the disease.

REFERENCES

Anderson D, Blobel G 1981 *In vitro* synthesis, glycosylation and membrane insertion of the four subunits of *Torpedo* acetylcholine receptor. Proc Natl Acad Sci USA 78:5598-5602

Crumpton MJ 1974 In: Sela M (ed) The antigens. Academic Press, New York, vol 3:1-78

Lefvert A-K, Bergström K 1978 Acetylcholine receptor antibody in myasthenia gravis; purification and characterization. Scand J Immunol 8:525-534

Lennon VA, Lambert EH 1981 Antigenicity of acetylcholine receptors. Ann NY Acad Sci, in press

McLachlan SM, Nicholson LVB, Venables G, Mastaglia FL, Rees Smith B, Hall R 1981a Acetylcholine receptor antibody synthesis in lymphocyte cultures. J Clin Lab Immunol 5:137-142

McLachlan SM, Bird AG, Weetman AP, Rees Smith B, Hall R 1981b Use of plaque assays to study thyroglobulin autoantibody synthesis by human peripheral blood lymphocytes. Scand J Immunol 14:233-242

Mendez B, Valenzuela P, Martial J, Baxter J 1980 Cell free synthesis of acetylcholine receptor polypeptides. Science (Wash DC) 209:695-697

Merlie JP, Hofler JG, Sebbane R 1981 Acetylcholine receptor synthesis from membrane polysomes. J Biol Chem 256:6995-6999

Merlie JP, Sebbane R, Tzartos S, Lindstrom J 1982 Inhibition of glycosylation with tunicamycin blocks assembly of newly synthesized acetylcholine receptor subunits in muscle cells. J Biol Chem 257:2694-2701

Pasquali JL, Fong S, Tsoukas CD, Slovin SF, Vaughan JH, Carson DA 1981 Different populations of rheumatoid factor idiotypes induced by two polyclomal B cell activators, pokeweed mitogen and Epstein Barr virus. Clin Immunol Immunopathol 21:184-189

Scadding GK, Vincent A, Newsom-Davis J, Henry K 1981 Acetylcholine receptor antibody synthesis by thymic lymphocytes: correlation with thymic histology. Neurology 31:935-943

Rosenthal AS 1978 Determinant selection and macrophage function in genetic control of the immune response. Immunol Rev 40:136-152

Atopy, autonomic function and β-adrenergic receptor autoantibodies

LEN C. HARRISON, JUDY CALLAGHAN, J. CRAIG VENTER,* CLAIRE M. FRASER* and MICHAEL L. KALINER**

*The Endocrine Laboratory, Royal Melbourne Hospital, P.O. 3050, Victoria, Australia, *State University of New York, Buffalo, New York 14214 and **National Institutes of Health, Bethesda, Maryland 20205, USA*

Abstract Atopic individuals (with asthma, allergic rhinitis or atopic eczema) have impaired sensitivity to β-adrenergic agents. After the finding of antibodies to the β-adrenergic receptor in the serum of a subject with allergic rhinitis, coded sera from atopic and control subjects were assayed for immunoglobulins that inhibited the specific binding of ^{125}I-labelled hydroxybenzylpindolol to β-receptors in mammalian lung membranes. Antibodies were present in nine of 60 subjects: 3/19 normal control subjects, 1/9 pre-allergic, 4/17 asthma, 0/8 allergic rhinitis, and 1/7 cystic fibrosis patients. Antibodies of the IgG class in these sera were also demonstrated by indirect precipitation of solubilized lung β-receptors. The autonomic sensitivity of the nine antibody-positive subjects (Ab⁺) was compared with that of antibody-negative subjects (Ab⁻). The Ab⁺ subjects required 15.0 ± 1.9 ng isoprenaline (isoproterenol) kg⁻¹ min⁻¹ i.v. to increase pulse pressure by at least 22 mmHg (Ab⁻, 7.7 ± 0.4; $n = 20$; $P < 0.001$), and 12.4 ± 1.8 ng isoprenaline kg⁻¹ min⁻¹ i.v. to increase plasma cyclic AMP concentrations by 50% (Ab⁻, 8.08 ± 0.62; $n = 13$; $P < 0.02$). Ab⁺ subjects required 2.06 ± 0.3% phenylephrine to dilate their pupils (Ab⁻, 2.55 ± 0.08; $n = 57$; $P < 0.05$) and 0.61 ± 0.08% carbachol to constrict their pupils (Ab⁻, 0.78 ± 0.03%; $n = 57$; $P < 0.05$).

A role for autoantibodies as β-receptor antagonists was further supported by showing that human lung cells (VA-13 line) cultured in the presence of globulins from Ab⁺ subjects had a markedly impaired cyclic AMP response to isoprenaline. These results suggest that autoantibodies to β-receptors play a pathogenetic role in asthma and related disorders. They have important implications for the concept of autoimmunity.

Atopy (Greek: 'strange disease'), a term introduced by Coca & Cooke (1923), now denotes a state characterized by: (1) familial predisposition to asthma, allergic rhinitis ('hay fever'), eczema, or urticaria (skin weals), (2) increased levels of serum immunoglobulin E (IgE), and (3) abnormal autonomic reactivity. The latter encompasses decreased sensitivity to β-

1982 Receptors, antibodies and disease. Pitman,London (Ciba Foundation symposium 90) p 248-262

adrenergic agonists and increased sensitivity of α-adrenergic and cholinergic agonists (Szentivanyi 1980).

Coca & Cooke (1923) reported the clinical and familial association between the above-mentioned diseases and suspected a common immunopathological basis. Consistent with this notion was the fact that the 'immediate hypersensitivity' of (atopic) individuals to extrinsic 'allergens' could be passively transferred by blood or serum (Prausnitz & Küstner 1921). However, the effector role of the immune system in atopy has not been well defined, beyond the demonstration that IgE provoked by allergens triggers the release of smooth muscle constrictors such as histamine from mast cells. What of the autonomic abnormalities in atopy, and their relationship to immune function? A possible connection between allergy and immunity is our discovery of autoantibodies to the β_2-adrenergic receptor in an atopic subject (Venter et al 1980), and the subsequent demonstration that such antibodies are associated with autonomic dysfunction (Venter et al 1981).

Atopy and autonomic function

Studies performed *in vivo*, beginning two decades ago, have established that asthmatic subjects have an impaired response to β-adrenergic agonists. The reduced effect of adrenaline (epinephrine) or isoprenaline (isoproterenol) on plasma levels of glucose, free fatty acids and cyclic AMP or on pulse pressure in asthmatics is correlated with an enhanced effect of acetylcholine or histamine on bronchial constriction (reviewed by Parker 1973, Szentivanyi 1980). In the late 1960s Szentivanyi (1968) proposed the β-adrenergic theory of asthma: an imbalance in autonomic control due to decreased β-adrenergic sensitivity of bronchial smooth muscle, mucous glands and mucosal vessels. During the next several years this hypothesis gained support from studies showing impaired cyclic AMP responses specifically to β-adrenergic agents in leucocytes from asthmatics (Logsdon et al 1972, Parker & Smith 1973, Conolly & Greenacre 1976, Makino et al 1977; for further discussion see Szentivanyi 1980). These findings raised the question of whether there was an intrinsic defect in the β-receptor.

Attempts to directly define β-receptors by the binding of the tritiated form of the natural agonist, adrenaline, were fraught with technical problems, but with the advent of the high affinity antagonists, [³H]dihydroalprenolol and ¹²⁵I-labelled hydroxybenzylpindolol (IHYP), it became possible in the mid-1970s to identify sites that fulfilled the criteria for specific β-adrenergic receptors (reviewed by Hoffman & Lefkowitz 1980). In keeping with the previous studies on biological responses it was then shown that cells from asthmatics did indeed show a reduction in the apparent number of β-receptors

(Kariman & Lefkowitz 1977, Galant et al 1978, Brooks et al 1979), although this was attributed solely to the down-regulation of receptors following the administration of β-adrenergic drugs for the treatment of asthma. Drug-induced down-regulation of receptor concentrations (and desensitization of post-receptor pathways) certainly occurs, but the evidence from studies in untreated and asymptomatic subjects clearly indicates that a defect in β-receptor binding is a primary feature of asthma (see Szentivanyi 1980). Similar conclusions apply also to subjects with atopic eczema and are consistent with the impaired catecholamine responses in skin from such subjects (Busse & Lee 1976).

Recently, the decrease in β-receptor binding in atopic subjects has been linked with an increase in α-adrenergic receptor binding, and Szentivanyi has expanded his theory to a 'dual receptor' hypothesis (Szentivanyi 1980).

Atopy, autonomic function and autoimmunity

In 1978 one of us (LC.H.) began a search for autoantibodies which might stimulate the parathyroid glands in patients with primary hyperparathyroid-ism—by analogy with the thyroid-stimulating antibodies found in patients with Graves' disease. Isolated bovine parathyroid cells obtained from Dr Edward Brown of the National Institutes of Health were incubated with dilutions of sera from patients or control subjects. After washing, the cells were exposed to an excess of ^{125}I-labelled protein A (Goding 1980) and specific uptake of radioactivity was used to indicate the presence of residual surface-bound IgG. Two of the sera tested were positive, in that they contained IgG to a component of bovine parathyroid cell membrane, but neither was from a patient with hyperparathyroidism. One was from a control subject suffering from asthma. The parathyroid cells were known to possess β-adrenergic receptors and these findings, coupled with our interest in autoimmune receptor disease, led us to speculate that asthmatics might produce autoantibodies to the β-adrenergic receptor. Subsequently, the ^{125}I-protein A assay, using human placental membranes, was applied to the screening of coded sera from atopic patients under the care of M.L.K. Three sera that were positive in the protein A assay, seven negative sera and four control sera were coded and sent to J.C.V. and C.M.F. to test for antibodies that might specifically immunoprecipitate solubilized lung β-receptors. Three of the 14 samples contained IgGs which indirectly immunoprecipitated Triton-solubilized canine lung β-receptors pre-labelled with IHYP (Venter et al 1980). These three samples, one from a patient with allergic rhinitis and two from patients with asthma, were those that had been positive in the protein A assay (human placental membranes used for the protein A screening assay were shown to contain 30 fmol of IHYP binding sites per mg protein).

In the initial report of these findings (Venter et al 1980) IgG from the patient with allergic rhinitis also inhibited the binding of IHYP to lung and placenta but not cardiac membranes (Fig. 1), indicating that at least some of

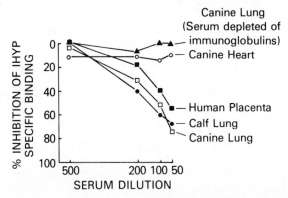

FIG. 1. Effect of serum no. 10 (subject R.W.) on binding of ^{125}I-labelled hydroxybenzylpindolol (IHYP) to membrane-bound β-adrenergic receptors. Purified membranes were incubated with dilutions of serum no. 10 or control serum in binding assay buffer (50 mM-Hepes, 4 mM-MgSO$_4$, pH 8.0), for 60 min at 30 °C. Canine lung membranes were also incubated with dilutions of serum no. 10 depleted of gamma globulins by immunoprecipitation with sheep anti-human globulin. The membranes were washed once in assay buffer and specific IHYP binding was measured as previously described (Venter et al 1980). Percentage inhibition of specific IHYP binding was determined from the ratio of IHYP bound in the presence of serum no. 10 to that bound in the presence of control serum. Binding with control serum at dilutions > 1:100 was the same as with buffer alone.

the antibodies recognized determinants on β$_2$-receptors *in situ*, at or near the ligand-binding site. The inability to totally immunoprecipitate all available IHYP-labelled receptors, and the lower titre with immunoprecipitation than with binding inhibition, suggested that the antibodies in this one serum were predominantly directed at the IHYP-binding site in the solubilized receptor.

In a follow-up study, specific, anti-β-receptor IgG antibodies were detected in nine of 60 coded sera: from 3/19 normal control subjects, 1/9 pre-allergic, 4/17 asthma, 0/8 allergic rhinitis, and 1/7 cystic fibrosis patients (Fraser et al 1980). Most importantly, we showed that the presence of these antibodies was associated with autonomic abnormalities (Fraser et al 1980, Venter et al 1981). Subjects with these antibodies require higher doses of isoprenaline to be infused to raise their pulse pressure or plasma cyclic AMP concentration. Moreover, this evidence for β-adrenergic resistance was accompanied by increased sensitivity to the effects of the α-adrenergic agonist, phenylephrine,

TABLE 1 Association between β-adrenergic receptor antibody status and autonomic sensitivity

	Antibody positive	Antibody negative	Significance[a]
Infusion rate of isoprenaline (ng kg^{-1} min^{-1}) to increase: pulse pressure by > 22 mmHg	15.0 ± 1.90 (n = 9)	7.7 ± 0.40 (n = 20)	$P < 0.001$
plasma cyclic AMP by > 50%	12.4 ± 1.80 (n = 9)	8.1 ± 0.62 (n = 13)	$P < 0.02$
Phenylephrine (%) to dilate pupils by >0.5 mm	2.06 ± 0.30 (n = 9)	2.55 ± 0.08 (n = 57)	$P < 0.05$
Carbachol (%) to constrict pupils by >0.5 mm	0.61 ± 0.08 (n = 9)	0.78 ± 0.03 (n = 57)	$P < 0.05$

[a] Student's t test.

on pupillary dilatation and by increased sensitivity to the effects of the cholinergic agent, carbachol, on pupillary constriction (Table 1). It is also interesting to note that the three control subjects with anti-receptor antibodies required a greater dose of isoprenaline to raise their pulse pressure (12.0 ± 1.73 ng kg^{-1} min^{-1}) than the 16 control subjects without antibodies (7.5 ± 0.55 ng kg^{-1} min^{-1}).

Our further studies on the molecular actions of β-adrenergic receptor autoantibodies are consistent with a role as β-receptor antagonists. Thus, we have shown that after preincubation of cultured human lung cells (VA-13 line) with anti-receptor IgG there is a marked decrease in the sensitivity and responsiveness of cyclic AMP to stimulation by isoprenaline (Fig. 2). It remains to be shown whether this effect is due to blockade at the receptor level only, or whether other mechanisms, such as desensitization at a post-receptor step or accelerated receptor loss, are also involved.

A unified hypothesis?

Our findings are consistent with a primary role for β-receptor autoantibodies in mediating autonomic dysfunction in at least some atopic subjects. The simplest interpretation is that the antibodies impair β-receptor-mediated relaxation of airways smooth muscle and unmask the opposing influence of other mediators, such as α-receptor agonists and acetylcholine. However, it will be important also to delineate the relationship of β-adrenergic function to other features of atopy, such as the triggering of histamine release from mast

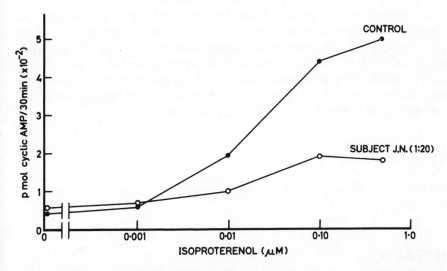

FIG. 2. Inhibition of the cyclic AMP response to isoprenaline (isoproterenol) in human lung fibroblasts exposed to serum globulins from an asthmatic subject, J.N. Human lung fibroblasts (WI 38, subline VA-13) were grown to confluence on plastic wells in RPMI 1640 medium supplemented with 2 mM-glutamine, 10% fetal calf serum and 25 mM-Hepes. Serum from subject J.N. or control serum (heat-inactivated for 30 min at 56 °C) was added to the culture medium for 90 min at 37 °C, in a final dilution of 1:20. The medium was then decanted and replaced with assay buffer (50 mM-Hepes, 2 mM-MgSO$_4$, 20 μM-Ro, a phosphodiesterase inhibitor) and the indicated concentrations of isoprenaline. After incubation for 30 min at 37 °C, boiling 50 mM-sodium acetate (pH 6.2) was added to each well. Detached cells were boiled for a further 3 min, the suspension was centrifuged, and an aliquot of the supernatant was taken for measurement of immunoreactive cyclic AMP using the New England Nuclear kit.

cells by IgE, and to determine whether autoantibodies to other receptors are involved. Furthermore, we do not understand what determines the anatomical localization of atopic manifestations—to the lower airways in asthma, the upper airways in allergic rhinitis, and the skin in urticaria and atopic eczema. There are also implications for the treatment of atopic diseases. Corticosteroids and immunosuppressive drugs, used occasionally for intractable asthma or atopic eczema, might impair autoantibody production. Plasmapheresis, reported to be effective in a single case of severe asthma (Gartmann et al 1978), also warrants appraisal.

Atopy must now be placed within the spectrum of autoimmune disorders. This concept is supported by the demonstration of defective suppressor T lymphocytes in atopic subjects (Rola-Pleszczynski & Blanchard 1981). Clearly, 'forbidden clones' that recognize self antigens may be more pervasive than was hitherto suspected. On the other hand, if autoimmunity is a naturally regulated state (Jerne 1974), perhaps it should be viewed as a continuum:

from a normal state of regulated autoimmunity, through the emergence of (?)non-pathogenic autoantibodies with advancing age or after exposure to certain drugs, to the emergence of pathogenic autoantibodies in classic autoimmune states. The latter autoantibodies usually mediate tissue destruction in conjunction with mononuclear cells or complement, but there may be less extreme situations, exemplified by atopy, where the manifestations are due solely to the specific effects of autoantibodies.

Acknowledgements

We are grateful to Mrs Linda Stafford for secretarial assistance.

REFERENCES

Brooks SM, McGowan K, Bernstein IL, Altenau P, Peagler J 1979 Relationship between numbers of beta adrenergic receptors in lymphocytes and disease severity in asthma. J Allergy Clin Immunol 63:401-406

Busse WW, Lee TP 1976 Decreased adrenergic responses in lymphocytes and granulocytes in atopic eczema. J Allergy Clin Immunol 58:586-596

Coca AF, Cooke RA 1923 On the classification of the phenomena of hypersensitiveness. J Immunol 8:163-168

Conolly ME, Greenacre JK 1976 The lymphocyte beta-adrenoceptor in normal subjects and patients with bronchial asthma: the effect of different forms of treatment on receptor function. J Clin Invest 58:1307-1316

Fraser CM, Harrison LC, Kaliner MC, Venter JC 1980 Autoantibodies to the β-adrenergic receptor are associated with β-adrenergic hyporesponsiveness. Clin Res 28:236A (abstr)

Gartmann J, Grob P, Frey M 1978 Plasmapheresis in severe asthma. Lancet 2:40 (letter)

Galant SP, Duriseti L, Underwood S, Insel PA 1978 Decreased beta-adrenergic receptors on polymorphonuclear leukocytes after adrenergic therapy. N Engl J Med 299:933-936

Goding JW 1978 Use of staphylococcal protein A as an immunological reagent. J Immunol Methods 20:241-253

Hoffman BB, Lefkowitz RJ 1980 Radioligand binding studies of adrenergic receptors: new insights into molecular and physiological regulation. Annu Rev Pharmacol Toxicol 20:581-608

Jerne NK 1974 Towards a network theory of the immune system. Ann Immunol (Paris) 125C:373-389

Kariman K, Lefkowitz RJ 1977 Decreased beta adrenergic receptor binding in lymphocytes from patients with bronchial asthma. Clin Res 25:503A (abstr)

Logsdon PJ, Middleton E, Coffey RG 1972 Stimulation of leukocyte adenyl cyclase by hydrocortisone and isoproterenol in asthmatic and nonasthmatic subjects. J Allergy Clin Immunol 50:45-56

Makino S, Ikemori K, Kashima T, Fukada T 1977 Comparison of cyclic adenosine monophosphate response of lymphocytes in normal and asthmatic subjects to norepinephrine and salbutamol. J Allergy Clin Immunol 59:348-352

Parker CW 1973 Adrenergic responsiveness in asthma. In: Austen KF, Lichtenstein LM (eds)

Asthma. Physiology, immunopharmacology, and treatment. Academic Press, New York, p 185-210

Parker CW, Smith JW 1973 Alterations in cyclic adenosine monophosphate metabolism in human bronchial asthma. I. Leukocyte responsiveness to β-adrenergic agents. J Clin Invest 52:48-59

Prausnitz C, Küstner H 1921 Studein über die überempfindlichkeit. Zentralbl Bakteriol Parasitenkd Infektionskr Hyg Abt I Orig 86:160-165

Rola-Pleszczynski M, Blanchard R 1981 Abnormal suppressor cell function in atopic dermatitis. J Invest Dermatol 76:279-283

Szentivanyi A 1968 The β-adrenergic theory of the atopic abnormality in bronchial asthma. J Allergy 42:203-231

Szentivanyi A 1980 The radioligand binding approach in the study of lymphocyte adrenoceptors and the constitutional basis of atopy. J Allergy Clin Immunol 65:5-11

Venter JC, Fraser CM, Harrison LC 1980 Autoantibodies to β$_2$-adrenergic receptors: a possible cause of β-adrenergic hyporesponsiveness in allergic rhinitis and asthma. Science (Wash DC) 207:1361-1363

Venter JC, Fraser CM, Harrison LC, Kaliner M 1981 Autoantibodies to β$_2$-adrenergic receptors correlate with autonomic nervous system abnormalities. Fed Proc 40:355 (abstr 697)

DISCUSSION

Venter: Dr Fraser and I have now looked at much wider groups of allergy patients than previously. The incidence of antibodies, assessed by receptor immunoprecipitation and inhibition of ligand binding, is becoming consistent at around 10–15% of allergic subjects (J. C. Venter & C. M. Fraser, unpublished).

Kahn: How specific is the antibody for asthma?

Venter: I think the three 'normal' control subjects who were positive in our first follow-up study may be a red herring. Of all the assays we have done so far, those three were the only controls to have anti-receptor antibodies. We have looked at larger populations including non-asthmatic patients and normal subjects. We have found these antibodies so far only in asthma, cystic fibrosis and other atopic patients, for example with allergic rhinitis.

Engel: Have you looked at subjects who are 'normal' and have antibodies, to see whether they have decreased responsiveness to β-adrenergic stimuli?

Venter: Those three controls had no apparent clinical symptoms yet they show changes in their physiological responses to catecholamines, namely decreased responsiveness of β-receptors. Out of a few hundred patients, they are the only three 'normal' controls in whom we have documented antibody. However, from the information coming out on the other autoimmune diseases, it is not particularly surprising to find antibody but no clinical symptoms.

Harrison: I would expect to find that maybe 5% of the normal population have these antibodies, in accord with the prevalence of latent autonomic abnormalities, as judged for example from methacholine or histamine sensitivity testing.

Roitt: You seem to find different percentages for the incidence of antibodies in the different groups of patients studied. Is that so?

Harrison: The group studied by Michael Kaliner at NIH were patients with a milder degree of atopy, and three out of 14 were positive. We have since studied patients in Australia who come to the respiratory clinics because of asthma and many are still receiving treatment. (This wasn't controlled for.) Our study used a different assay: whole lung cells incubated at 37°C for 90 minutes with patients' globulins.

Venter: The immunoprecipitation assays are difficult because the lung β-receptor is unstable and we are dealing with a reversible complex. As I mentioned earlier, we are now attempting to use the monoclonal antibodies that Dr Fraser has raised to the β-receptor to set up a competitive assay. We may then find a better correlation between different assays.

Roitt: Is the feeling, then, that we are looking at the tip of an iceberg? This antibody might be very common in asthma, and if your tests were more sensitive or done in more severely affected patients, it might be easier to see this. You could also argue that in the less severely ill patients there is a neutralization of antibody which prevents its detection, because of the widespread receptors. If you were, for example, to take peripheral blood cells from asthmatics and stimulate them with pokeweed mitogen, you might find antibody, even though the serum was negative.

Venter: We are dealing with a very large patient population—there are on the order of 20 million asthmatics in the USA. I am not prepared to say that all these people have autoantibodies to the β-receptor. However, what you are saying is not unreasonable.

Jacobs: I am interested in the properties of the antibodies. Have you looked to see whether these anti-β-adrenergic receptor antibodies are agonists—that is, stimulating antibodies? You might have to use a very short incubation, if so, since if you expose β-receptors to agonists *in vitro* they may become desensitized very rapidly.

Venter: There is a very little information on this point. We are now screening all our antibodies for both agonist and antagonist properties.

Harrison: We have some evidence on this. We studied a patient with the Type B syndrome of insulin-resistant diabetes and acanthosis nigricans—Drs Flier and Kahn's first patient, in fact. She came into hospital several times and most recently has had hypoglycaemia. At the end of a glucose tolerance test she fell into a stupor and was revived with oral glucose while semi-conscious. She had no evidence of sympathetic overactivity at this time but her adrenaline level, subsequently measured, was elevated. It turns out that she has an immunoglobulin, or at least a factor in her serum, that inhibits cyclic

AMP production. We think she has both insulin receptor antibodies and β-receptor antibodies, and that blockade or desensitization of her β-adrenergic responses might impair 'counter-regulation' by catecholamines to hypoglycaemia. When we preincubated her serum with cultured VA-13 lung fibroblasts for a shorter time than usual, 30 minutes, there was a small but consistent increase in the basal level of cyclic AMP over the control, by 10–15%. That suggests an agonist effect but it hasn't been studied any further. We saw this with sera from several of the asthma patients too.

Rodbell: Have you tested these antisera against cyclic AMP production, say in the frog erythrocyte as compared to the turkey erythrocyte (with β_2 and β_1 receptors respectively)? Was there any cross-reactivity with other animal species?

Venter: There is no cross-reactivity between β_1- and β_2-receptors even in the same species with the autoantibodies that we have tested so far. It appears as if the autoantibodies are specific for the β_2-receptor and do not affect the β_1- or α-adrenergic receptor, EGF receptors, insulin receptors or other membrane receptor functions.

Blecher: Is it an unreasonable suggestion that the hyper-α-adrenergic and hypercholinergic sensitivity in allergic asthma may be due to a mimetic antibody, as in Graves' disease? Have you looked at the binding of α-adrenergic agonists in the presence of the patient's serum?

Venter: We have not yet looked for α-adrenergic receptor autoantibodies although, as you point out, this work opens up a lot of possibilities. For example, if autoantibodies exist in a large segment of individuals to a variety of membrane receptors, it makes me wonder whether these autoantibodies could be physiological regulators of membrane receptor density and function rather than just mediators of pathology. Because of the existence of anti-idiotypic antibodies, there are enough levels of control to provide a possible regulatory function. Pathology may result when the autoantibody concentration becomes unregulated.

Drachman: Many patients with asthma are treated with adrenergic agents. Does the treatment contribute to antibody production, or to the β-adrenergic hyposensitivity?

Venter: Relatively mild asthmatics were chosen for our study, so that they were not on any medication for at least a month, to rule out any possibility of drug-induced artifacts. Treatment with high concentrations of agonist can produce hyposensitivity.

Harrison: Adding isoprenaline to the serum before fractionation doesn't affect the cyclic AMP assay or the immunoprecipitation assay, but we can't rule out the possibility that the autoimmune response might be initiated by the ligand itself. If a drug ligand stimulated antibody production against its binding site region, these antibodies might 'see' the ligand like the receptor. If antibodies to these first antibodies were produced they might have 'anti-receptor' properties.

Dr Gurnam Basran and Professor Margaret Turner-Warwick at the Brompton Hospital (London) have screened sera from a large group of asthmatics for β-adrenoceptor blocking activity and have confirmed some of our findings (Basran et al 1981). They studied the effect of sera from both normal control and asthmatic subjects on the specific binding of the radio-ligand, [^{125}I]iodohydroxybenzylpindolol (125-I-HYP), to guinea-pig and human lung membrane preparations. The results were expressed as 'relative binding' which was defined as a ratio of the specific binding of 125-I-HYP in the presence of test serum compared with the specific binding in the presence of a reference serum. They showed that sera from the asthmatic group produced significantly greater inhibition of binding than the sera from the control group of normal non-atopic subjects ($P < 0.001$) (Fig. 1).

More interestingly, sera from a proportion (15–25%) of their asthmatic subjects gave a value of relative binding which fell outside the statistical normal range defined by the 99% confidence limit for the normal control group (Fig. 1). This would be consistent with the presence of a circulating β-adrenoceptor blocking factor in this subgroup of asthmatics.

Davies: Is there any information on the IgG extracts from these sera?

Venter: Yes, but on only four patients. To validate his data, Dr Basran took two serum samples which showed high β-adrenoceptor blocking activity in his system (called 'abnormals') and two samples which showed binding inhibition within the normal range (called 'normals') and sent these blind-coded to our laboratory. Using IgG extracts from these samples we found inhibition of binding in our system in his two 'abnormal' samples and no significant inhibition with his two 'normals'. He further validated his data by using Dr Anders Hedberg's system in his laboratory in Göteborg, Sweden, and hence showed that there was a consistency in the findings in the various laboratories. Dr Basran is now doing further studies on the asthmatic patients with reference to their clinical classification, together with functional studies on β-adrenoceptor systems to evaluate the clinical relevance of the circulating β-adrenoceptor blocking factor and its possible role in the pathogenesis of asthma.

Hall: In many autoimmune diseases one feels more secure in the diagnosis if there are overtones of other autoimmune diseases as well. For example, in myasthenia gravis one often finds anti-nuclear factor or thyroid autoanti-bodies. In Graves' disease there are many associations. One form of insulin-resistant diabetes with acanthosis nigricans has many features of SLE-like syndromes. Have you looked for such things in your asthmatic patients? Deborah Doniach, Margaret Turner-Warwick and I looked at a series of patients with intrinsic asthma and found an increased frequency of

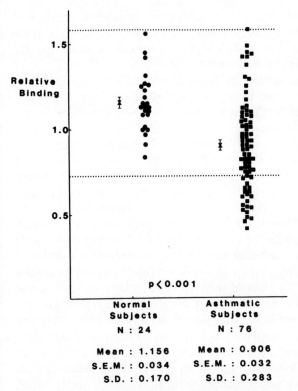

FIG. 1. (Harrison). Specific binding of [^{125}I]iodohydroxybenzylpindolol to guinea-pig lung membranes in the presence of sera from normal and asthmatic subjects. Results are expressed as 'relative binding' defined as specific binding in the presence of test serum compared with specific binding in the presence of reference serum. The mean for the asthmatic group is significantly lower than that for the control group ($P < 0.001$). The 99% confidence limit for the normal group is shown by the dotted lines. (Results of G. S. Basran & M. Turner-Warwick.)

thyroid autoantibodies (Hall et al 1966). This might mean that you are in the acceptable area for autoimmune diseases. We were looking at iodide goitre in patients with asthma and we found an increased frequency of thyroid autoantibodies. We thought there was an underlying defect in the organification of iodine, associated with autoimmune thyroid disease, in these patients, and that is why they developed goitre.

Venter: We haven't done any systematic investigation, but there seems to be an overlap. For example, the patient mentioned by Len Harrison with insulin-resistant diabetes also has autoantibodies to the β-receptor.

Hall: This association might not be true of all asthmatics, but there might be a subgroup with an autoimmune 'tendency', and the majority of this subgroup might have antibodies but very few in other subgroups.

Venter: We have also studed one patient with myasthenia gravis and asthma. She was treated with glucocorticoids, and the asthma, the myasthenia and the anti-β-receptor antibodies all disappeared around the same time (J. C. Venter & W. Busse, unpublished work).

Bottazzo: We are looking at the prevalence of allergic disorders, including asthma, eczema, hay fever, and drug and food allergies, in thyroid auto-immunity. We are surprised by the high incidence of these conditions in our thyroid patients and their families.

Venter: The work of Hall, Turner-Warwick and Deborah Doniach (1966) referred to by Professor Hall was followed by another study from Professor Turner-Warwick's unit, showing the presence of circulating smooth muscle antibodies (of the IgG class) in patients with intrinsic asthma (Turner-Warwick & Haslam 1970). Dr Basran with Professor Turner-Warwick and co-workers have extended this study to see if the presence of the smooth muscle antibody correlated with the presence of the β-adrenoceptor blocking factor. They have shown that although smooth muscle antibody was detected in 18 and reproducible β-adrenoceptor blocking activity (observed on at least two separate occasions) in nine out of their 76 mixed atopic and non-atopic asthmatic subjects, there was no overlap of patients in these two subgroups.

Vincent: What is known about the structure of the β_2-adrenergic receptor?

Venter: I discussed this briefly earlier (p 76). The mammalian lung β_2-receptor has been purified by my laboratory from human, dog and calf lungs and appears to have a basic subunit of M_r 50 000–59 000, depending on the species. We have evidence for larger structures on the order of M_r 90 000–100 000 of which the M_r 59 000 subunit is clearly one component. Our data indicate that the 59 000 unit may be disulphide-cross-linked, either to a second 59 000 subunit, which would make the receptor a dimer of identical units, or to a second, yet to be identified subunit. Our hydrodynamic data on β_2-receptors (Table 1, p 75) indicate that the intact receptor has an M_r of 90 000.

Vincent: What concentrations can you reach in your assays? Comparing titres with the thyroid antibodies is not very relevant if you are looking at quite different antigen concentrations which might be below the K_d values for antibody binding.

Venter: Lung membranes have the highest density of β_2-receptors, on the order of 300 fmol/mg of protein. In the heart we find only around 30 fmol/mg protein. In the soluble immunoprecipitation assays we generally add 1–3 fmol of receptor per assay.

Vincent: If you used more receptor in the assay, would you detect antibodies in more patients?

Venter: It is possible. We hope to devise more sensitive assays using monoclonal antibodies. The immunoprecipitation assay is a difficult one to use. However, we feel that this assay is highly specific. We prefer to be certain of having identified a few patients where we can clearly demonstrate immunoprecipitation, rather than relying totally on binding or biological response as an indication of autoantibodies. Immunoprecipitation tells us that we have an antibody which is specific for the β-receptor molecule.

Mitchison: How much of the iodohydroxybenzylpindolol binding is specific?

Venter: The label is very hot (2200 Ci/mmol) so we can easily measure less than one fmol of receptor. Perhaps 20–30% of the binding is non-specific in the lung. In the heart it is much worse—50% of the binding is non-specific.

Harrison: There is approximately 40% non-specific binding in the VA-13 human lung cells. The label also binds to serotonin and to α-adrenergic receptors. The specificity is determined by competition with isoprenaline.

Kahn: I am concerned about the apparent difference between the bioassay results and the immunoprecipitation results. It is possible that what is being measured in the bioassay may not strictly be an antibody activity; you are working with an ammonium sulphate precipitate and the patients are receiving drugs which could be protein-bound and might alter bioactivity. Have you any additional bioassay data that ascribe the activity you measure to an IgG, or some other known class of Ig? Can you be sure that the results are not due to drug co-precipitation or an endogenous chemical which co-precipitates and might have a certain affinity for serum proteins?

Harrison: If we add isoprenaline, 0.5 μM, to the serum before doing the ammonium sulphate precipitation there is no effect. Also, in two of our original patients, the index patient and patient J.N. whom I mentioned, the IgG has been purified on protein A-Sepharose, and the inhibitory effect is retained. The sera were not 'immunodepleted'. In the globulin studies one cannot exclude other things; a 45% ammonium sulphate precipitation will bring down a range of globulins, including transport proteins.

Kahn: Could you use another agent (a prostaglandin, perhaps) which stimulates adenylate cyclase in these systems and is still effective after antibody treatment, to show that the cyclase has not been altered?

Harrison: We have not done that.

Friesen: In general the biological response *in vitro* to a hormone occurs at concentrations 10-fold lower than are required to stimulate cyclic AMP and 100-fold lower than are required to inhibit binding of a ligand in a receptor assay (Catt & Dufau 1973). Thus I would expect the bioassay to be the more sensitive by an order of magnitude or more.

Venter: From the results of Dr Basran and Professor Turner-Warwick, it is evident that the sera from a proportion of their asthmatic population showed significant β-adrenoceptor blocking activity (personal communication, G. S. Basran). We are going to do immunoprecipitation assays on these patients to see if we identify the same patients.

REFERENCES

Basran GS, Ball AJ, Hanson JM, Turner-Warwick M 1981 Circulating beta-adrenoceptor blocking factor in asthma? Thorax 36:712

Catt KJ, Dufau ML 1973 Spare gonadotrophin receptors in rat testis. Nat New Biol 244:219-221

Hall R, Turner-Warwick M, Doniach D 1966 Autoantibodies in iodide goitre and asthma. Clin Exp Immunol 1:285-296

Turner-Warwick M, Haslam PL 1970 Smooth muscle antibody in bronchial asthma. Clin Exp Immunol 7:31-38

Prolactin and growth hormone receptors

H. G. FRIESEN, R. P. C. SHIU, H. ELSHOLTZ, S. SIMPSON and J. HUGHES

Department of Physiology, University of Manitoba, 770 Bannatyne Avenue, Winnipeg, Canada R3E OW3

Abstract The two hormones prolactin and growth hormone exhibit considerable structural homology as well as exerting similar biological effects, especially the primate hormones. One effect of prolactin that deserves greater attention is its action on the immune system including the stimulation of growth of experimental lymphomas, both *in vivo* and *in vitro*. One cultured lymphoma cell line has proved to be a very useful model system in which to examine prolactin receptor synthesis and turnover as well as post-receptor mechanisms of action.

Prolactin and growth hormone receptors from rabbit mammary gland and liver respectively have been partially purified and characterized. Polyclonal antibodies to prolactin and growth hormone receptors have been generated. The antibodies have been shown to cross-react with prolactin or growth hormone receptors from a number of species, indicating structural homology among receptors as well as hormones. The polyclonal antisera inhibit the action of prolactin *in vivo* as well as *in vitro*. In addition, several of the same antisera also mimic the action of prolactin. As yet the presence of autoantibodies to prolactin or growth hormone receptors in human serum samples has not been recognized.

The extensive structural homology between the two pituitary hormones, growth hormone (GH) and prolactin, as well as their overlapping spectrum of biological effects, prompted us to examine the receptors for these two hormones. The ontogeny, distribution, regulation, purification and characterization of the two receptors has been one focus of our research for almost a decade. In this symposium selected aspects of our work will be reviewed with particular emphasis on the characterization of the receptors and the use of antibody probes to examine the two receptors. Despite the accumulation of considerable information about these two receptors, their precise role in mediating hormone action and the mechanisms involved remain obscure. An emerging concept that deserves more scrutiny is that prolactin itself may have an immunoregulatory role. The data on this last point are derived from a

1982 Receptors, antibodies and disease. Pitman, London (Ciba Foundation symposium 90) p 263-278

series of isolated and unrelated reports which taken together provide compelling evidence for this point of view.

Prolactin and the immune system

In keeping with the symposium's title of 'Receptors, Antibodies and Disease', we wish first to address the role of prolactin in immunoregulation. Prolactin is a fascinating hormone with many and varied actions ranging from stimulation of milk-protein synthesis to action as a luteotropic agent to the promotion of growth. In one review more than 80 biological effects of prolactin were documented but no mention was made of any action on lymphoid tissue or immune mechanisms (Nicoll 1974). The first example of the effect of prolactin on lymphoid tissues relates to the mammary gland and IgA-secreting cells. Weisz-Carrington et al (1978) reported that the migration of IgA immunoblasts into the mammary gland is a hormonally mediated event, with prolactin greatly enhancing the entry of IgA-secreting plasma cells. An immunoregulatory role for prolactin has also been suggested by experiments by our colleagues at the University of Manitoba; and this is the second example we wish to cite. Berczi & Nagy (1981) have shown that antibody production, delayed hypersensitivity to dinitrochlorobenzene, rejection of skin grafts and the development of adjuvant arthritis are all impaired either after hypophysectomy or after the pharmacological suppression of prolactin secretion with bromocriptine.

The third example derives from the remarkable and specific growth-stimulating effect of prolactin on an experimental rat lymphoma (Noble et al 1980). This tumour has proved to be of considerable interest, since the lymphoma cells derived from the tumour begin to proliferate in a dose-dependent manner when prolactin is added to the culture medium. These cells form the basis of an exquisitely sensitive bioassay for prolactin (pg/ml), have receptors for prolactin and are useful for examining the mechanism of action of prolactin (Tanaka et al 1980). The growth rate of lymphomas *in vivo* is accelerated in proportion to the elevation of serum prolactin levels. Thus during pregnancy the growth of tumour to a 10 g size takes only 10 days compared to 38 days in a control rat. Parenthetically, it is interesting that when Burkitt's lymphoma occurs during pregnancy it often presents with extensive mammary gland infiltration. This association raises the question whether prolactin in some manner influences the proliferation of lymphoma cells at this site. Of some interest is the fact that several human lymphomas that we have examined have prolactin and growth hormone receptors and, perhaps of even greater interest, appear to concentrate prolactin and human growth hormone (hGH) in their cytosol (Table 1). The growth of leukaemic

TABLE 1 Prolactin and growth hormone-like activity in extracts of human lymphomas

| | Nb2 cell count × 10³ | | | PRL(ng/g) | |
Specimen	Tissue Extract	Extract + anti-hPRL	Extract + anti-hGH	Bioassay	RIA
1	41.4	32.1	27.0	7.5	7.5
2	104.0	61.0	50.5	55.0	10.0
3	58.6	42.5	34.9	15.0	15.0

The lymph nodes from three patients were homogenized in 0.3 M-sucrose in ratio of 1 to 5 (w/v) and centrifuged at 100 000 × g. The supernatant (50 µl added to 2 ml culture media) was assayed by Nb2 cell bioassay. These assays were repeated in the presence of either anti-hPRL or anti-hGH. The cell count in the control in the absence of prolactin was 21.1 × 10³ cells. It is apparent that all three lymphomas stimulate growth of the Nb2 cells. Not all the mitogenic activity is neutralized by anti-hPRL or anti-hGH. In the case of lymphoma 2 the bioassay estimate of PRL is five-fold greater than the radioimmunoassay (RIA) estimates.

cells and an increase in colony-forming units under the influence of hGH also has been reported (Desai et al 1973, Golde et al 1980).

Prolactin and the Nb2 lymphoma cell

The Nb2 cell is a poorly differentiated lymphoblastic cell with a high mitotic index. Electron microscopy indicates the absence of phagocytic vacuoles, suggesting that this tumour is not of macrophage origin. Immunocytochemical studies have revealed an absence of both surface and cytoplasmic IgG. It is worth noting that most (perhaps as many as 75% of) human lymphoblastic lymphomas are of B cell origin, yet some tumours may express surface immunoglobulins poorly. No detectable α-naphthyl-acetate esterase activity, a marker for T cells, was found on the Nb2 cells. Further characterization with antibodies to IgA, IgM and IgE and antibodies to T cell helper and non-helper cells is under way.

Fig. 1 shows the dose–response curve and the specificity of Nb2 node lymphoma cells in culture. The mitogenic response appears to be specific for lactogenic hormones. In addition, as shown in Fig. 2, prolactin receptors on the Nb2 cell exhibit the same specificity and affinity as was previously reported for the rabbit mammary epithelial cell (Shiu et al 1973). In an experiment examining the prolactin concentration required for half-maximal receptor occupancy and half-maximal stimulation of lymphoma cell growth it was shown that 5.8 pM prolactin concentrations stimulated growth to 50% of maximum while 50% receptor occupancy occurred only at 75 pM. Similarly, the minimal effective concentration to inhibit prolactin binding was 10- to 15-fold greater than required to stimulate cell growth, with a maximal effect on growth observed at 30% receptor occupancy. These results are very

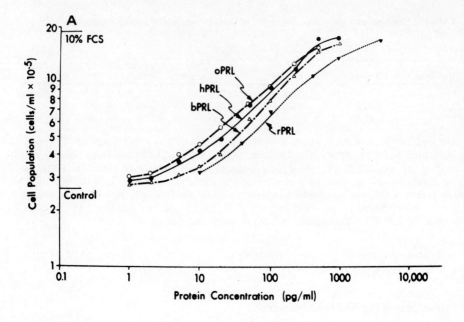

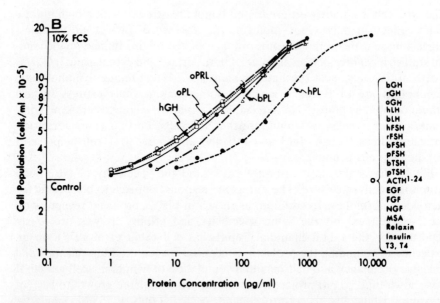

FIG. 1. The increase in lymphoma cell number over a three-day incubation period. A. The effect of purified prolactin from four species (ovine, bovine, rat, human). B. Lactogenic hormones, including primate growth hormone, cause an increase in cell number whereas other peptides and hormones do not.

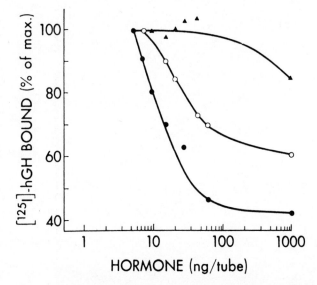

FIG. 2. The inhibition of binding of ^{125}I-labelled hGH to lymphoma cells by human prolactin (●—●) and ovine prolactin (○—○). Ovine growth hormone (▲—▲) or other non-primate growth hormones do not inhibit the binding of ^{125}I-hGH to receptors. Thus ^{125}I-labelled hGH is binding to prolactin receptors. Note that only primate growth hormones show both lactogenic and somatogenic activity.

similar to those reported for other hormones and receptors where a biological response is elicited by a concentration of hormone which is at least an order of magnitude less than that which leads to measurable occupancy (Dufau & Catt 1976).

When incubated in calf serum the lymphoma cells continue to proliferate, as a result of the mitogenic effect of endogenous prolactin and placental lactogen. Under these circumstances down-regulation of receptors occurs. When Nb2 cells are incubated in the presence of horse serum the cell number remains constant but the number of receptors increases at least twofold (Fig. 3). This increase in receptor number is abolished when the culture medium contains 100 ng/ml cycloheximide, and as little as 10 ng/ml partially prevents the increase. After binding of [125]-I-labelled prolactin to the surface of Nb2 cells, the tracer is internalized and degraded. Maximal binding of ^{125}I-prolactin is achieved about one hour after incubation at 37 °C, after which time the quantity of cell-bound radioactivity decreases with incubation time.

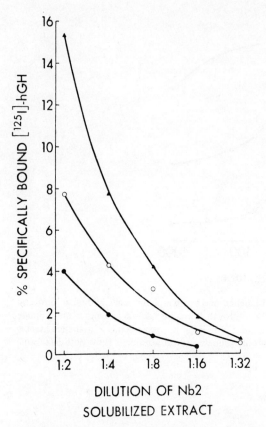

FIG. 3. When lymphoma cells are incubated for extended periods in 10% horse serum (stationary growth phase) there is a gradual increase in binding of ^{125}I-labelled hGH to receptors. ●—●, 4 h in horse serum. ○—○, 8 h in horse serum. ▲—▲, 24 h in horse serum. The increase in binding is presumed to be a return to a basal state after down-regulation of receptors by exposure to prolactin present in calf serum.

Biosynthesis and turnover of receptors

The biosynthesis and turnover of prolactin receptors in Nb2 cells has been examined using density-labelling methods. Lymphoma cells were incubated with ^{2}H- and ^{13}C-labelled amino acids. After 12 hours the cells were solubilized and the extracts were subjected to density equilibrium ultracentrifugation using caesium chloride gradients. Fractions of the gradients were assayed for prolactin receptors. Newly synthesized prolactin receptors were recognized by a density shift in the receptors in caesium chloride gradients. The refractive index at which the prolactin receptor banded when cells were in the usual culture media was 1.3575 while the ^{2}H-, ^{13}C-labelled receptor had a refractive index of 1.361—a downward shift of 0.004 to 0.005 ηD units.

After 12 hours of exposure to heavy amino acids, virtually all the prolactin receptor was density-labelled, implying the fairly rapid turnover of these receptors. This approach to the study of the synthesis of the prolactin receptor circumvents the methodological difficulty inherent in studies using radioactive isotopes which demand the purification and/or specific identification of labelled receptors. It also makes it feasible to investigate the regulation of synthesis, transport to the cell surface and degradation of prolactin receptors in cultured prolactin-responsive cells.

Characterization of prolactin and growth hormone receptors

The purification and characterization of rabbit mammary gland prolactin receptors has been reported (Shiu & Friesen 1974). Rabbit mammary glands were homogenized and centrifuged and a $100\,000 \times g$ pellet was obtained containing the bulk of prolactin receptors. The particulate membrane fraction was solubilized with Triton X-100 and prolactin receptors were purified by affinity chromatography. An approximate 2000-fold purification was achieved. Isoelectric focusing of purified receptor protein reveals several bands with maximal binding in eluants with a pH of 6 to 7. Complete purification of membrane receptors is complicated by the presence of detergents which retain contaminating membrane lipids and proteins in micelles along with the receptor.

Similar approaches have been used to purify and characterize the growth hormone receptors from rabbit liver (Waters & Friesen 1979a, b). Instead of using 5 M-MgCl$_2$ to elute GH receptors we used 2.5 to 4 M-urea. Under these circumstances GH receptors but not prolactin receptors, which are also present in rabbit liver, were eluted. Subsequently the latter could be eluted with 5 M-MgCl$_2$. Table 2 summarizes some of the known characteristics of prolactin and GH receptors.

Antibodies to receptors

The purified GH or prolactin receptors were used for immunizing guinea-pigs to generate antibodies to receptors. The antibodies were detected by the inhibition of binding of ^{125}I-prolactin or GH to particulate membrane fractions containing receptors for prolactin and GH (Shiu & Friesen 1976b, Waters & Friesen 1979b). Antibodies to rabbit prolactin receptors inhibit the binding of this hormone to rabbit mammary gland receptors, and, to varying

TABLE 2 Properties of rabbit mammary gland prolactin and rabbit liver growth hormone receptors

	Prolactin	Growth hormone
Composition	Glycoprotein	Sialoglycoprotein
Relative molecular mass (M_r) in Triton	220 000	300 000
Subunit size (M_r)	64 000 and 75 000	70 000 tetramer
pI	6.5	4.7
K_a	3.16×10^9 M^{-1}	2×10^9 M^{-1}
Common antigenic sites	rabbit, rat, human	rabbit, rat, mouse, sheep, human

degrees, to prolactin receptors located on target tissues from several different species. Thus not only are the amino acid sequences of hormones conserved among species, but homology of receptors for the same hormones in different species is also evident.

The antisera have been shown not only to inhibit binding of these hormones to receptors but also, in the case of prolactin, to block hormone-mediated events *in vitro* and *in vivo*. In mammary gland explants one of the guinea-pig antisera inhibits prolactin stimulation of casein synthesis and aminoisobutyric acid transport while not interfering with glucose utilization by the explants (Shiu & Friesen 1976a). When antisera to the prolactin receptor was administered to lactating rats, milk production was inhibited, as judged by a decreased weight gain of pups suckling dams that were injected daily with antisera to the prolactin receptor (Bohnet et al 1978).

Antibodies to the GH receptor do not inhibit the binding of prolactin to the mammary gland prolactin receptor and vice versa (Fig. 4). As yet, antibodies to the GH receptor have not been shown to inhibit any biological effects stimulated by growth hormone. One attempt to inhibit the weight gain in GH-treated hypophysectomized rats by anti-GH receptor antisera proved unsuccessful.

More recently, we have examined the effects of antisera to prolactin receptors on the stimulation of Nb2 cell growth. A number of antisera inhibit the full expression of the mitogenic effect of prolactin on cell growth, while themselves exerting a modest proliferative effect on the growth of Nb2 cells (Fig. 5). The IgG fraction as well as the bivalent F(ab')$_2$ fragments derived from the IgG of these antisera cause these effects while the univalent Fab fragments fail to stimulate growth of the Nb2 cell. Thus the cross-linking and clustering of surface prolactin receptors appears to be a prerequisite for triggering hormone-mediated events, which is similar to the effects of other hormones. In addition, these experiments, together with comparable experi-

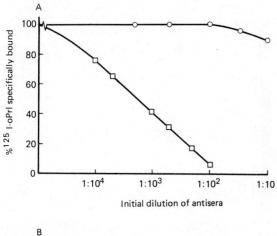

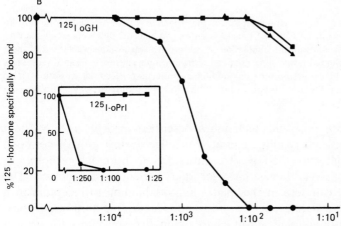

Gamma globulin dilution (initial antiserum dilution equivalents)

FIG. 4. A. Antibodies to the prolactin receptor inhibit binding of ^{125}I-labelled ovine prolactin (^{125}I-oPrl) to rabbit mammary gland receptors (□—□) but antibodies to GH receptor do not (○—○). B. Effect of anti-receptor IgG fraction on binding of ^{125}I-oGH to GH receptor purified by affinity chromatography (urea fraction). ●—●, anti-GH receptor. ■—■, anti-prolactin receptor IgG. ▲—▲, normal guinea-pig IgG fraction. The inset shows the effect of the IgG on binding of ^{125}I-oPrl to the same purified receptor. Anti-GH receptor but not anti-prolactin receptor antibodies inhibit binding of ^{125}I-oPrl. Therefore, we conclude that ^{125}I-oPrl does bind to GH receptor.

ments for other hormones, provide compelling evidence that the protein sequence embraced by the prolactin molecule is not a mandatory structural requirement for initiating and mediating the action of prolactin.

We have begun to generate monoclonal antibodies to prolactin and growth

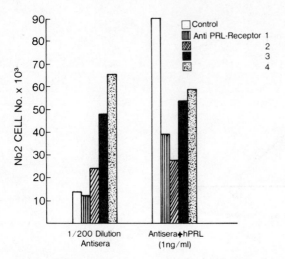

FIG. 5. Effect of antisera to prolactin receptors on the growth *in vitro* of Nb2 cells. (The antisera were generated in goats by Dr P. Kelly, Laval University.) When Nb2 cells were incubated with four different antisera a significant stimulation of cell growth was evident with three of them (left-hand columns). Similar results were obtained with guinea-pig antisera to prolactin receptors (results not shown). In the presence of 1 ng/ml human prolactin (hPRL), all antisera at 1/200 dilution inhibited the proliferative response of the Nb2 cells to prolactin, whereas control sera did not (right-hand columns).

hormone receptors using the techniques described by Köhler & Milstein (1975). Antibodies are readily generated in mice against growth hormone receptors. The detection of low titre antibodies to hormone receptors in culture media from hybridomas, however, does present some problems. The presence of fetal calf sera in the media inhibits binding to receptors to a considerable extent because of the endogenous lactogenic hormones. Thus, we have covalently coupled ^{125}I-hGH to rabbit liver receptors for growth hormone using disuccinimidyl suberate. The conjugate was partially purified to remove free hGH and test antisera were examined for their ability to precipitate the ^{125}I-hGH–GH receptor complex (Table 3). Subsequently we have been successful in propagating several hybridomas that secrete antibodies which inhibit the binding of ^{125}I-hGH to particulate receptors from rabbit liver. We are now in the process of characterizing the specificity and IgG class of the antibody produced.

Conclusion

The objective of studies on growth hormone and prolactin receptors has been to gain an understanding of the mechanism of action of each of these

TABLE 3 Immunoprecipitation of ^{125}I-hGH–GH receptor complex

| | Radioactivity in immunoprecipitate (c.p.m.) (antiserum dilution) | | |
	1:100	1:200	1:500
Control	865 ± 47[a]		
Antiserum 1	1039 ± 8	1070 ± 115	1090
Antiserum 2	1676 ± 18	1418 ± 61	1143

Rabbit liver was solubilized in 1% Tris-Triton, pH 7.6. A fraction was incubated overnight with ^{125}I-hGH and the bifunctional cross-linking reagent disuccinimidyl suberate (0.25 mM) was added for 30 min at room temperature the next morning. The mixture was added to a Con A column and the unbound ^{125}I-hGH removed. The eluted ^{125}I-hGH–GH receptor was then used as label to assess the presence of antibodies in mouse sera: 50 μl of serum at 1:100, 1:200 and 1:500 dilution was incubated with 25 μl of label (^{125}I-hGH coupled to GH receptor) and 50 μl of buffer or normal mouse serum to give a 1 100 serum concentration and 430 μl of buffer (1% bovine serum albumin in phosphate-buffered saline, pH 7.5). Normal mouse serum served as a control. After incubation at room temperature for 3 h, 100 μl of goat anti-mouse IgG at a dilution of 1:2 was added to precipitate mouse IgG. This mixture was left overnight at 4 °C. The mixture was centrifuged, the supernatant decanted and the pellet counted.
[a] Mean ± SD.

hormones. Some progress on this path has been achieved but much remains to be discovered. The isolation and complete characterization of the receptors must be accomplished, and the mediators of hormone action that are generated after the hormone–receptor interaction remain to be identified. It is our view that the lymphoma cell offers an excellent model system in which to study these questions.

Acknowledgements

The research was supported by grants from MRC of Canada and NCI of Canada, and by USPHS grant HD07843-08.

REFERENCES

Berczi I, Nagy E 1981 Immunodeficiency in hypophysectomized rats: Restoration by prolactin. Fed Proc 40:1031 (abstr 4541)
Bohnet HG, Shiu RPC, Grinwich D, Friesen HG 1978 In vivo effects of antisera to prolactin receptors in female rats. Endocrinology 102:1657-1661
Desai LS, Lazarus H, Li CH, Foley GE 1973 Human leukemic cells. Effect of human growth hormone. Exp Cell Res 81:330-338
Dufau ML, Catt KJ 1976 Gonadal receptors for luteinizing hormone and chorionic gonadotropin

in cell membrane receptors for viruses, antigens and antibodies In: Polypeptide hormones and small molecules. Beers, RF Jr, Bassett EG (eds) Raven Press, New York, p 135-170

Golde DW, Bersch N, Kaplan SA, Rimoin DL, Li CH 1980 Peripheral unresponsiveness to human growth hormone in Laron dwarfism. N Engl J Med 303:1156-1159

Köhler G, Milstein C 1975 Continuous culture of fused cells secreting antibody of predefined specificity. Nature (Lond) 256:495-497

Nicoll CS 1974 Physiological actions of prolactin. In: Greep R, Astwood EB (eds) The pituitary gland and its endocrine control, part 2, p 253-292. Williams & Wilkins, Baltimore (Handb Physiol sect 7: Endocrinology, vol IV)

Noble RL, Beer CT, Gout PW 1980 Evidence in vivo and in vitro of a role for the pituitary in the growth of malignant lymphomas in Nb rats. Cancer Res 40:2437-2440

Shiu RPC, Kelly PA, Friesen HG 1973 Radio-receptor assay for prolactin and other lactogenic hormones. Science (Wash DC) 180:968-971

Shiu RPC, Friesen HG 1974 Solubilization and purification of a prolactin receptor from the rabbit mammary gland. J Biol Chem 249:7902-7911

Shiu RPC, Friesen HG 1976a Blockade of prolactin action by an antiserum to its receptors. Science (Wash DC) 192:259-261

Shiu RPC, Friesen HG 1976b Interaction of cell membrane prolactin with its antibody. Biochem J 157:619-626

Tanaka T, Shiu RPC, Gout PW, Beer CT, Noble RL, Friesen HG 1980 A new sensitive and specific bioassay for lactogenic hormones: measurement of prolactin and growth hormone in serum. J Clin Endocrinol Metab 51:1058-1063

Weisz-Carrington P, Roux ME, McWilliams M, Phillips-Quagliata JM, Lamm ME 1978. Hormonal induction of the secretory immune system in the mammary gland. Proc Natl Acad Sci USA 75:2928-2932

Waters MJ, Friesen HG 1979a Studies with anti-growth hormone receptor antibodies. J Biol Chem 254:6826-6832

Waters MJ, Friesen HG 1979b Purification and partial characterization of a nonprimate growth hormone receptor. J Biol Chem 254:6815-6825

DISCUSSION

Kahn: Thinking of screening human diseases for anti-prolactin receptor antibodies, there are many patients with idiopathic galactorrhoea, gynaeco-mastia, and some women with macromastia which can be unilateral, some-times almost mimicking autonomous growth. One wonders if any of these breast diseases could be associated with anti-prolactin receptor antibodies.

Friesen: We have looked at selected examples of some of these conditions, particularly patients with hyperprolactinaemia and galactorrhoea. So far we have not found any patients with autoantibodies to the prolactin receptor.

Bitensky: Have you looked at patients with prolactin-producing micro-adenomata? Could these pituitary tumours be driven by a prolactin receptor antibody?

Friesen: Yes; we looked at 25 or 30 of these patients, and haven't found any prolactin receptor antibodies.

Jacobs: Does prolactin have any effect on the turnover of its receptor?

Friesen: Density-labelling studies, currently under way, should provide an answer to that question.

Harrison: What is the evidence that this growth factor, which is not prolactin itself, because it is not inhibited by antibodies to prolactin, is not an activated prolactin receptor, by analogy with the effects of steroids in activating their receptors? You are looking at a growth effect, which presumably is mediated inside the target cell by an action at the nucleus. Is there any evidence that it is 'activated' receptor that you are looking at, or a piece of it?

Friesen: We have no direct evidence that the putative mediator is or is not part of the prolactin receptor. If it were the receptor, or a component of it, it would have to be released from the liver membranes which are co-cultured with the lymphoma cells, enter these lymphoma cells and trigger the mitogenic response in them.

Harrison: The 'factor' would have to do that anyway?

Friesen: Yes, but very little receptor is shed from particulate cell membranes into culture media, so on that basis the factor is unlikely to be part of the receptor. But of course it could be a small fragment derived from it.

Mitchison: It would be of considerable interest if any of your antisera had an agonist action. Have you looked for this effect at high concentrations of the antibody? Do you have an assay which would pick up a growth hormone agonist effect?

Friesen: We have tested our anti-growth hormone receptor antisera to see whether they block the effect of growth hormone in a hypophysectomized rat. In that study, they had no effect; but perhaps we didn't give enough antiserum. We didn't see any stimulating effect of the growth hormone receptor antisera on growth in this model.

Drachman: In your studies where bromocriptine (which suppresses prolactin secretion) altered immune responses, did it abolish an existing response or did it prevent the subsequent development of immune responses?

Friesen: The drug was given concurrently with the immunization. We haven't yet looked to see whether bromocriptine abolishes an established immune response.

Mitchison: Have you looked at the antisera to the prolactin receptor for immunosuppressive activity? The prediction from your results is that these antisera should be immunosuppressive.

Friesen: Provided that the antibody titre generated passively is of sufficient magnitude, yes. We haven't done this yet.

Roitt: Could bromocriptine or its analogues be given to patients with lymphoma?

Friesen: Bromocriptine is primarily used clinically to reduce prolactin secretion in patients with hyperprolactinaemia. We haven't used it in lymphoma patients or as an immunosuppressant in other patients.

Harrison: In the prolactin adenoma patients you find no antibodies to the prolactin receptor, but antibodies to pituitary tissue have been reported by Franco Bottazzo and Deborah Doniach in such patients. Do these antibodies stimulate the pituitary to make prolactin? If there are such antibodies, is their production being inhibited by bromocriptine?

Friesen: That hypothesis has not escaped us, but I don't know the answer.

Bitensky: In patients treated with bromocriptine for microadenomata, there is no clinical evidence for immunosuppression, so far as I know.

Friesen: No, but to my knowledge no one has looked for this.

Hall: It is an interesting idea that prolactin might be involved in attracting immune cells to the breast so that these cells can produce the specific secretory immunoglobulins (IgA). Has anyone looked at this, in animals or in patients, where there is hyperprolactinaemia or bromocriptine suppression of prolactin, and measured the specific immunoglobulin content of the milk?

Friesen: Not to my knowledge.

Mitchison: These experiments could be interpreted entirely in terms of changes in the breast tissue rather than in the plasma cells. Is there evidence, in the experiment on the accumulation of plasma cells in the breast tissue, of an effect on the plasma cell rather than on the breast tissue?

Friesen: The data of Weisz-Carrington et al (1978) indicate an increase in the number of IgA-secreting plasma cells and in the amount of IgA in the mammary gland of virgin mice treated with prolactin. These increases appear to be due to the enhanced capacity of the gland to attract or retain precursors of IgA plasma cells derived from gut-associated lymphoid tissue.

Vincent: Have you compared the prolactin receptor on lymphocytes with the receptor you isolate from rabbit mammary glands?

Friesen: The prolactin receptor on the Nb2 rat lymphoma cells cross-reacts with antibodies generated against rabbit mammary gland prolactin receptors. Antigenically therefore they appear to be the same.

Jacobs: Is there any increased incidence of lymphomas in patients with hyperprolactinaemia?

Friesen: Not that I'm aware of, but I am also unaware of anyone who has examined that question.

Davies: How about prolactin receptors on normal lymphocytes? Have you had any luck with isolating those?

Friesen: The concentrations that we have found are very low.

Kahn: The lymphocyte lines that we have haven't been screened systematically for prolactin receptors, only for growth hormone receptors. The hGH receptors are present in varying amounts on different cultured human lymphoblastoid cells.

Davies: In the normal human, do you then think there are high affinity prolactin receptors in low concentrations, on the lymphocytes?

Friesen: Yes.

Roitt: It would be interesting to look at blast cells, induced by mitogen stimulation of lymphocytes. Often the blast cells express surface molecules that are not abundant on the resting lymphocyte, because it is not very interested in doing anything at that stage.

Harrison: Could this growth stimulation be a heterologous effect of prolactin—an indirect effect mediated by another receptor for a growth factor in the medium in which you grow the lymphoma cells? In other words, could prolactin up-regulate receptors for other growth factors in the medium?

Friesen: There are no data to suggest that possibility. However, the mechanism of action of prolactin on casein synthesis by the mammary gland has been clarified by Djiane et al (1982). They have done similar studies to ours; namely, incubating prolactin with plasma membranes from target tissues to determine whether a mediator of the action of prolactin is generated. They report that only plasma membranes from target tissues of prolactin release a mediator. The signal generated from the plasma membrane appears to be a small molecular weight peptide. They postulate that this peptide activates the nuclear mechanisms leading to an increase in the transcription of casein gene mRNA.

Mitchison: Are antisera against prolactin itself also powerful immunosuppressive agents *in vivo*?

Friesen: They haven't been examined for this effect but from the results I presented, one would predict that they should be.

Bottazzo: Are patients treated with bromocriptine more susceptible to viral infections than normal?

Hall: No, but this is at a crude clinical level. There could be more subtle evidence of immune deficiency.

Friesen: It is also important to recognize that in the clinical setting when bromocriptine is used, circulating levels of prolactin are never decreased to zero. In most conditions for which bromocriptine is given, prolactin levels are reduced from 100–1000 ng/ml to concentrations of 10–20 ng/ml or even somewhat greater. These levels are well into the normal range and hardly a state of prolactin deficiency. Moreover, serum human growth hormone levels are unaltered after bromocriptine treatment. In human subjects, hGH is a potent lactogenic as well as somatogenic hormone. Thus patients on bromocriptine are rarely if ever seriously prolactin-deficient.

Davies: One might even predict lymphomas in patients on chronic bromocriptine therapy?

Hall: There has been no evidence of neoplasms in patients treated with bromocriptine.

Mitchison: The hypothesis that prolactin is a powerful immunoregulatory agent would be greatly strengthened by antisera experiments. The same point was made about interferon, and when antisera were tested *in vivo* they did in fact confirm the prediction.

Vincent: What happens to the animals in which you raise the antibody to prolactin receptor? Do they develop any immunodeficiency?

Friesen: This hasn't been tested.

Kahn: Thinking of the possible clinical conditions in which one might look for antibodies to growth hormone receptors, there are patients with immunological disease and growth retardation. Have you screened for the possibility that growth deficiency in these diseases is due to antibodies to the growth hormone receptor?

Friesen: No.

REFERENCES

Djiane J et al 1982 In: Tolis G (ed) Proc 3rd International Symposium on Prolactin, Athens, October 1981. Raven Press, New York, in press

Weisz-Carrington P, Roux ME, McWilliams M, Phillips-Quagliata JM, Lamm ME 1978 Hormonal induction of the secretory immune system in the mammary gland. Proc Natl Acad Sci, USA 75:2928-2932

Speculations on potential anti-receptor autoimmune diseases

MELVIN BLECHER

Department of Biochemistry, Georgetown University Medical Center, Washington, DC 20007, USA

Abstract Many autoimmune disorders have a strong tendency to cluster in a single patient or type of patient. Therefore, in those cases in which anti-receptor antibodies are known to be responsible for one of the diseases in the cluster, it is logical to proceed investigatively on the presumption that the aetiology of other members of the cluster may also have an anti-receptor autoantibody basis. This logic is examined by considering examples of clustering in human diseases involving both organ-specific and non-organ-specific autoimmunities. The strong relationship between clustering among autoimmune diseases and the HLA-B8/DRw3 haplotype may provide a marker for anti-receptor autoimmune diseases.

Ten years ago, Lennon & Carnegie (1971) developed, on the basis of data derived from studies of experimental autoimmune encephalomyelitis, a hypothesis of 'immunopharmacologic block'. The hypothesis proposed that, in certain organ-specific autoimmune diseases, antibodies or 'immunocytes', produced against cell surface receptors for peptide hormones or neurotransmitters, would complex with such receptors, thereby blocking the normal function of those—and related—cells. Although they applied the hypothesis specifically to human multiple sclerosis, Lennon & Carnegie suggested that it could apply equally well to myasthenia gravis and a wide variety of autoimmune diseases of secretory organs. Four years later, Carnegie & Mackay (1975) described the validation of their hypothesis by evidence then emerging on an autoimmune anti-receptor aetiology for myasthenia gravis, Graves' disease and acanthosis nigricans with insulin resistance.

There are two main theses to this paper. One, that Carnegie was quite correct, and that the relatively few anti-receptor autoimmune human diseases so far identified may represent just the tip of the iceberg. Secondly, there is a

---

1982 Receptors, antibodies and disease. Pitman, London (Ciba Foundation symposium 90) p 279-300

tendency for autoimmune diseases to cluster in a single patient or in a single type of patient; therefore, in those cases in which anti-receptor antibodies are known to be, or suspected of being, responsible for one member of the constellation of diseases, it is logical to proceed investigatively on the presumption that other members may have a similar aetiology. The question arises as to whether all anti-receptor autoantibody disorders participate in clustering. Although a review of the literature suggests an affirmative answer, patients with bronchial asthma or allergic rhinitis appeared to be an exception to the general rule. Although blocking antibodies to β_2-adrenergic receptors have been found (Venter et al 1980), there was no suggestion in early studies that other types of anti-receptor autoantibodies were present. More recently, however, Venter and his collaborators (J. C. Venter, personal communication) have found a patient with bronchial asthma and myasthenia gravis who produced both anti-β-adrenergic and anti-cholinergic receptor antibodies, and another asthmatic with ataxia telangiectasia who produced anti-insulin receptor antibodies, in addition to anti-β-adrenergic receptor antibodies. Furthermore, it is possible that the concurrent α-adrenergic and cholinergic hypersensitivities observed in these patients (Venter et al 1980, C. M. Fraser, J. C. Venter & M. Kaliner, unpublished observations) are due to the autoimmune production of mimetic antibodies; assays for such anti-receptor antibodies have not yet been done (M. Kaliner, personal communication). From this evidence it appears clear that anti-β-adrenergic receptor antibody disorders are not exceptions to the 'cluster' rule.

I shall now give some examples of polyautoimmune disorders in which searches for additional antibodies against receptors and other informational proteins may be fruitful.

Diabetes mellitus

A clinical association between insulin-dependent diabetes mellitus (IDDM, or Type I diabetes mellitus) and autoimmune disorders has been repeatedly documented. The disease cluster may involve the adrenal cortex, neuro-muscular junctions, parathyroid, thyroid, liver and gastrointestinal tissues (Table 1). In addition, IDDM is frequently associated with autoantibodies to pancreatic islet cells (Bottazzo et al 1974, Lendrum et al 1975, MacCuish et al 1974) and to insulinoma cells (Huang & Maclaren 1976, Maclaren et al 1975). Furthermore, examination of sera from IDDM patients with polyendocrine disorders by an immunofluorescence technique revealed organ-specific auto-antibodies against pancreatic islets, adrenal cortex, thyroid microsomes and thyroglobulin, gastric parietal cells, gastric intrinsic factor, smooth muscle, mitochondria, and nuclei (Bottazzo et al 1974). Since, in the immunofluor-

TABLE 1 Autoimmune disorders associated with insulin-dependent diabetes mellitus

Disorder	Reference
Idiopathic Addison's disease	Irvine & Barnes 1972
Idiopathic hypoparathyroidism	Blizzard 1969
Hashimoto's thyroiditis, thyrotoxicosis, primary hypothyroidism	⎰Perlman 1961 ⎱Crome et al 1967 Ganz and Kozak 1974
Myasthenia gravis	Osserman 1969
Pernicious anaemia (anti-intrinsic factor, anti-parietal cell antibodies)	⎰Irvine et al 1970 ⎱Ungar et al 1968
Schmidt's syndrome (Addison's disease with chronic lymphocytic thyroiditis, sometimes with pernicious anaemia, ovarian failure, IDDM)	⎰Schmidt 1926 ⎱Carpenter et al 1964
Polyendocrine disorders (rheumatoid arthritis, chronic ulcerative colitis, idiopathic thrombocytopenic purpura, bronchial asthma, thyrotoxicosis, acute hepatitis, etc.)	Whittingham et al 1971

escence technique used by Bottazzo and colleagues (1974), islet cell antibodies reacted with both α and β pancreatic cells, it is just possible that, in autoimmune insulitis, a reduced production of both insulin and glucagon will occur.

In all autoimmune disease clusters in which diabetes mellitus is a component, the presence of anti-insulin receptor antibodies in sera is, of course, readily testable by well-established methods (cf. Kahn et al, this volume). In IDDM, sera containing anti-β islet cell antibodies might well block the response of isolated islet cells to glucose, in a manner mimicking the pharmacological action of somatostatin, thereby providing a functional assay for this antibody (Okamoto et al 1975).

The presence of organ-specific antibodies against thyroid, adrenal cortical and gastric parietal tissues in patients with polyautoimmune disease could be tested by assays based on the presumption that, among the antibodies being produced, will be those directed against cell surface receptors in these tissues. Thus, methods for assaying for Graves' disease immunoglobins could be adapted for anti-thyroid antibodies. Methods to assay for anti-adrenal cortex antibodies might be based on the blockade of the binding of radiolabelled ACTH to isolated adrenal cortical plasma membranes (Lefkowitz et al 1970) or impairment of the ability of ACTH to activate adenylate cyclase or stimulate steroidogenesis in suspensions of adrenal cortical cells (Finn et al 1976).

Diabetic patients with parietal cell autoantibodies tend to present with diffuse Type A gastritis. When chronic, this syndrome includes, among other characteristics (Table 2), hypergastrinaemia and autoantibodies to intrinsic

BLECHER

TABLE 2 Features of Type A chronic atrophic gastritis

General: Autoimmune characteristics
  Hypergastrinaemia
  Pernicious anaemia, impaired B_{12} absorption
  Hashimoto-type thyroid lesions
Autoimmune: Antibodies to parietal cells (90%), intrinsic factor (75%), thyroid epithelial cells
  (66%), nuclei (26%), adrenal cortex and parathyroid (minor)
Associated with: Major—Hashimoto's thyroiditis, IDDM, vitiligo
  Minor—Addison's disease, hypoparathyroidism

The percentages refer to the frequency of appearance of these features in this disorder.

factor and thyroid epithelial cells (Strickland & Mackay 1973). The course of hypergastrinaemia can be followed by radioimmunoassay (Yalow & Straus 1977). Autoantibodies to the intrinsic factor glycoprotein might be assayed by: (a) impedance of the binding of cobalamin (vitamin B_{12}) to intrinsic factor, or (b) inhibition of the binding of the intrinsic factor–cobalamin complex to ileal plasma membrane receptors.

Connective tissue diseases

Insulin resistance can be associated with a variety of connective tissue diseases (Table 3). Dr Kahn (p 91) has already described the anti-insulin

TABLE 3 Connective tissue diseases associated with insulin resistance

Acanthosis nigricans	Congenital lipodystrophy
Diffuse scleroderma	Rheumatoid arthritis
Sjögren's syndrome	Systemic lupus erythematosus

receptor antibody basis for the insulin resistance in acanthosis nigricans, Sjögren's syndrome and diffuse scleroderma, and has remarked on the seemingly anomalous absence of such antibodies in the sera of several patients with lipoatrophic diabetes plus acanthosis nigricans, as tested by both binding inhibition and immunoprecipitation assays (Wachslicht-Rodbard et al 1981).

Systemic lupus erythematosus (SLE) is a product of an aberrantly regulated immune response. A suppression of cell-mediated immunity is accompanied by enhanced humoral immunity. These abnormalities may account for the multitude of antibodies to nuclei and other cellular components found in these patients (Table 4). Complexes between these antibodies and their antigens, depositing in renal glomerular and vascular basement membranes, contribute to the pathogenesis of the renal and skin lesions typical of SLE.

TABLE 4 Immunological abnormalities associated with systemic lupus erythematosus

Antinuclear antibodies (90%)
Positive SLE cell test (66–80%)
Hypocomplementaemia (75%)
Rheumatoid factors (20%)
False-positive syphilis test (15%)

Data from Mannik & Gilliland (1977). The percentages refer to the frequency of appearance of the abnormalities.

The polyantibody characteristics of this complex disease make it a prime candidate for investigations into the presence of anti-receptor antibodies. Pedersen et al (1981) recently reported on a young female patient with SLE accompanied by acanthosis nigricans and massive insulin resistance. Present in her serum were low titres of a factor that inhibited the binding of labelled insulin to isolated normal human fat cells, and also reduced the sensitivity of such cells to the biological effects of insulin. Immunofluorescence studies suggested that the factor may be an IgG. Undoubtedly, future studies will establish whether or not the factor is an anti-insulin receptor antibody.

Typically, patients with Sjögren's syndrome present with hypergammaglobulinaemia, elevated IgM concentrations and symptoms of several autoimmune diseases (Table 5). Although, as described by Dr Kahn (this volume),

TABLE 5 Autoimmune disorders associated with Sjögren's syndrome

Usually:	Hypergammaglobulinaemia with elevated IgM levels
	Antibodies to nuclei, thyroglobulin, salivary ducts
	Leukopenia
	Accelerated red blood cell sedimentation rate
Often:	Rheumatoid arthritis
	Thrombocytopenic purpura
	Chronic active hepatitis
Rarely:	Systemic lupus erythematosus
	Diffuse scleroderma
	Polymyositis
	Periarteritis nodosa

anti-insulin receptor antibodies were found in the one such patient studied (Kawanishi et al 1977), no endocrinological abnormalities other than extreme insulin resistance were observed. However, if this syndrome is indeed a member of the autoimmune, anti-receptor antibody cluster phenotype, further studies with additional patients may uncover other such antibodies.

In rheumatoid arthritis, patients frequently produce 'rheumatoid factors', which are immunoglobins (IgG, IgM, IgA) produced against the patient's own, probably altered, IgG (Table 6). Such rheumatoid factors may also be found in patients with IDDM (see Table 1), progressive systemic sclerosis (Table 7), SLE, chronic active hepatitis (Table 8), as well as in a recently discovered autoimmune disease complex—namely, rheumatic disease with anti-lipomodulin antibodies (Table 9; Hirata et al 1981). Although anti-receptor antibodies have not yet been reported in rheumatoid arthritis, the polyautoimmune nature of this complex disorder suggest that such a phenotype is very likely.

Vitiligo hypomelanosis is, in the majority of cases, idiopathic. Typical vitiligo, however, is known to occur in conjunction with a variety of autoimmune diseases, namely, idiopathic Addison's disease, hyperthyroidism, hypoparathyroidism, pernicious anaemia and alopecia areata. It is

TABLE 6 Immunological features of rheumatoid arthritis

Rheumatoid factors (IgG, IgM and IgA, specific against IgG)
Antinuclear/anti-DNA antibodies
Rheumatoid factors are also found in: insulin-dependent diabetes mellitus, diffuse scleroderma, systemic lupus erythematosus, chronic active hepatitis, rheumatic disease with anti-lipomodulin antibodies

TABLE 7 Diffuse scleroderma or progressive systemic sclerosis

Hypergammaglobulinaemia (IgG and IgM)
Same antibodies as found in: systemic lupus erythematosus
                              rheumatoid arthritis
                              myositis
                              Raynaud's syndrome
                              Sjögren's syndrome

TABLE 8 Characteristics of autoimmune chronic active hepatitis

Lesions containing small lymphocytes and plasma cells
Elevated IgG, IgM and IgA (50–70%)
Antibodies to: smooth muscle (40–80%)
               mitochondria (10–20%)
               gastric/thyroid/adrenal tissues (5%)
               rheumatoid factors (10–20%)
Associated autoimmune diseases: Hashimoto's thyroiditis
                                Sjögren's syndrome
                                rheumatoid arthritis
                                arthralgias
                                insulin resistance
                                glomerulonephritis
                                ulcerative colitis
Positive effects with immunosuppressive therapy

The percentages refer to frequencies of appearance in this disease.

TABLE 9 Anti-lipomodulin antibodies in patients with connective tissue diseases

	Patient distribution of anti-lipomodulin antibody[a]
Control subjects	0/20
Systemic lupus erythematosus	16/26
Rheumatoid arthritis	7/13
Dermatomyositis	2/5
Periarteritis nodosum	2/5

[a] Anti-lipomodulin antibody was detected by the ability to counteract the inhibitory effect of lipomodulin on phospholipase A_2. (Adapted from Hirata et al 1981.)

possible that vitiligo hypomelanosis in such cases is due to the autoimmune production of anti-melanocyte antibodies directed specifically against the cell surface receptor for melanocyte-stimulating hormone (MSH). This hypothesis can be tested by a binding assay for such an antibody using cultured Cloudman melanoma cells and a binding competition assay for MSH binding (Di Pasquale et al 1977).

Cardiomyopathies are diseases in which the presenting signs and symptoms result entirely or predominantly from dysfunction of the myocardium. They may result from primary involvement of the myocardium or from involvement secondary to a generalized disease. The latter is known to occur in settings of connective tissue diseases such as SLE, diffuse scleroderma, polyarteritis and dermatomyositis, as well as with diabetes mellitus, hepatic cirrhosis and vitiligo hypermelanosis (Glick & Braunwald 1977). Because of this clustering, an anti-receptor autoimmune aetiology to secondary cardiomyopathies is a distinct possibility, that can be readily tested.

Addison's disease

Organ-specific autoantibodies have been demonstrated repeatedly in idiopathic autoimmune Addison's disease (Besser et al 1971, Elder et al 1981). The pattern of reduced production of corticosteroids in response to ACTH, in the face of elevated plasma concentrations of the hormone, seen in this type of Addison's disease is similar to that observed in tubercular Addison's disease or congenital adrenal hyperplasia; however, the basis for the autoimmune version may be different.

A clue to this difference may be found in those patients with autoimmune Addison's disease who also present with a constellation of autoimmune endocrine disorders (Table 10). Neufeld et al (1980) have discerned two patterns: the Type I autoimmune polyglandular syndrome that may result

TABLE 10 Autoimmune Addison's disease and associated autoimmune endocrine disorders

Adrenal cortex antibodies (50–75%)
Gonadal steroidal cell antibodies (40%)
Thyroid and parathyroid antibodies with hypothyroidism and hypoparathyroidism
Schmidt's syndrome: primarily Addison's disease with chronic lymphocytic thyroiditis; secondarily with IDDM (7%), ovarian failure, pernicious anaemia.

Incidence data in parentheses, from Elder et al (1981).

from a thymic dysfunction (Arulanantham et al 1979) and that is characterized by adrenal insufficiency, hypoparathyroidism and chronic mucocutaneous candidiasis, frequently in association with chronic active hepatitis, early-onset pernicious anaemia, alopecia and primary hypogonadism; and the Type II version, characterized by adrenal insufficiency, thyroid autoimmune disease and/or IDDM. The Type II syndrome, which has a broad age of onset and a marked increase in incidence of the HLA-B8 antigen (Type I exhibits no consistent association with HLA antigens), is essentially Schmidt's syndrome (Schmidt 1926) expanded to include IDDM (Carpenter et al 1964).

In a recent study of 37 patients with autoimmune Addison's disease (including two with IDDM), Elder et al (1981) found that 27 had adrenal cortex autoantibodies; of the latter group, 11 also had steroidal cell autoantibodies (SCA). SCA were found mainly (86% of cases) in patients with the Type I autoimmune polyglandular syndrome, and to a small extent (13%) in patients with the Type II syndrome.

The nature of the antigens producing the autoantibodies in the Types I and II syndromes is not known. It should not be difficult to determine whether hormone receptors are the antigens. The lack of tissue or sex specificity for serum SCA found in the Type I syndrome (Elder et al 1981) could be due to the heterogeneous nature of the immunoglobulins in the sera used. Indeed, tissue adsorption studies showed that there were two distinct kinds of adrenocortical autoantibodies in some patients with Addison's disease: one type was specific for the adrenal cortex and the other was cross-reactive with all steroid-producing tissues (Elder et al 1981). It might, therefore, be possible to fractionate the SCA immunoglobulins by specific tissue adsorption techniques, or by isoelectric focusing. Of additional interest is the possibility that the cross-reactivity among a variety of steroid-producing cells observed in SCA could be due to an antigenic structure or protein common to all of these cell types.

Hashimoto's thyroiditis

This is a chronic inflammatory disorder of the thyroid in which autoimmune

TABLE 11 Autoimmune features associated with Hashimoto's thyroiditis

Hypergammaglobulinaemia
Anti-thyroglobulin and anti-thyroid microsome antibodies
Lymphocytic infiltration of the thyroid gland
Sjögren's syndrome
Pernicious anaemia
Progressive hepatitis
Idiopathic Addison's disease
Graves' disease
Rheumatoid arthritis
Systemic lupus erythematosus

factors are thought to play a prominent role in the production of hypothyroidism. Evidence for this includes lymphocytic infiltration of the thyroid, hypergammaglobulinaemia, and circulating antibodies directed against several components of thyroid tissue (Table 11). In addition, this disorder coexists with inordinate frequency with a variety of other diseases of a presumed autoimmune nature. These coexisting diseases, as well as Hashimoto's disease itself, also appear with unusual frequency in family members of patients with Hashimoto's disease. This panoply of autoimmune diseases, presenting to various extents in patients with Hashimoto's thyroiditis, provides a fertile field of investigation into the natures of both the antigens and the autoantibodies produced.

Hypoparathyroidism

The association of many atrophic diseases (idiopathic Addison's, pernicious anaemia, Hashimoto's thyroiditis, hypothyroidism, thyrotoxicosis, alopecia, moniliasis) with idiopathic hypoparathyroidism, the demonstration that lymphocytic infiltration occurs when animals are injected with isologous parathyroid tissue, and the demonstration of organ-specific circulating antibodies specific for parathyroid tissue in a significant number of patients with idiopathic hypoparathyroidism, all adds up to incriminating evidence that this entity is attributable to, or associated with, an autoimmune process (Blizzard 1969). The mechanism and induction of this disease remains unknown. It is not known if the reduced production of parathyroid hormone (PTH) in autoimmune hypoparathyroidism is due to the generation of antibodies directed against the β-adrenergic agonist or the calcium 'receptor' (which are linked to the production of cyclic AMP), or against intracellular components of the biosynthetic system for the hormone. One could conceive of an assay for the former type of antibody based on its ability to impede the activation of adenylate cyclase in parathyroid cells or plasma membranes by PTH secretagogues such as isoprenaline (isoproterenol).

Pernicious anaemia

Patients with pernicious anaemia frequently have circulating antibodies against their gastric mucosal parietal cells (cf. Table 1). They also frequently present with antibodies characteristic of other autoimmune disorders, such as Hashimoto's disease, Addisonian adrenal atrophy, and hypoparathyroidism. In addition, the chronic gastric inflammatory lesions seen in such patients resemble those seen in the thyroid in Hashimoto's disease. Clearly, the autoimmune production of antibodies directed against receptors for thyrotropin, adrenocorticotropin and parathormone, as well as against intrinsic factors, are distinct possibilities in such patients.

HLA-B8/DRw3 haplotype

The association between certain HLA antigens and an increased risk for specific diseases has been known for several years (Sasazuki et al 1977). One such association is that of the HLA-B8 and HLA-DRw3 antigens with diseases involving immunological dysfunction. For example, chronic active hepatitis, coeliac disease, myasthenia gravis, Graves' disease, sicca syndrome, SLE, Addison's disease, dermatitis herpetiformis (a defect in the Fc receptor in cells of the reticuloendothelial system), and Type II autoimmune polyglandular syndrome are all associated with the HLA-B8/DRw3 haplotype (Ganda & Soeldner 1977, Sasazuki et al 1977, Lawley et al 1981). Indeed, examination of a population of 'normal' subjects, unique only in that they were Rh-positive and possessed the HLA-B8/DRw3 antigens, revealed that half of this group had defective reticuloendothelial system Fc receptor function similar to that seen in patients with dermatitis herpetiformis (Lawley et al 1981). Thus, it might be fruitful to examine patients with autoimmune dysfunction in conjunction with the marker HLA-B8/DRw3 haplotype for a possible defect in the expression of Fc receptors on a number of circulating and fixed tissue cells. It may be that the Fc receptor defect renders it likely that IgG-containing immune complexes will not be cleared and destroyed normally, but will remain in the circulation and be deposited in tissues, producing tissue damage. At the same time, an Fc receptor abnormality on immunoregulatory cells may greatly increase the likelihood of an aberrant immunological response to some antigen, leading to the development of an autoimmune disease.

Affective disorders

Affective disorders might also be considered as candidates for an anti-receptor autoimmune explanation. If individuals were to produce antibodies against their own neurotransmitter receptors, one might expect the waxing and waning of severe psychotic symptoms not unlike the spontaneous relapses and remissions that mark the course of the known autoimmune receptor diseases previously discussed. Using currently available techniques for direct binding assays for neurotransmitter receptors, it should be possible to detect circulating and tissue antibodies directed against receptors for opiates, γ-aminobutyric acid (GABA), dopamine, α- and β-adrenergic agonists, muscarinic cholinergic agents, and so on, if such antibodies are, indeed, produced in some psychotic patients. By limiting the search for neurotransmitter receptor autoantibodies to the sera of patients with severe recurrent affective disorders and a history of autoimmune disease, one might increase the odds of finding such antibodies (Pert 1977). This approach is given credence by a report from Heath & Krupp (1967) that psychotic behaviour was produced in rhesus monkeys by the cerebroventricular injection of an IgG fraction isolated from sera from sheep immunized against human septal–caudate tissue. Furthermore, IgG isolated from the serum of patients with acute schizophrenia (but not from control subjects), when injected intraventricularly or intravenously into monkeys, caused abnormalities in EEGs recorded from the septal region and basal caudate nucleus, concomitant with catatonic behaviour.

This promise has not yet been fulfilled. Dr Candace Pert (personal communication) has screened about 100 sera from various in-patients from the psychiatric services of the Clinical Center at the National Institutes of Health for antibodies against a variety of neuroreceptors, with all negative results. These patients did not, however, exhibit concurrent autoimmune clustering, thereby increasing the odds against finding an autoimmune neuropathy. Nevertheless, the hypothesis continues to be worthy of exploration, particularly in the light of E. Heilbronn's work with acetylcholine receptor antibodies which suggests that these immunoglobulins may have central as well as peripheral effects, and the results accumulated by W. E. Bunney's group over many years which suggest that alterations in central neurotransmitter and drug receptor states lead to fluctuations in mood state.

Miscellaneous

Information, less definitive than that described above, is available for several other disorders. The severe dermatological lesion of necrobiosis lipoidica diabeticorum (NLD) is characterized by microangiopathy and collagen disorganization with granulomatous changes typical of autoimmune phenomena. Cultured skin fibroblasts derived from diabetic patients with NLD lesions exhibited an insulin receptor-binding defect (Cheung et al 1978), and the authors suggested that, since the lesions appeared before glucose intolerance in these patients, the basis for the reduction in insulin binding may be anti-receptor autoantibodies or altered insulin receptor. The definitive experiments are yet to be reported.

Antibodies (IgG) that interact strongly with fibrinogen and the fibrin monomer and inhibit the polymerization of fibrin monomers to form the fibrin gel have been found in the sera of two patients with SLE (Galanakis et al 1978) and of a patient with the cluster of chronic active hepatitis, postnecrotic cirrhosis, ulcerative colitis, and a coagulation defect (Hoots et al 1981). In the latter studies it was shown that the antibody inhibited neither the cleavage of fibrinopeptides nor the formation of covalent cross-linking bonds, but instead appeared to be specifically directed against the polymerization site in the E domain of the fibrin macromolecule. Since the polymerization site, like hormone and neurotransmitter receptor sites, may be considered to be informational in nature, the antibody to this site could be placed in the category of anti-receptor antibodies.

Finally, in an as-yet-unconfirmed report Jüppner et al (1978) detected species-specific IgG antibodies that blocked the binding of parathyroid hormone (PTH) to membrane receptors on cultured human lymphoblastoid cells in the sera of 49 out of 50 uraemic patients with secondary hyperparathyroidism (high levels of C-regional PTH). If confirmed, this finding may help to explain PTH resistance in the presence of 'inappropriately' high concentrations of C-regional PTH (Massry 1977).

Conclusion

On the basis of clustering among autoimmune disorders, plus additional evidence, upwards of 20 potential anti-receptor autoantibody diseases have been identified. These suggestions are all testable, using existing or newly derived assays for specific anti-tissue site antibodies.

REFERENCES

Arulanantham K, Dwyer JM, Genel M 1979 Evidence for defective immunoregulation in the syndrome of familial candidiasis. N Engl J Med 300:164-168

Besser GM, Cullen DR, Irvine WJ et al 1971 Immunoreactive corticotropin levels in adrenocortical insufficiency. Br Med J 1:374-376

Blecher M, Bar RS 1981 Speculations regarding potential anti-receptor autoimmune diseases. In: Receptors and human disease. Williams & Wilkins, Baltimore, Md, p 259-265

Blizzard RM 1969 Idiopathic hypoparathyroidism: a probable autoimmune disease. In: Miescher PA, Müller-Eberhard HJ (eds) Textbook of immunopathology. Grune & Stratton, New York, vol 2:547-550

Bottazzo GF, Florin-Christensen A, Doniach D 1974 Cell antibodies in diabetes mellitus with autoimmune polyendocrine deficiencies. Lancet 2:1279-1282

Carnegie PR, Mackay IR 1975 Vulnerability of cell-surface receptors to autoimmune reactions. Lancet 2:684-686

Carpenter CJC, Solomon N, Silverberg SG, et al 1964 Schmidt's syndrome (thyroid and adrenal insufficiency): a review of the literature and a report of 15 new cases including 10 cases of coexisting diabetes mellitus. Medicine 43:153-180

Cheung HS, Machina T, Nimni M 1978 Fibroblast insulin receptors in necrobiosis lipoidica diabeticorum. Abstracts of the Endocrine Society Meeting (abstr 160)

Crome L, Erdohazi M, Rivers RPA 1967 Fulminating diabetes with lymphocytic thyroiditis. Arch Dis Child 42:677-681

DiPasquale A, McGuire J, Carga JM 1977 The number of receptors for β-MSH in Cloudman melanoma cells is increased by dibutyryl cyclic AMP or cholera toxin. Proc Natl Acad Sci USA 74:601-605

Elder M, MacLaren N, Riley W 1981 Gonadal autoantibodies in patients with hypogonadism and-or Addison's disease. J Clin Endocrinol Metab 52:1137-1142

Finn FM, Johns PA, Nishi N, et al 1976 Differential response to ACTH analogs by bovine adrenal plasma membranes and cells. J Biol Chem 251:3576-3585

Galanakis DK, Ginzler EM, Fikrig SM 1978 Monoclonal IgG anticoagulants delaying fibrin aggregation in two patients with systemic lupus erythematosus. Blood 52:1037-1046

Ganda OP, Soeldner SS 1977 Genetic, acquired, and related factors in the etiology of diabetes mellitus. Arch Intern Med 137:461-469

Ganz K, Kozak GP 1974 Diabetes mellitus and primary hypothyroidism. Arch Intern Med 134:430-432

Glick G, Braunwald E 1977 The cardiomyopathies and myocarditides. In: Thorn G et al (eds) Harrison's Principles of internal medicine. McGraw-Hill (Blakiston), New York, p 1289-1295

Heath RG, Krupp IM 1967 Schizophrenia as an autoimmune disorder. Arch Gen Psychiatr 16:1-33

Hirata F, Del Carmine R, Nelson CA et al 1981 Presence of autoantibody for phospholipase inhibitory protein, lipomodulin, in patients with rheumatic diseases. Proc Natl Acad Sci USA 78:3190-3194

Hoots WK, Carroll NA, Wagner RH et al 1981 A naturally occurring antibody that inhibits fibrin polymerization. N Engl J Med 304:857-861

Huang SW, Maclaren NK 1976 Insulin-dependent diabetes: a disease of autoaggression. Science (Wash DC) 192:64-66

Irvine WJ, Barnes EW 1972 Clinics Endocrinol Metab 1:549-594

Irvine WJ, Clarke BF, Scarth L, Cullen DR, Duncan LJP 1970 Thyroid and gastric autoimmunity in patients with diabetes mellitus. Lancet 2:163-168

Jüppner H, Bialasiewicz AA, Hesch RD 1978 Autoantibodies to parathyroid hormone receptor. Lancet 2:122-124

Kahn CR, Kasuga M, King GL, Grunfeld C 1982 Autoantibodies to insulin receptors in man: immunological determinants and mechanisms of action. This volume, p 91-105

Kawanishi K, Kawamura K, Nishina Y, et al 1977 Successful immunosuppressive therapy in insulin resistant diabetes caused by anti-insulin receptor antibodies. J Clin Endocrinol Metab 44:15-21

Lawley TJ, Hall RP, Fauci AS et al 1981 Defective Fc receptor functions associated with the HLA-B8/DRw3 haplotype. N Engl J Med 304:185-192

Lefkowitz RJ, Roth J, Pastan I 1970 Prototype of a radioligand-cell membrane receptor assay system: the ACTH receptor assay system. Science (Wash DC) 170:633-635

Lendrum R, Walker G, Gamble OR 1975 Islet cell antibodies in juvenile diabetes mellitus of recent onset. Lancet 2:880-883

Lennon VA, Carnegie PR 1971 Immunopharmacological disease: a break in tolerance to receptor sites. Lancet 1:630-633

MacCuish AC, Barnes EW, Irvine WJ et al 1974 Antibodies to pancreatic islet cells in insulin dependent diabetes with coexistent autoimmune disease. Lancet 2:1529-1531

Maclaren NK, Huang, SW, Fogh J 1975 Antibody to cultured human insulinoma cells in insulin-dependent diabetes. Lancet 1:997-1000

Mannik M, Gilliland BC 1977 Systemic lupus erythematosus. In: Thorn GW et al (eds) Harrison's Principles of internal medicine. McGraw-Hill (Blakiston) New York, p 426-430

Massry SG 1977 Is parathyroid hormone a uraemic toxin? Nephron 19:125-130

Neufeld M, Maclaren NK, Blizzard RM 1980 Autoimmune polyglandular syndromes. Pediatr Ann 9:154-162

Okamoto HY, Noto Y, Miyamoto S et al 1975 Inhibition by somatostatin of insulin release from isolated pancreatic islets. FEBS (Fed Eur Biochem Soc) Lett 54:103-105

Osserman KE 1969 Muscles (myasthenia gravis). In: Miescher PA, Müller-Eberhard HJ (eds) Textbook of immunopathology. Grune & Stratton, New York, p 607-623

Pedersen O, Hijlund E, Beck-Nielsen H 1981 Diabetes mellitus caused by insulin receptor blockade and impaired sensitivity to insulin. N Engl J Med 304:1085-1088

Perlman LV 1961 Familial incidence of diabetes in hypothyroidism. Ann Intern Med 55:796-799

Pert CB 1977 A request for serum samples from psychiatric patients with associated autoimmune disease: is some psychosis caused by an autoimmune response to neurotransmitter receptors? Commun Psychopharmacol 1:307-309

Sasazuki T, McDevitt HO, Grumet FC 1977 The association between genes in the major histocompatibility complex and disease susceptibility. Annu Rev Med 28:425-452

Schmidt MB 1926 Eine biglanduläre Erkrankung (Nebennieren und Schilddrüse) bei morbus Addisonii. Verh Dtsch Ges Pathol 21:212-220

Strickland RG, Mackay IR 1973 A reappraisal of the nature and significance of chronic atrophic gastritis. Digest Dis 18:426-440

Ungar B, Stocks AE, Martin FIR 1968 Intrinsic factor antibody, parietal cell antibody, and latent pernicious anaemia in diabetes mellitus. Lancet 2:415-418

Venter JC, Fraser CM, Harrison LC 1980 Autoantibodies to β_2-adrenergic receptors: a possible cause of adrenergic hyporesponsiveness in allergic rhinitis and asthma. Science (Wash DC) 207:1361-1363

Wachslicht-Rodbard H, Muggeo M, Kahn CR et al 1981 Heterogeneity of the insulin receptor interaction in lipoatropic diabetes. J Clin Endocrinol Metab 52:416-425

Whittingham S, Matthews JD, Mackay IR et al 1971 Diabetes mellitus, autoimmunity, and ageing. Lancet 1:763-767

Yalow RS, Straus E 1977 Heterogeneity of gastrointestinal hormones. In: Bonfils S et al (eds) Hormonal receptors in digestive tract physiology. Elsevier/North-Holland Biomedical Press, Amsterdam, p 79-93

DISCUSSION

Possible autoimmune origin of Eaton-Lambert syndrome

Newsom-Davis: We have recently presented evidence for an autoimmune aetiology in another disorder of neuromuscular transmission, the myasthenic Eaton-Lambert syndrome (Lang et al 1981). This syndrome is characterized by an impaired release of acetylcholine quanta from the nerve terminal in response to a nerve impulse; that is, the quantal content of the end-plate potential is reduced. Some patients have associated bronchial carcinoma but others do not, and in these cases autoimmune diseases may be associated, which first suggested to us its possible autoimmune origin. Pernicious anaemia, coeliac disease, vitiligo or past thyrotoxicosis have been present in five of our patients. Clinically, the patients show pronounced proximal muscle weakness. A 5–10-day course plasma exchange caused clinical and electromyographic improvement which reached its peak about 15 days after the last exchange, suggesting that a humoral factor was interfering with ACh release. We prepared IgG fractions from the plasma of seven patients and injected these fractions intraperitoneally (10 mg/day) into groups of mice for periods of 37–99 days. At the end of the experiment, levels of human IgG in the sera of these animals were in the same range as in man. Electrophysiological studies on the diaphragm *in vitro* showed a highly significant reduction in the quantal content of the end-plate potential compared to mice injected with control IgG. Thus the pathophysiological features of the disorder in man can be transferred passively to mice. We therefore suggest that in the Eaton-Lambert syndrome there is an IgG autoantibody to antigenic determinants on structures at the nerve terminal that are concerned with ACh release.

Kahn: Do these patients with the Eaton-Lambert syndrome also have various types of cancer?

Newsom-Davis: We have studied only one patient with bronchial carcinoma. It is especially interesting that his IgG fraction transferred the disease to mice, for this suggests that the tumour may act as a neoantigen, inducing production of an autoantibody that cross-reacts with nerve terminal determinants. However, we have not yet excluded the possibility that a peptide was transferred in the IgG fraction.

Kahn: Isn't Eaton-Lambert syndrome normally identified in patients with underlying tumours?

Newsom-Davis: It is difficult to say. The incidence in association with carcinoma may be higher but, because of the poor prognosis in this group, the prevalence could be lower. Patients with the apparently non-carcinomatous form of the disease have been followed for 20 years or more.

Mitchison: I believe that Reg Kelly hopes to enumerate the synaptosomal membrane proteins. He should eventually have a library of monoclonal antibodies against all the proteins. Shouldn't those include the target proteins that you have in mind?

Newsom-Davis: Yes. In addition, botulinum toxin poisoning produces an illness not unlike the Eaton-Lambert syndrome, and with Dr Oliver Dolly at Imperial College we have been investigating whether IgG from these patients with Eaton-Lambert syndrome can interfere with toxin binding.

Vincent: The botulinum-binding protein in the presynaptic terminal, if there is one, hasn't yet been identified, and is probably present as a small number of sites per nerve terminal; this may make it difficult to say where the Eaton-Lambert IgG, or other protein, is binding.

Newsom-Davis: Dr Engel, have you ever used your electron microscopic techniques to look for immunoglobulins at the presynaptic region in this syndrome?

Engel: I looked at the light microscopic level at three cases of this type of myasthenic syndrome in 1977, using protein A and rabbit anti-human C3 labelled with peroxidase as immunocytochemical probes. I detected no immune complexes at the end-plate. More recently, I repeated this study in 12 additional cases and saw no antibody at the end-plate in any of the biopsy specimens. This, however, does not mean that the myasthenic syndrome is not antibody-mediated. Let us assume that an autoantibody is formed against a specific protein which can affect the probability of ACh release—such as, for example, a protein associated with the calcium channel in the presynaptic membrane. A predictable effect of the autoantibody would be to reduce the number of antigen molecules on the presynaptic membrane. Consequently, the number of antibody molecules bound to the presynaptic membrane would also decrease. If the numerical density of the antigen was low to begin with, its concentration would become extremely low during the course of the disease (possibly fewer than 50 molecules per μm^2). Even if each molecule of antigen bound more than one autoantibody molecule, the concentration of the latter would fall below the sensitivity of the immunoperoxidase method.

Newsom-Davis: The number of botulinum-binding sites at the nerve terminal seems to be small, so that might be true for Ig also.

Mitchison: What is one to make of Brian Lacey's finding (unpublished) that in various pathological conditions, human sera contain antibodies which can stain frozen sections of rat cerebellum?

Newsom-Davis: One would want to be sure that binding is not non-specific.

Mitchison: The diversity of the patterns of staining seems to suggest something more than that.

Newsom-Davis: The cerebellar observations might be important in the context of the Eaton-Lambert syndrome. Cerebellar disorder can occur as a 'remote effect' of bronchial carcinoma, and was in fact present in our patient with this syndrome, raising the possibility that the disordered neuromuscular transmission and the cerebellar deficit might have a similar aetiology.

Drachman: We have plasmapheresed one patient with carcinomatous cerebellar degeneration, with the same idea in mind. We found no change in cerebellar ataxia. We have not yet tried passive transfer of the serum from this patient to experimental animals.

Fundamental aetiology of autoimmune disease

Rodbell: As a general comment, I came to this symposium not knowing anything about autoimmune disease, and I am not sure how much more I understand now, but one thing that has struck me (and was brought into focus by Mel Blecher's paper) is the question of disease clustering. What is the survey mechanism that picks up these different changes in receptors (or non-receptors, or informational proteins) and causes several diseases to be apparently associated, and is that clustering really correct? I say this because I am left with the feeling that not everyone is happy about associative autoimmune diseases. In some cases it appears to be proven, in some cases not. Also, the survey mechanism appears to pick up surface membrane proteins only, but has anyone looked for internalized proteins that have important regulatory aspects? There may be other proteins which are normally not accessible to the immune system and for some reason become exposed. Has that been tested for?

Kahn: This brings us back to the question that Franco Bottazzo raised earlier, and is something which I don't understand. If we summarize the data (Fig. 1), it seems that there is a large group of generalized autoimmune diseases, by which we mean diseases in which there are antibodies to intracellular antigens (anti-DNA antibodies, or anti-ribonucleoprotein antibodies) which stain the nuclei or DNA from all cells. We also have anti-receptor antibody diseases, which can be conceived of as a series of entities overlapping the large group to more or less extent. Our Type B, insulin-resistant patients mostly fall into the category of generalized autoimmune disease, whereas patients with Graves' disease or myasthenia gravis or atopic syndromes overlap to a much lesser extent.

There is also another large group of autoimmune conditions, which overlaps with the generalized diseases to a very small extent, that would be called organ-specific autoimmunity diseases. They are often endocrine diseases, such as autoimmune adrenal insufficiency, Hashimoto's thyroiditis, or insulin-dependent diabetes mellitus, Type I; or diseases involving the gastrointestinal tract, like hepatitis or coeliac disease. They can also be diseases of the skin, such as vitiligo. Very few of these occur in patients with

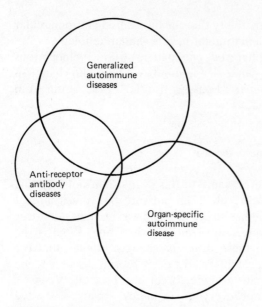

FIG.1. (Kahn). Suggested relationships between types of autoimmune diseases.

generalized autoimmune diseases, and they overlap the other autoimmune syndromes (with anti-receptor antibodies) to only a small extent. If we want to elucidate the fundamental aetiology of autoimmune diseases, and if we agree on this breakdown, it would suggest that there are different mechanisms which operate in these different classes of autoimmune diseases.

Mitchison: I would like to clarify what Martin Rodbell, and perhaps molecular biologists in general, mean when they say they don't understand autoimmune diseases.

I think they mean that this scheme of Dr Kahn's is not a theory of how autoimmune disease works, but a portmanteau of what the facts are, and that won't satisfy the molecular biologists. They want a simple explanation of *why*. We should make it clear to Martin Rodbell that he will leave this meeting without that theory—and that leaves the rest of us still in business!

Knight: I think that Dr Kahn's breakdown of these diseases clouds the issue, rather than clarifies it. I suggest that if we look at the incidence of all these possible autoimmune conditions, we shall probably find that about 20% of the population have one or other of them. If you put them together in the kind of spectrum you depicted, this is confusing the situation.

Kahn: If one just takes the clinical observations, the diseases do cluster, but they do not cluster randomly. The organ-specific types of autoimmune disease quite often cluster with one another, so that patients with insulin-independent diabetes do have an increased incidence of Graves' disease,

Hashimoto's thyroiditis or autoimmune adrenal failure, but rarely have systemic lupus erythematosus. I don't know if there is an increased incidence of diabetes mellitus in patients with SLE. It seems that if we are looking for immune regulation mechanisms and how they can be perturbed, there must be different mechanisms operating in these various diseases.

Knight: Surely all this tells us is that the genes that predispose to one of these conditions, whatever they might be and however they may act, happen to predispose to certain other diseases?

Kahn: It could be under genetic control, but at present we don't know that it is all under genetic control. The difference could also be controlled by environmental factors. We would need to know the genetics underlying each disease category. Perhaps the genetic control differs in the different categories.

Bottazzo: I would like to make three final points regarding the heterogeneity of organ-specific autoimmune responses.

(1) In the majority of endocrine autoimmune disorders antibody production continues for many years, even when the target organ is atrophied. In juvenile, Type I (insulin-dependent) diabetes, however, islet cell antibodies disappear quite soon after diagnosis and persist in no more than 10–15% of cases (Bottazzo et al 1981). This is reminiscent of the transient appearance of smooth muscle antibodies after several types of viral infection. Our recent studies on the natural history of diabetes confirmed that islet cell antibodies are present several years before the clinical expression of the diseases in predisposed sibs. More surprising still was the finding that a proportion of these individuals also showed pituitary cell antibodies (Mirakian et al 1982).

(2) Endocrine antibodies vary in their degree of cell specificity (Bottazzo et al 1980). There are 'common' antigens in thyroid adrenal cortex and pancreatic islets; on the other hand, there are cell-specific antibodies to parietal cells, to glucagon cells and somatostatin cells in the endocrine pancreas, and also specific antibodies to gut-related paracrine cells, for example GIP or secretin (S) cells. In the pituitary we see specific antibodies to the prolactin cells or the growth hormone cells, but in juvenile diabetes and in the prediabetic phase of predisposed relatives, pituitary antibodies appear to react with several cell types.

(3) Finally, there is the question of intracellular antigens which are also present on the cell surface. The 'microsomal' thyroid, gastric and adrenal antigens are also represented on the cell surface. The growth-stimulating and blocking antibodies are entirely directed to cell surface receptors.

The long latency period observed in most of the endocrine autoimmune disorders may well be explained by the simultaneous presence of destructive and regenerative phenomena in the glands. In the polyendocrine syndromes there may be a more extensive disturbance of the self-regulating mechanisms than in autoimmunity affecting a single organ.

Harrison: I want to disagree with Dr Kahn's scheme. I think it's a false classification which conceals our ignorance, in fact. What we are ignorant about, firstly, is the specificity of the autoantibodies found in these conditions; we also have no idea of what happens prospectively in any of these diseases. We know only what the available tests tell us. The specificity of the autoimmune reaction is, to my mind, a separate problem that will not be helped by studying clinical situations. For example, once we know that there are antibodies to the gastrin receptor, and that they appear before antibodies that are detected by immunofluorescence to something inside the gastrin-producing cell, we shall immediately place pernicious anaemia in the anti-receptor class as opposed to the organ-specific class, and the whole perspective will change. We don't know the prime effectors of autoimmune disease, but I would guess that we ought to be looking at autoantibodies directed at cell surface antigens, as likely candidates. Their molecular specificities and functional effects must be defined and a temporal profile built up. At this level of analysis we can compare diseases and do genetic studies in human families to elucidate relationships. I don't think it helps us to make clinical divisions at this stage. I suspect that antibodies to DNA in SLE may be a red herring. Is there a surface antigen or receptor involved in SLE? The problem is what determines why one person gets one expression of autoimmunity and someone else gets another expression. I don't think the scheme you present (Fig. 1) helps us with that.

Kahn: Maybe I'm wrong! I haven't been convinced, though, that there is much overlap between the generalized autoimmune diseases and the organ-specific autoimmune diseases. To me, they are fairly distinct groups. This seems to suggest that either they are genetically predetermined to be different, or the recognition of different types of antigens is being modulated in different ways. Is there anything we know immunologically about why different types of antigens may be preferentially dealt with in different ways?

Drachman: In this meeting at least two possible explanations for the initiation of an autoimmune reaction have been suggested: (1) alteration of the antigen, and (2) a defect of immunoregulation. However, it is now apparent that patients with autoimmune diseases often show evidence of a rather widespread autoimmune response—that is, a clustering of autoimmune diseases. Doesn't this tend to favour the immunoregulatory defects hypothesis?

Mitchison: Yes.

Roitt: There is very little evidence for structurally altered antigen in autoimmune conditions. If the anecdotal evidence accumulated by the clinicians that the organ-specific and non-organ-specific diseases cluster separately is confirmed, then what is probably causing these two different groups of diseases to cluster is something like the concentrations and forms in which the antigens tend to circulate and are presented to the immune system. It is more likely that factors such as these, rather than similarities in the individual shapes of the autoantigens concerned, provide the common thread within each cluster. If their presentation to the immune system in terms of concentration, and association with MHC, is what is critical for the control of autoreactivity, the association of diseases could be related to defects in immunoregulation; however, the lack of overlap of organ-specific and non-organ-specific disorders would imply that different regulatory mechanisms operate in respect of the antigens concerned in these two groups.

Drachman: We have heard two different points of view on susceptibility to autoimmune diseases, namely that inherited traits may be the most important predisposing factors, or that other alterations that are not understood may play a role. What non-genetic mechanisms could predispose to autoimmune disorders? Is it possible that groups of suppressor cells can be depleted, so as to allow a cluster of autoimmune disorders to develop?

Knight: The simple answer is the fact that when multiple autoimmune conditions occur in one patient, it has been observed that there is a tendency for them not to appear together. There is a discordance in the time of onset, and this does not fit with the depletion of a range of suppressor cells (Solomon et al 1965).

Blecher: I should like to put into perspective the discussion that has been generated by my wide-ranging and speculative paper.

The discussants have been of essentially three points of view: those who think that the approach I suggested would not get at the fundamental aetiology of anti-receptor autoimmune diseases; those who believe that the chief value of testing for autoantibodies is the information about pathogenesis that such assays may provide; and, those who consider it possible that the approach based on the second viewpoint might provide us with basic information about the aetiology question.

Mine is essentially the second point of view. That is to say, whatever the aetiology of autoimmune diseases, and whatever the relationships between generalized, organ-specific, non-organ-specific and anti-receptor autoimmune diseases, data leading to an understanding of the pathogenesis of a variety of autoimmune diseases may be generated simply by testing for hitherto unsuspected antibodies directed against receptors and other informational macromolecules. The other major aspect of my thesis was that the tendency for autoimmune diseases to cluster in a single patient or single type of patient may provide a rational basis upon which to proceed in investigations of the genesis of the clinical symptoms, not necessarily the genesis of the autoimmunity.

These caveats should be kept in mind when considering the approaches suggested in my paper.

REFERENCES

Bottazzo GF, Vandelli C, Mirakian R 1980 The detection of autoantibodies to discrete endocrine cells in complex endocrine organs. In: Pinchera A et al (eds) Autoimmune aspects of endocrine disorders. Academic Press, London, p 367-377

Bottazzo GF, Pujol-Borrell R, Doniach D 1981 Humoral and cellular immunity in diabetes mellitus. Clinics Immunol & Allergy 1:139-159

Lang B, Newsom-Davis J, Wray D, Vincent A, Murray N 1981 Autoimmune aetiology for myasthenic (Eaton-Lambert) syndrome. Lancet 2:224-226

Mirakian R, Cudworth AG, Bottazzo GF, Richardson CA, Doniach D 1982 Autoimmunity to anterior pituitary cells and the pathogenesis of insulin-dependent diabetes mellitus. Lancet 1:755-759

Solomon N, Carpenter CCJ, Bennett IL, Harvey AM 1965 Schmidt's syndrome (thyroid and adrenal insufficiency) and coexistent diabetes mellitus. Diabetes 14:300-304

Index of contributors

*Entries in **bold** type indicate papers; other entries refer to discussion contributions*

Indexes compiled by John Rivers

Subject index